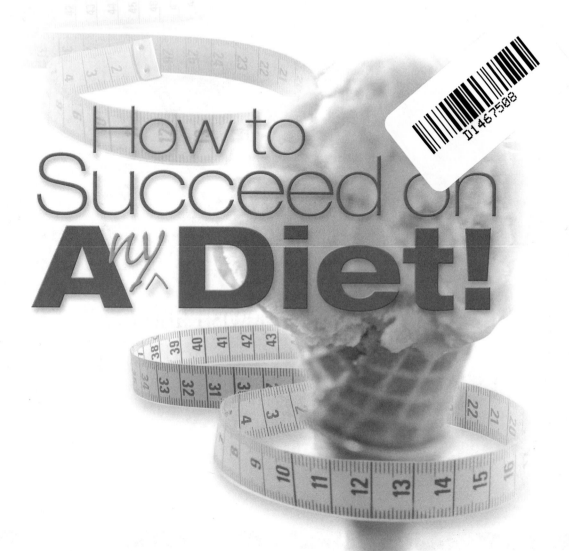

How to Succeed on A͜ny Diet!

A Jewish and *Friendly* Guide to Dieting & Exercise

How to Succeed on

A Jewish and *Friendly* Guide
to Dieting & Exercise

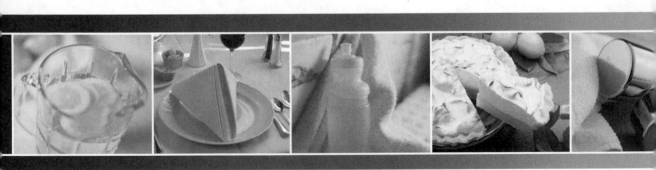

A ny ^ Diet!

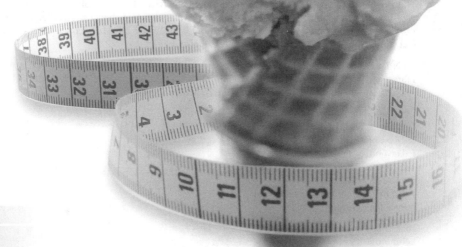

hava Goldman

FOREWORD BY
Rabbi Dr. Abraham J. Twerski

This book is not intended to replace sound medical advice. If you are taking a prescription medication, you should never change diets without consulting your physician, because any dietary change may effect the way your medicine works in your body. In addition, as we have mentioned in this book, please consult your physician before starting any new exercise regime.

ISBN 1-931681-70-8
Library of Congress Control Number: 2005925131
Manufactured in the USA by Malloy, Ann Arbor MI

Distributed by
Israel Book Shop
501 Prospect Street #97
Lakewood, New Jersey 08701
Tel 732-901-3009
Fax 732-901-4012
Isrbkshp@aol.com
www.israelbookshop.com

Distributed in Europe by
Lehmanns
Unit E, Viking Business Park
Rolling Mill Road
Jarrow, Tyne and Wear
NE32 3DP England

Cover design by DC Design

A Tribute

One of the wisest, warmest, and most far-sighted leaders of the Jewish world in our generation was HaRav HaGaon Rabbi Betzalel Rakow zt"l. For forty years he stood at the helm of the citadel of Torah learning and observance known to the world as Gateshead. Under his watchful eye, Gateshead developed into a powerhouse of Torah scholarship and religious observance. Rabbi Rakow zt"l was one of the undisputed leaders of English Jewry over the last two decades.

Several years ago, with a vision ahead of its time, this great sage saw the need for an increased awareness of health and fitness in the Jewish world. To this end, he encouraged the author of this book to write a diet, nutrition, and exercise column for Jewish women every week in a national English newspaper. After several years of writing this column, Rabbi Rakow suggested that the author reach further afield and write a book on the subject. Week after week he gently persuaded, encouraged, and motivated until the project began to take shape. Whenever the author or her husband came to the Rav for advice (on other matters), he would always take the time to ask, "How is the book coming along?" He was looking forward to writing his approbation for it. But that was not in the plans of Heaven. Rabbi Rakow zt"l returned his pure soul to his Maker before the author was able to finish the project.

It is with great sadness that we have had to write a tribute in place of an approbation, but without the Rav zt"l, this book may never have been written. He believed in it and he encouraged it, and for that alone, we will be eternally indebted. We hope and pray that in his merit this book will find favor in the eyes of all who read it.

In Memory

In memory of my late father-in-law Aryeh Nachum (Lloyd Nathaniel) ben Avraham Yitzchok Goldman z"l.

His yearning for truth, love of wisdom, and passion for teaching and writing were cut short in the prime of his life. His legacy lives on in his son and grandchildren.

Acknowledgments

Although it's the writer's name that you see on the front cover, there's a whole bunch of people who helped turn this dream into a reality.

Thanks go to:

Bubba and Zeida Spitzer, for always being there;

Charlotte Friedland, for taking on the unofficial role of mentor/overseer/mother hen and generally believing in me;

Cherry Baker (National Presenter, Instructor of the Year 1994, nominee for Lifetime Achievement Award 2002), for teaching me, reviewing the exercise section of this book, and for always being there to answer my questions.

Deenee Cohen (of DC Design), for designing the lip-smacking front cover;

Dovid and Ruthie Morgan, whose enthusiasm and advice helped spring-board this project;

Elissa Epstein, for proofreading so professionally and efficiently (and at such short notice!);

HaRav Shlomo Brevda, for his sagacious wisdom, his heartfelt blesssings, and his constant support and encouragement;

Michele DeFilippo (of 1106 Design), for crafting the interior design and layout of this book so skillfully, and for holding my hand throughout the entire process;

Moshe Kaufman (of Israel Book Shop), for taking me under his wing, guiding me every step of the way, and sharing in my excitement;

MIL (Mother-In-Law), for her unwavering support, unconditional love, and never-ending belief in everything I do;

Mum and Dad, for all that they have invested in me;

My brother, (the best bro' in the world,) for supporting me through courses, crises and catastrophes;

My husband, who, one night, "a lifetime ago," remarked "You've got so much in your head — you should write a book!". From dream to reality, this book is the culmination of his constant belief in me. He has been my cheerleader, confidante, chief-encourager and very best friend. But besides his emotional support, without his hard work there would simply be no book. Not only did he see there was a book in my head, (long before anyone else did), he helped to draw it out, craft it, organize it, edit it, and proofread it. He found our publisher, chief editor, layout designer, and printer. And then he supervised the entire publishing process, from beginning to end. I thank him from the bottom of my heart for the hours that he spent on this book (often till 4am!), for his uncompromising professionalism, and for his patience with me — as I resisted all those red pen slashings! I thank him for looking after the children on so many occasions when I was busy at the computer, and for looking after me as well. He was always there when I needed him, in whatever capacity I needed. Truly, this book is his book;

My sister, the most positive "you-can-do-it!" person I know;

Rabbi Dr. Abraham J. Twerski, for taking the time out of his busy schedule to write the Foreword to this book.

Rabbi Yacov Abenson, for his warmth, his caring, and his guidance;

The kids, for putting up with "abridged version" bedtime stories, "emergency" one-pot meals, and only half a listening ear when I was working on the book. Although they didn't know what we were doing, they were great!;

Tova Ovits, whose skillful editing turned an English manuscript into an American book.

And finally, no thank you would be complete without acknowledging the One behind it all.

Thank you **Hashem (G-d)**, for bringing it all together and allowing me to be part of it.

Dedication

I dedicate this book to anyone who wants to lose weight.
I believe you can do it. Now it's your turn to believe it.

General Table of Contents

Foreword 1

Introduction 3

About This Book 3

About the Author 4

How This Book is Organized 7

How To Use This Book 9

Section 1: On Your Marks — How To Get Started 11

Chapter 1: How Do I Choose A Diet? 13

Chapter 2: Are You Ready? 45

**Section 2: Get Set — Taking Charge of Your Eating
Habits** 59

Chapter 3: Twenty-Four Reasons Why We Eat And What We Can
Do About Them 61

Section 3: Go! — Tips To Keep You on Track 89

Chapter 4: Practical Tips 91

Chapter 5: Enlisting External Support 123

Chapter 6: Friday a.k.a. Erev Shabbos 139

Chapter 7: Shabbos 161

Chapter 8: Yom Tov — General 173

Chapter 9: Yom Tov — Specific Yomim Tovim 191

Chapter 10: Summer Vacations 221

Chapter 11: Eating Right When Eating Out 239

Section 4: Runner's Cramp — Oh No, I've Hit a Plateau! 253

Chapter 12: Re-Motivation 255

Chapter 13: Blasting The Plateau 261

Section 5: Keep Going — Exercise 267

Chapter 14: Exercise — Why Bother? 269

Chapter 15: Which Exercises Do What? 283

Chapter 16: What's An Exercise Class All About? 301

Chapter 17: Do's And Don'ts Of Exercise 313

Chapter 18: Exercise Tips 317

Chapter 19: Debunking Fitness Myths 327

Section 6: The Finishing Line — Life After Weight Loss . . 343

Chapter 20: The Winner's Circle: How To Stay There for Life 345

The Last Word 359

Section 7: Appendices 361

Appendix 1: Reasons To Lose Weight 363

Appendix 2: What's A Healthy Weight For Me? 377

Appendix 3: Calculating Calories 385

Appendix 4: Debunking Dieting Myths 389

Appendix 5: Fiber: What's It Really All About? 395

Appendix 6: Drinking 407

Appendix 7: Dieting And Kids 411

Appendix 8: Eating Disorders — When Dieting Goes Too Far 417

Index 425

Detailed Table of Contents

Foreword 1

Introduction 3

About This Book 3

About the Author 4

How This Book is Organized 7

How To Use This Book 9

Section 1: On Your Marks — How To Get Started 11

Chapter 1: How Do I Choose A Diet? 13

  Eat Healthy, Live Healthy 13

    A Healthy Diet — The Two Essential Rules 13

    What Makes a Diet Healthy? 14

    What About Negative Long-Term Health Aspects? 16

  The Equation (What Makes a Diet Work?) .17

  Let's Get Personal (How To Analyze Yourself Before Choosing a Diet) . . .19

    My Personality 20

    Personal Preferences 20

    Outside Influences/Lifestyle 20

  A World of Choice (Which Diet Should I Choose? An Analysis) 21

    Weight Watchers 21

    The Complete Scarsdale Medical Diet 23

    Dr. Atkins' New Diet Revolution 25

    The Zone 27

    The "Eat More, Weigh Less" Diet 30

    Slimming World 31

    The Original Hay Diet/Food Combining for Health 34

    Fit for Life 35

Meal Replacements (Liquids, Cookies, Formulas, Etc.) 36
Diet Pills 37
Fad Diets (Quick-Fix Diets) 38
Yo-Yo Dieting 40
The "I'm Just Being Careful" Diet ("IJBC" Diet) 41
Additional Points To Ponder 43

Chapter 2: Are You Ready? . . . . **.45**
Correct Attitudes 45
Who's Responsible Anyway? 45
Willpower 46
Be Realistic 47
Focusing on Yourself 47
Take Pride in How You Diet 49
Money Matters 51
Rewards 51
The Practical Side of Being Ready 54
Avoiding False Starts (Is Now the Right Time?) 54
Study Your Chosen Diet 56
Clean-Up Time 56
Stock Up on Staples 56

Section 2: Get Set — Taking Charge Of Your Eating Habits 59

Chapter 3: Twenty-Four Reasons Why We Eat And What We Can Do About Them . . . . **.61**
Why Do We Eat? 61
Hunger 61
Tayvah/Desires 62
Eating By the Clock 63
Stress 64
Comfort 64
Lonely 64
Nerves/Worry 64
Boredom 64
Social Pressures 65
Socializing 65
Celebrating 65
Procrastination 66
Boring Job 66
Unawares 66
Tired 66
Conditioned Response 67
Mitzvos 67
Making a Transition 67
Thirsty 67

Medicine 67
Weather 68
Why Do You Eat? (A Tick-the-Box Questionnaire) .68
What We Can Do About the Reasons We Eat 70
Hunger 70
Tayvah/Desires 71
Eating By the Clock 71
Stress 72
Comfort 75
Lonely 76
Nerves/Worry 77
Boredom 80
Social Pressures 80
Socializing and Celebrating 81
Procrastination 83
Unawares 84
Tired 84
Conditioned Response 85
Mitzvos 85
Making a Transition 85
Thirsty 85
Medicine 86
Weather 87

Section 3: Go! — Tips To Keep You On Track 89
Chapter 4: Practical Tips 91
Food, Glorious Food 91
Fill Up on Plant Food 91
Dressing Down Salad 92
Slurp Soup 93
New-Size French Fries 94
Milk Your Milk for What it's Worth 95
Snack Attack 95
Prepare for Snack Attacks 96
Take Cereal Seriously 96
Halt Salt 96
Spice Up Your Life with Spices 97
Banish Booze 97
Sweet Treats 98
Don't Choke on Chocolate 99
Fighting Fats 99
Clarifying Cholesterol 102
Subject Yourself To Substitution 104
BLT: Bites, Licks, and Tastes 105

Non-Food Advice 106
  The Weighing Way (At the Scale) 106
  Monitor and Motivate 107
  Dear Diary 108
Out and About 110
  Shopping When Hungry 110
  Shopping When in a Rush 111
  Food Labels 111
  On the Town 117
Day-To-Day Advice 117
  Weigh To Go (Weighing Food) 117
  Serving: Here and There 118
  Cooking Methods That Start with "B" 119
  Downsize Portions 119
  Small is Beautiful 119
  Eat From a Plate 119
  Short-Circuit Binges 120
  How To Eat 120

Chapter 5: Enlisting External Support **123**
What Types of Support Are There? 125
  Nearest and Dearest 125
  Let's Be Partners (A Dieting Partner) 132
  Troop To Group (Going To a Weight Management Group) 133
  Find a Mentor 136

Chapter 6: Friday a.k.a. Erev Shabbos **139**
Avoiding an Erev Shabbos Dieting Disaster 140
  Busy Bee 140
  Hunger 146
  Tastes 'N' Testers 149
  Lunchtime 151
Erev Shabbos: Avoiding a Shabbos Dieting Disaster 157
  Be Prepared 157
  Alternative "Healthyotherapy" 158
  Thinking of You 158
  Automatic Pilot 159
  Save Up 159
  Beautiful Fruitful 160
  Last Minute Morsels 160

Chapter 7: Shabbos **161**
Friday Night 161
  The Twilight Zone 161
  At the Ready 162
  Mine, All Mine 162
  At Arm's Length 162
  More Please 163

The Return of the Chicken Soup 163

Chock-A-Block At Chicken Time 163

Kugel Time 164

Dessert Time 165

After the Meal 166

Sofa Settlers 166

Shabbos Day 167

To Kiddush Or Not To Kiddush — That is the Question 167

Looking At Lunch 168

Horsey Dorsey Coursey — Hors D'oeuvre 168

Cholent Quotient 169

Meeting the Meat 169

Desert Dessert 170

Seudah Shilishis 170

How Full is Full? 171

Melaveh Malkah 171

Chapter 8: Yom Tov — General **173**

Before Yom Tov 173

Save Up 173

Be Prepared 174

Sensational Seasonal Fruits 174

Think-Drink 174

Freezer Teasers 174

Cool Food 174

Plan of Action 175

Erev Yom Tov 176

Eat! 176

Sleep 176

Mind Set 176

One Course Less 176

Treat Yourself Versus Blowing it 177

Listen To Your Body 177

Stay in Control 178

Enjoy 178

On Yom Tov Itself 179

Move 179

After the Schloff 179

Chocolate 179

Nibbly Bits 179

Trick Your Tummy 180

Seudah Shilishis 180

The Second-Night Seudah 180

Menus Under Scrutiny 181

Kiddush 182

Challah 182

Honey 182

Mayonnaise 183
Hors D'oeuvres 183
Soup 183
Soup Nuts/Croutons 183
Matzah Balls 184
Roast Beef 184
Tzimmes 184
Potato Kugel 184
Coleslaw 184
Apple Pie 185
Ice Cream 185
Chocolate Syrup 185
Drinks 186
Get Back on Track 187
After Yom Tov Pick-Me-Up 187
No Big-Time Yom Tov Approaching 189
Yummy Fruits 'N' Veggies 189
Light Makes Light 189
Long Days-y, No Lazy 189
A "Spring" in the Step 189
Looking Good, Feeling Good 190
Take Up a New Activity .190

Chapter 9: Yom Tov — Specific Yomim Tovim **191**
  After Rosh Hashanah 191
    Fasting After Feasting 191
  Erev Yom Kippur 192
    Look After Yourself 192
    Listen To Your Body 193
    What To Eat (and What To Avoid) Before the Fast 193
    Drink 195
    Bites, Licks, and Tastes .196
    Fasting and Weight Loss 196
    All Change 196
  After Yom Kippur 197
    Eat Slowly 197
    Chew 197
    Pause 197
    Stop When You Are Full .197
  Nine Tips for Chanukah: One for Each Candle 198
    (Plus One for the Shammash)
    Time-Bound Sit-Around .198
    Rewording Rewarding 199
    Daylight Saving 199
    Caution: Portion 200
    Fill Up During the Day 200
    Drink Something First 201

Have a Mini Snack Before the Goodies 201
Look After Yourself 201
Leave the Leftovers 203
Purim 203
The Day Before Tanis Esther 204
Tanis Esther 207
Purim Day 210
Pesach 213
Before Pesach 214
Seder Nights 217
Motzei Pesach 219
Shavuos 219
Cheesecake 219

Chapter 10: Summer Vacations **221**
The Theory Side 221
Expecting To Lose 222
Aiming To Stay the Same/Small Gain 223
Blowing the Diet 224
The Practical Side 225
Advice for All Vacation Scenarios 225
Advice for Different Summer Vacation Scenarios 227
Boost for After the Summer Vacation 236

Chapter 11: Eating Right When Eating Out **239**
Psyching Up To Go Out 240
Planning Ahead 240
Adapting the Menu To Your Diet 241
Potential Problem Areas 241
Confusion, Confusion 242
I'm Staaaaaaarving! 243
The Portion Sizes Are Too Big 244
Hidden Extras 248
There's Just Too Many Courses 250

**Section 4: Runner's Cramp — Oh No, I've Hit
A Plateau!** **253**

Chapter 12: Re-Motivation **255**
Lose Weight 255
Review Your Reasons 255
Lax Versus Exact 256
Fill Out a Food Diary 256
Monitor Your Weight Loss 256
Variety — The Spice of Life 257
Build Up a Stockpile 258
Surround Yourself with Success 258
Use Your External Support 258

Make Sure You Are Rewarding Yourself 258
Complying with Complacency 259
Change Diet 259
Learn To Learn 259
Get Back on Track 260

Chapter 13: Blasting The Plateau **261**
All Change 262
Time for More Change 262
Yet More Change 263
Choose Your Fruits and Veggies Wisely 263
Eat Enough 264
Make Fiber Your Friend 264
Exercise Your Exercise Options 265
Drink 265
Limit Freebies 265
A Change is As Good As a Rest 266

Section 5: Keep Going — Exercise **267**

Chapter 14: Exercise — Why Bother? **269**
150 Reasons To Exercise 269
Talking Heart To Heart 270
Better for Diabetics 271
Inside Out (Internal Organs, Lungs, Intestines, and Stuff) 271
Body Bits (Bones, Muscle, Cartilage, etc.) 272
Oops-A-Daisy Injury (Prevention and Recovery) 273
Weight Loss Wonders 274
Mirror, Mirror on the Wall, Who's the Fairest of Us All? (Appearance) .275
The Feel-Good Factor 275
Living it Up (Quality of Life) 276
Spiritual Reasoning 279
Perks of the Job (Side Benefits) 280

Chapter 15: Which Exercises Do What? **283**
Aerobics 284
What is Aerobics? 284
Why Should I Do Aerobic Exercise? 284
How Do You Work Aerobically? 285
Different Types of Aerobic Exercises 286
Stretching 287
What is Stretching? 287
Why Should I Stretch? 288
How Do I Stretch? 290
Different Stretching Classes 291
Strength Training 292
What is Strength Training? 292
Why Should I Do Strength Training? 293

How Do I Perform Strength Training? 293
Different Strength Training Classes/Activities 296
Mind-Body Exercise 296
What is Mind-Body Exercise? 297
Why Should I Do Mind-Body Exercises? 297
How Do I Access the Benefits of a Mind-Body Exercise? 299
Different Types of Mind-Body Classes 299

Chapter 16: What's An Exercise Class All About? **301**
The Warm-Up 301
What is a Warm-Up? 302
A Stitch in Time Saves Nine 303
Going it Alone 303
The Class 303
Aerobic Classes 305
The Cooldown 309
How To Cool Down 310
A Word About Stretching 311

Chapter 17: Do's And Don'ts of Exercise **313**
Eating 313
Drinking 314
Nausea 314
Insomnia 315
Physical Conditions 315
Shmoozing 316

Chapter 18: Exercise Tips **317**
Benefits Are Sure (When You Endure) 317
No Pain, No Gain 318
Tune in To Yourself 318
Falling Off the Bandwagon 318
Staying Motivated 318
Do Less 319
Log it 319
Work Out with a Friend 319
Keep Your Goals in Sight — Literally 319
Train for an Event 319
Keep Yourself Entertained 320
The Right Gear 320
Clothing 320
Water Bottles 321
Watches 321
Footwear 321

Chapter 19: Debunking Fitness Myths **327**
Who Needs Exercise? 327
Exercise is a Modern Invention for the Bored — My Grandmother
Managed Very Well Without it — I Can Too. 327

Exercise Is Not for Me. I'm Too Old. 328

Exercise Is Not for Me. I'm Too Fat. 329

Exercise Is Not for Me. I'm Too Skinny. 330

I Can't Exercise. I've Never Done it Before. 330

I Can't Exercise Because I Get Dizzy. 330

I Can't Exercise Because it's Too Expensive. 331

I Can't Exercise Because I Am Pregnant. 331

I Can't Exercise Because I've Just Had a Baby. 332

I Can't Exercise Because I Suffer From Stress Incontinence. 333

What Exercise Can and Can't Do 334

I Need To Lose Weight, Therefore I Need To Exercise (Read: Without
Dieting). 334

I Don't Need To Go To a Gym Or Exercise Class — I'm on the
Move All Day. 335

I Was Really Fit Three Months Ago. Now That I Want To Start
Exercising Again, I'm Going To Continue From Where I Left Off. . . .335

Exercise Will Cure All Aches and Pains. 336

Exercising Once a Week is Useless. 336

Exercising Once a Week is Enough. 337

I Have To Exercise for Thirty Consecutive Minutes in Order
To Benefit. 337

If I Stop Exercising, My Muscles Will Turn To Fat. 337

By Focusing on Abdominal Exercises I Will Get Rid of My
Excess Midriff. 338

The Class/Session Itself 338

Exercise is Boring. 338

I Can Only Join a Gym If I've Got the Latest Gear. 339

I Can't Go To an Aerobics Class Because I Won't Be Able To Follow
All the Moves (and Therefore I Won't Benefit). 339

I'm Really Fit So I Can't Go To a Regular (Easy) Aerobics Class. 340

Going for "the Burn" is the Way To Go. 340

I Can't Go To the Class Because I Can't Keep Up with the Instructor. . . .341

Section 6: The Finishing Line: Life After Weight Loss 343

Chapter 20: The Winner's Circle: How To Stay There For Life 345

Prioritizing Priorities 345

A New Perspective 345

Plan of Action 346

Experiment 346

A Stitch in Time Saves...Pounds 347

Weighing 347

Other Monitors 347

Pop-Up Party Time 348

The 90-10 Rule 348

The "T" Factor 349

Beware the Dragon of Boredom 349

Be Flexible 350
Activate Yourself 350
Never Say Never 350
Focus on the Benefits Acquired 351
Keep in Touch 352
Step Forward 352
Having Babies 352
Don't Listen To Other People 352
Watch Out for the Downward Spiral 353
Keep Rewarding Yourself 354
Set Up a Club 354
Enjoy Being at Goal 354
    Reassess Your Wardrobe 354
    Take Up New Interests 355
    Enjoy Eating 356

The Last Word **359**

Section 7: Appendices 361

Appendix 1: Reasons To Lose Weight 363
Long-Term Health Problems 364
    Heart Disease 364
    Atherosclerosis 364
    Hypertension (High Blood Pressure) 365
    High Blood Cholesterol 365
    Diabetes 366
    Gallstones 366
    Cancer 366
    Respiratory Problems 367
    Joint Diseases 367
    Immobility 367
Short-Term Health Problems 368
    Back Pain 368
    Varicose Veins 368
    Shortness of Breath 368
    Skin Complaints 368
    Infertility 369
    Pregnancy Problems 369
Appearance 369
Clothes 370
Relationships 371
    Shidduchim (Dating) 371
    Husbands 371
    At Work 372
    Socially 372
Everyday Life 373

Financial 373
Short-Term Motivators 374
Negative Motivators 374
   I'm Doing it for You 374

Appendix 2: What's A Healthy Weight For Me? **377**
  The Height-Weight Chart 377
  BMI: Body Mass Index 379
  Waist-Hip Ratio/Body Type 382
     How To Find Out If You're an Apple Or a Pear 382
     Risk Factors 383

Appendix 3: Calculating Calories **385**
  How Many Calories Does Your Body Need? .385
     The Shortcut Method To Calculate How Many Calories Your
     Body Needs 385
     The More Scenic Long Route To Calculate How Many Calories
     Your Body Needs 386

Appendix 4: Debunking Dieting Myths **389**
  I've Been on Every Diet Going and None of Them Work 389
  I Don't Have To Diet — I'll Go To the Gym Instead 390
  I Won't Lose Weight if I Eat Late at Night 390
  If Eating Less Doesn't Work, I Have To Eat Less…and Less…and Less . .391
  If I Ignore My Cravings They'll Go Away 391
  To Lose Weight I Must Not Eat in Between Meals 391
  Skipping Breakfast Saves Calories 391
  The Quickest and Surest Way To Lose Weight is To Fast 392
  You Can Eat As Much As You Want of a Fat-Free Food and Still
    Lose Weight 392
  Drinking Flushes Away Excess Calories 393
  My Whole Family is Fat — Therefore it's My Destiny To Be Fat, Too 393

Appendix 5: Fiber: What's It Really All About? **395**
  Digestion — The "Ins" and "Outs" 396
  What is Fiber? 397
     What is Insoluble Fiber? 397
     What is Soluble Fiber? 397
  What Does Fiber Do? 397
     What Does Insoluble Fiber Do? 397
     What Does Soluble Fiber Do? 398
  Health Benefits 398
     Health Benefits of Insoluble Fiber 398
     Health Benefits of Soluble Fiber 399
  Benefits To a Weight Loss Program 400
  How Much Fiber Does a Person Need? 401
  Fiber Contents of Foods 401
  How Do We Increase Fiber in Our Diet? 406

Appendix 6: Drinking . . . . **.407**
  So How Much Do I Need To Drink Each Day? 408
    The Formula 408
  A Word About What Not To Drink 408

Appendix 7: Dieting And Kids . . . . **.411**
  Physical Factors 412
    Changing Height 412
    Inaccurate BMI Readings 412
    Growth Spurts 412
    Changing Shape 412
    Activity Levels 412
  Emotional Factors 413
    Choose Your Battlefield 413
    Hormones 413
    Self-Esteem 413
    Stress for Mom 414
    Adolescent Immaturity 414
    Mental Health 414
    Responsibility 414
    Peer Pressure 414
  When Will My Child Be Old Enough To Diet? .416

Appendix 8: Eating Disorders — When Dieting Goes Too Far . . . . **.417**
  Anorexia 417
  Bulimia 418
  Binge Eating Disorder 419
  Who Gets Eating Disorders? 419
  What Causes Eating Disorders? 419
    Personality Factors 419
    Emotional Factors 419
    Family Factors 420
    Society Factors 420
    Triggers 420
  Physical Consequences of Eating Disorders 420
  Where To Find Help 421
  Help and Treatment 421
    What is the Best Treatment for an Eating Disorder? 421
  Are You at Risk? Take a Self-Test 422

Index . . . . **.425**

Foreword

by Rabbi Dr. Abraham J. Twerski

I know precious little about nutrition, and I am not an authority on dieting. Why, then, am I writing a foreword to a book about dieting?

Every month, without fail, there are several new, *guaranteed to work*, miracle diets boldly announced on magazine covers, some of which even assure you that you can eat to your heart's content and lose weight. Over the years, there have been *hundreds* of such miracle diets that will enable one to lose thirty pounds in four weeks without any effort.

Just a bit of common sense would indicate that if any one of these diets had any merit, why would there be a need for new ones every month? Certainly, over the years, a successful diet would have proven itself.

The answer is that all these diets do work…for a short period of time. Then the weight is regained plus some, so it's time to try another *guaranteed to work* miracle diet, and it, too, will take off pounds quickly and put them back on just as quickly. The result is the "yo-yo syndrome." No miracle diet is sustainable over the long term.

I once saw a hostess reprimand her seven-year-old child for licking the gravy off his fingers. "Stop eating like an animal!" she said. I could not help being aware of her obesity and thinking, "My dear lady, if only you *did* eat like an animal, you would not be overweight." Animals in the wild are neither obese nor bulimic. They eat to provide their bodies with essential nutrients, and when they have enough, they stop eating.

In contrast, we humans eat more than our bodies require. We have found that eating can soothe our nerves. We can use food as a tranquilizer. Let's face it. When we eat more than the body requires, food becomes a drug. We may not like to think of ourselves as being drug addicts, but there is no getting away from it. So it is a "legal drug," bought at the supermarket rather than from a dealer, but the deleterious effects are the same.

If you are looking for a "quick fix" diet, don't read this book. Pick up one of the magazines that sports a diet that will let you take off thirty pounds in four weeks and put on forty pounds in the next eight weeks. **If you really want to keep your weight down for the long term, read this book and follow the recommendations faithfully.** It will require dedication, effort, and perseverance, but the result will be well worth it.

Introduction

About this Book

Why Do I Need Another Diet Book? (What Makes This Book So Different?)

Whether you are a first-time dieter or an old pro, the planet of weight loss can be a very confusing, overwhelming, and frustrating world.

In the United States alone, it is a $33 billion dollar industry. From weight loss centers and diet gurus to diets and diet products; from health clubs and personal trainers to in-home gym equipment and private exercise classes — the options available today are mind-boggling.

And that's all before we even start with the information (and misinformation) that accompanies all these options.

There are literally millions of diet and exercise books, all professing to possess that ultimate elixir, that one sure way to lose it all. Where does anyone start, let alone navigate all the way through to a happy ending?

And even when people do find a starting place, who can understand what they're reading? Half the time the information is presented in medical jargon or technical terms by some doctor or professor, or both, and the other half of the time, the information may be readable — but what a bore it is to read. The style is so off-putting, dry, and wordy — who can be bothered to read it from start to finish?

And if you eventually do find something that is well-written, for-the-layman, informative, and enjoyable-to-read, it often seems to be out of touch with how a woman thinks, feels, functions, and basically lives. Let's be realistic: Who has the time or inclination to dirty three pots, cooking three different ways for a recipe — and that's only the main course?

After all is said and done, and one actually finds the "perfect" weight loss book, just how much of it is suitable for a Jewish lifestyle? How much of it is in tune with where we are coming from? Does it help for Shabbos? Yom Tov? Sheva Brochos? The way we take vacations?

That's why this book is so needed (and different) — because this book is:

✔ **Not** another diet book. It is a **handbook** on how to succeed on **any** sensible, healthy eating plan. It's a guide for the confused with lots of clearly written and clearly laid-out information, in addition to oodles and oodles of well-tested practical tips.

✔ Written in simple-Simon-easy-to-understand layman's terms, in a down-to-earth yet upbeat, snappy style, because I want you to read the whole book and not get bored halfway through.

✔ Written for women by a woman who has helped many women over the years to reach their weight loss goals and stay there. It's in tune with a woman's psyche and the way she lives.

✔ Applicable, practical, and sympathetic to a Jewish lifestyle. It will even guide you through the weight loss issues involved in the life cycle of the Jewish year.

✔ Designed to help you choose a healthy diet, motivate you to stick to it, and help you carry it through to a successful conclusion. It will also teach you what to do after you have arrived at your goal weight to ensure you stay there for as long as you want.

✔ Full of relevant information on weight loss, nutrition, and exercise as they relate to the Jewish woman in our times.

Now that you know what makes this book so unique, the next question is, who wrote it?

About the Author

Her Qualifications

Chava Goldman holds a BA in Business Administration and is a qualified Weight Management Consultant. She has run her own Diet and Exercise Consultancy for nearly a decade and has designed and currently supervises a Weight Management Group. Over the years, Chava has helped many women reach and maintain their dieting goals. She also advises fellow diet consultants from around the world.

Chava is also one of the premier Orthodox Jewish aerobics instructors in the world. She is a fully qualified RSA Aerobics and Body Conditioning Instructor, specially trained in Advanced Choreography and Antenatal and Postnatal Exercise. Chava regularly teaches classes (sometimes with nearly one hundred participants) to high schools, seminaries, and married ladies. She runs an Ante/Postnatal Exercise course for qualified instructors and will soon be training future aerobics instructors.

In addition, Chava has written a weekly column for a national newspaper on diet and exercise issues for the Jewish woman and is currently a freelance journalist and guest lecturer. The British Government recently commissioned her to write a short guide to dieting and exercise for Anglo Jewry.

Chava also loves photography, writing poetry, painting and creating modern art.

She somehow fits all this around her very busy schedule as a mother of a whole lot of lively children and as a wife of a husband in full-time Torah learning.

Chava says the secret to her busy schedule is to be well organized and not to breathe — there's no time for that!

Weight Management consultant. Aerobics instructor. Writer. Lecturer. Mother…Who else should write such a book? But if you ask Chava, she'll tell you that her real qualification for writing this book is that she was there…

Her Real Qualification

Chava jokes that she was born twenty-eight pounds overweight and just never managed to lose them. She tried every diet going. She even tried her own thing (starvation) and just as soon as she managed to reach her goal, she put it all back on again. She was sometimes thirty pounds overweight, sometimes fifty pounds overweight — she even reached sixty-four pounds overweight at one point.

Throughout her youth and into her early years of marriage, Chava Goldman was the perennial yo-yo dieter. On a diet, off a diet, on-off, on-off for years. If there was a report card for effort in weight loss Chava claims that she would have received straight As. But where it mattered most — to get it off and keep it off — she was a dismal failure.

Looking back, Chava understands what the problem was. She was never missing the will and desire to lose the weight — just the knowledge and real understanding of *how* to diet. She read books, she asked people, but in the end, the clarity just wasn't there. Until one day, she said, "Enough is enough," and set out to thoroughly research the entire subject of dieting and diets.

The book that you are holding in your hands is the culmination of that research, which involved a decade-long journey.

At about the same time as she started her diet research, a friend persuaded Chava to go to an aerobics class. Chava remembers vividly that she didn't want to go. After all, for her entire life, exercise had just made her hot and sweaty and had given her migraines. Her friend quite literally had to drag her to the class. But to Chava's great surprise, this beginner's class turned out to be a lot of fun. She was hooked. So hooked, in fact, that she went on to become a qualified aerobics instructor and create her own classes. The rest, as they say, is history.

With her increased awareness of weight loss management and exercise, Chava began to lose those stubborn pounds. And as the pounds came off and stayed off, a burning desire grew inside her to share her newly found secrets with anyone who would listen. To that aim, she became a qualified Weight Management Consultant, started her own Weight Loss Group, began to write a weekly column on diet and exercise, and eventually, "top-secretly," began to write this book.

So, if you'd ask…

Why Did She Write This Book?

That's simple. Chava wants to share with you all that she has learned on her long, hard journey. She wants you to have the knowledge and the tools that she wished she had had when she first started out so many years and pounds ago. Chava wants to save you from the pitfalls and stumbling blocks, annoyances and aggravations, and disappointments and waste of time, energy, and money that she went through over and over again.

And, most of all, now that Chava has made it and has tasted the sweet joy of being the shape and size that she really wants to be, she wants you to be able to get there and stay there as well.

As Chava remarks, if this book helps just one person live a healthier, happier, longer life, then it will all have been worthwhile.

We hope that person will be you.

How This Book is Organized

This book contains seven main sections. Although you can start at the very beginning ("a very good place to start…"), you don't have to. You can just dive into the section that contains the relevant information you need.

Section 1: On Your Marks — How To Get Started

Choosing a diet based on the book's front cover, or because Cousin Sarah lost weight on it, may seem like a good idea, but you run the risk of a return trip next month when you find out it didn't work.

This section takes an honest look at which diets do what and how to choose the most appropriate one for your lifestyle and needs. It attempts to prepare you to start your diet mentally, emotionally, and physically.

Section 2: Get Set — Taking Charge of Your Eating Habits

We don't always eat just because we're hungry. If we did, we wouldn't need diets. This section lists oodles of reasons why we choose food — whether for comfort, boredom, or out of habit — and gives you practical advice on how to counteract the urge to munch.

Section 3: Go! — Tips To Keep You on Track

Losing all those pounds without sacrificing your enjoyment of food is what this section is all about. Not only are there tons of tips relevant to food and the kitchen, but there are plenty of tips to help get your brain into dieting gear as well. And what about Shabbos, Yom Tov, vacations, and eating out? It's all in this section.

Section 4: Runner's Cramp — Oh No, I've Hit a Plateau

What happens when your dieting gets stale or you hit a plateau? Turn to this section — it's full of motivational and practical tips to re-energize you and blast that plateau to smithereens.

Section 5: Keep Going — Exercise

Dieting without exercising is like using only half your troops. You may win the "battle of the bulge," but it'll be harder and take longer. Or in more friendly terms, think of dieting and exercise as the Mr. and Mrs. of the Weight Loss World.

This section clarifies why exercising is so vital to successful, permanent weight loss and which exercises do what. It also takes you through a typical exercise class and gives you a fresh perspective on "classic" fitness myths.

Section 6: The Finishing Line — Life After Weight Loss

At last, you've made it. And now it's time to think ahead to how you can live a life without dieting (yes, it can be done…) while maintaining your new trim 'n' slender self.

This section provides practical tips on overcoming the hurdles to living the rest of your life in the winner's circle.

Section 7: Appendices

This section provides useful information on weight-related subjects. Topics range from reasons to lose weight to what's a healthy weight; from debunking dieting myths to calculating calories; from understanding fiber to the need to drink; from why children shouldn't be forced to diet to eating disorders.

How To Use This Book

There are basically three ways to read this book (no, not back-to-front or front-to-back, nor lying or sitting, not even upside down, …):

- Read from Cover to Cover
- Use the Table of Contents for Specific Subjects
- Use the Index to Find a Particular Topic

Read From Cover To Cover

If you are new to dieting and want the full works in terms of the science, background, tips, and skills involved in losing weight, there's no better way to read this book than from top to toe.

Glance through each chapter's contents first to get a bird's-eye view. You will probably be tempted to rush on to the next chapter — but don't. Take your time. If you are reading in order to apply the principles found within the pages of this book, then go back and **reread each chapter, with pen in hand, marking or underlining anything you would like to implement or note.** In the long run, this will mean saving time and getting results.

Use the Table of Contents for Specific Subjects

This book was organized in a way that allows you to easily refer to particular weight loss issues. If it's just not your nature to read a book methodically from cover to cover, or if you are pressed for time, you can still glean the specific information you need by using the table of contents to find the subject you require.

For example, if you are going on vacation to Miami and don't know how to tackle all that restaurant-hopping, glance at the table of contents and find "Chapter 11: Eating Right When Eating Out." Voilà! You've got something to read on the airplane.

Use the Index To Find a Particular Topic

If you want to find a specific topic, you can drag your finger through the Index. Topics such as "weighing yourself", "Atkins' diet", or "cholesterol", are listed there.

Now let's begin.

WARNING! STOP RIGHT THERE AND READ THIS FIRST.

One day as I was walking outside, deep in thought as to what to make for lunch, a woman I had not seen for quite a while drove up to the red light alongside me.

"Hey!" she exclaimed as she leaned towards me while pressing the electric window-down button. "How did you lose all your weight?" It was all I could do to control myself from laughing in her face at the sheer irony of the situation. I estimated that I had approximately thirteen and a half seconds — the time it would take the lights to change from red to green — to tell her of my experiences, research, and findings over the last ten years. I didn't think she had a week to spare, so I just pointed to the lights and to the heavens, threw my hands up, and laughed.

If you want a quick-fix, headlines only answer to all your weight problems; if you want to know the golden, magical bottom line way to shed all unwanted excess pounds and develop a perfectly toned, healthy body in seconds, then I have news for you. The bad news is there is no *quick* fix. But the good news is there are many *effective* ways to fix.

Once you have internalized this and you realize that it takes time to learn the ropes, then you are ready to begin. Take it slow and steady and enjoy your journey. There's plenty to see and do along the way.

On Your Marks – How To Get Started

*H*ere we are, poised at the starting line, braced and eager to begin losing unwanted weight. We are charged with enthusiasm and now feel inspired to either go on that diet we've been promising ourselves, or to get straight back onto the diet we've abandoned.

But, contrary to popular belief, dieting isn't all about willpower and waistlines. If you start a half-understood program that lacks nutritional basics, or one that's not suitable for your lifestyle, you'll find that your resolve has gone up in smoke after the first two weeks.

If you want to achieve success, you have to make informed decisions. This brings us to a few major questions about diets: What exactly is a "healthy diet?" What really makes a diet work? How do you choose a diet suitable for your personality and lifestyle? Which diet should *you* choose? These questions, and many more, are addressed in this section in Chapter 1.

But even after you've chosen the diet right for you, there is still a bit of pre-game preparation to do. You need to ensure that you are ready both mentally and physically. We'll help you take care of that in Chapter 2.

So let's begin the journey to Diet Land together.

If you want to be further motivated or convinced to go on a diet (for other reasons than your clothes don't fit anymore, etc.), then turn to "Appendix 1: Reasons To Lose Weight," before you continue. If you want to know your ideal target weight at any time, then turn to "Appendix 2: What's A Healthy Weight For Me?"

Chapter 1

— ◆ ◆ ◆ —

How Do I Choose A Diet?

Eat Healthy, Live Healthy

A Healthy Diet — The Two Essential Rules

Not every successful (i.e., weight-reducing) diet is a great diet for healthy living. There are lots of diets out there that will reduce body weight. Even starvation will reduce weight. But, and it's a BIG but, not all of them promote healthy living. (When was the last time you came across a healthy person suffering from starvation?)

At best, they can only be successfully implemented on a short-term basis. At worst, they can be detrimental to good health.

For a diet to be *truly* healthy, it must follow two cardinal rules:

    ✔ Provide us with all necessary nutrients;

    ✔ Not have any long-term, negative health ramifications.

> *By the end of this chapter you should be able to analyze any diet and decide if it's the right one for you.*

What Makes a Diet Healthy?

At the risk of reiterating what we have all heard a million times before, from any and all health professionals worth their salt, let's clarify what constitutes a healthy diet.

In short, just like a car needs gas and oil to run, so too, we need food to provide our bodies with energy, nutrients, vitamins, minerals, etc. In addition, we can't survive on unleaded gas alone — instead, we need a mixture of nutrients obtained from a variety of foods.

There are five basic food groups:

- ✔ Breads, cereals, pastas, and potatoes (commonly known as starches/carbohydrates);
- ✔ Fruits and vegetables;
- ✔ Milk and dairy foods;
- ✔ Meat, fish, and alternatives (also known as proteins);
- ✔ Foods containing fat and sugar-dense foods.

The ideal balance is to make the starchy foods (preferably whole-wheat varieties) the main part of your meals. These foods are high in essential vitamins, minerals, and fiber and are low in fat. They also help to fill you up. Next, we must aim to eat at least five portions of fruits and vegetables each day. These also provide essential vitamins, minerals, and fiber and are mostly low in fat (getting the message?). We also have to choose a variety of milk products and protein foods (although not as much as the starchy foods). These foods will provide you not just with valuable protein, but also with calcium, iron, and zinc. And lastly (and let's hope, leastly...) we should try to eat fatty[1] and sugary "no-no" foods sparingly[2] ("Elementary, my dear dieter...").

Foods in one group can't replace those in another. No one food group is more important than another — for good health, you need them all.

Below is a table showing a typical daily food intake before and after a policy of healthy eating has been implemented.

---

[1] See "Fighting Fats," page 99.
[2] Alcohol also comes under this heading.

BEFORE	AFTER
Breakfast	**Breakfast**
1 cup of coffee (with sugar and whole milk)	1 cup of decaffeinated coffee with skim milk and artificial sweetener
1 bowl of sugar-coated cereal with whole milk	1 piece of fresh fruit
	2 slices of whole-wheat toast with reduced-sugar jam
Lunch	**Lunch**
Pizza, french fries, full-fat coleslaw	Whole-wheat pasta with reduced-fat Cheddar cheese, tomato sauce, and spices
Chocolate ice cream	Sorbet/Popsicle
Large glass of Coke	Large glass of Diet Coke
Dinner	**Dinner**
Fried chicken cutlets in breadcrumbs	3 slices white roast chicken (without skin)
Roast potatoes (in oil)	Baked potato
Stir-fried vegetables (in oil)	Mixed vegetables (large portion)
Glass of wine	Canned pineapple in own juice
	Glass of diet lemonade
Snacks/Extras	**Snacks/Extras**
Cookies/nosh/candies & chocolate	Rice cakes/low-calorie crackers with reduced-fat/light cheese triangle
	1 Mini Milk Munch bar
	Fresh fruit

What About Negative Long-Term Health Aspects?

If you've only got a few pounds to lose before you hit that magical, ever-elusive goal, maybe you will decide to embark on a weird, you-realize-it's-unhealthy diet. It may work — and it may work quickly. If you're only going to be on it for a short time, no long-term health issues are likely to arise. But, if you are like most people and you have more than just a "few pounds" to go, or you're thinking about a long-term maintenance plan, then read further…

Before embarking on *any* diet, and certainly before embarking on a long-term diet, it is very important to ensure that you will, in effect, be doing your body more good than harm.

This means checking out the diet — big time. What is its history? What qualifications does the person who designed it possess? Does your doctor think it's a good, balanced, healthy diet? Sometimes the diet book itself will supply you with the information you need, and yes, sometimes it might take a little effort and research. Remember, you are setting yourself up to expend a lot of your time, energy, effort, and money (and hope) on this diet; doesn't it make sense to ensure that it's a healthy one?

Below (on page 21) in the section titled "A World of Choice (Which Diet Should I Choose? An Analysis)" we analyze some of the more common diets together with their premises, and the truths behind the diets. Even if your chosen diet is not listed, it might still be worth your while to read this section so that you can clarify what sort of questions can arise when choosing a diet.

IN CONCLUSION

We need a diet that will ensure we get the supply of nutrients our bodies need. In addition, we don't want to compromise our overall long-term good health by choosing an unbalanced diet.

Although there are many wild and wacky diets on the market these days, they do not all conform to these long-standing principles. Yes, they may well work, but they may also compromise your health in the long-term as well.

Following these two basic guidelines for a healthy diet will not only promote good health, but will also ensure a varied, satisfying choice of menu. No one wants to survive on carrot sticks alone. We want to scratch each tastebud's itch — be it in terms of having something sweet or something savory, something crunchy or something soft, etc. Following these principles will promote not only good health, but also happy health. And that's great news.

The Equation (What Makes a Diet Work?)

Even if we eat healthily (see previous section), we won't be guaranteed a weight loss (unless, of course, we've been living off snacks and sweets for years).

So I am going to tell you about the one, all-time unequivocal, write-it-in-stone equation that we need to know when we are talking about weight loss.

Weight Loss = Fewer Calories[3] Coming In Than Are Going Out

What does that mean?

In short, every person needs a certain number of calories per day to maintain his/her current weight. This number varies from person to person depending on his/her age,[4] build, metabolism,[5] weight,[6] and level of activity.[7]

If we consume more calories than we require, our bodies store those calories in the form of fat. If we consume fewer calories than we need, we lose fat — because the body eventually uses our fat as an energy source when it runs out of calories.

Let's get more specific: If we want to lose one pound in weight, we have to burn off 3,500 calories. We have two ways to achieve this:

> ✔ **We can cut down on the number of calories we consume to create this deficit.**

To give you a rough idea what that means in real, yummy-eating terms, let's look at a list of foods that, if resisted in the course of a week, would create this magical deficit:

---

[3] Calories are our body's source of energy. They come from the food we eat. This can be in the form of proteins, carbs, fats, or alcohol. Water, minerals, and vitamins do not produce calories. Neither, for that matter, do cholesterol or fiber.

[4] We need the most calories when we are about twenty-five and then it's a gradual but significant downhill from then on. I.e., the older you are, the fewer calories you need to keep your body functioning.

[5] Some people have naturally faster metabolic rates than others. Because children and adolescents are still growing, they also have relatively faster rates than adults.

[6] If you are obese or very overweight your body needs more energy (calories) to move its greater load. So you will burn more calories doing the same activity as Mrs. Average who has an average weight and build.

[7] See page 386.

Food	Calories
1 bag of potato chips	136
1 large chocolate Milk Munch bar	200
1 cup pistachio nuts	775
3 Tbsp. salad dressing (full fat)	312
10oz whole milk	180
1 beefburger in a bun	321
1 portion thin-cut french fries	462
1 vanilla ice cream bar	180
1 slice chocolate cheesecake	271
1 chocolate and walnut brownie	505
3 Tbsp. corn	122
4 jelly Beans	40
TOTAL	3,504 (Hey, that's near enough...)

Or,

✔ We can increase the rate at which calories are burned off.

The table below shows you how many calories are burned off by engaging in various continuous exercises for twenty minutes (for a person weighing roughly 150 pounds).

Activity	Calories Burned
Mild aerobics	150
Walking	115
Mopping the floor	85
Raking the leaves	80

To put this into perspective in terms of hard work, one hour's demanding aerobic class burns off 450 calories. It would take eight classes in one week to burn off 3,600 calories and therefore see yourself one pound lighter on the scales.

To sum it up in one sentence: **If we want to lose weight we either have to eat fewer calories or exercise more (or do a combination of both).** This equation is non-negotiable. You can't get around the facts. Eat more calories than your body needs and you gain weight, eat fewer calories, and…bingo.

Understanding this principle explains why we need a diet at all. Most diets are just different versions of the same theme: We want to lose weight, so we must eat fewer calories. Each diet has a different strategy toward achieving this goal. Where one might limit fats, another limits carbohydrates, etc. Each diet has been specifically designed to create this oh-so-important deficit in calories to guarantee the desired end product of losing those troublesome extra pounds. (And this is the case even for those diets that claim they are not a calorie-counting diet. That may be true — i.e., they won't make *you* count your calorie intake, but in the end, even *their* diets work by creating that impossible-to-avoid calorie deficit).

Let's Get Personal (How To Analyze Yourself Before Choosing a Diet)

Now that we have covered what constitutes a healthy diet, and the reason why a diet works, we are still left with the question of which diet is going to suit you best.

Ever felt the frustration of beginning a new diet and not being able to stick to it? Ever heard the term "yo-yo" dieting[8] and been able to relate? Have you ever felt that your life revolves around trying out the latest diet? Do you remember feeling frustrated because whatever weight you started a diet on, you always seemed to be either the same (or more) when you started the next one?

The problem is not necessarily you. The problem may be the compatibility between you and your diet.

I wish I had a dollar for every time someone has asked me to recommend "the best diet." You want to know the very best diet? The one that's foolproof, that'll help you get rid of those extra pounds *and* keep them off? There's a simple answer. **The best diet is the diet that works best for you.**

No two people think, feel, react, or eat exactly the same way. Some like large quantities of food because they have large appetites. Some like to graze all day, but don't mind small portions. A diet has got to work *for* you, not against you. It's no good deciding to start the latest craze or high protein diet when you don't even like meat or fish. It just isn't going to last. You need to choose a diet that is right for you because it fits in with *your* tastes, preferences, lifestyle, and habits.

If a diet can be easily incorporated into your lifestyle, it stands to reason that it'll endure the test of time. And, for that matter, so will you.

---

[8] On a diet, off a diet, on a diet, off a diet…

In order to choose the appropriate diet for your personality and lifestyle, a little self-analysis is required. Although you may well come up with many more (and please feel free to…), here's a checklist to help you get started.

My Personality

✔ Am I meticulous or slap-dash? (Will I mind weighing food, counting points, or writing things down?)

✔ Am I the type of person who likes to be methodical, organized, and prepared (a list-lover?), or spontaneous (whatever I feel like, I do/eat)?

✔ Am I usually calm and in control (if yes, tell me your secret…) or am I usually in a rush or facing another emergency?

Personal Preferences

✔ Do I actually like fruits and veggies? Or do I prefer meat and potatoes?

✔ Can I cope with restrictions — either in terms of quantity of food, or in terms of variety of food? (If you can't face either, forget about dieting.)

✔ Do I need to eat a lot because I am often hungry?

✔ Do I prefer lots of different types of food or do I tend to just stick to good old faithful favorites?

✔ Do I like to cook and prepare food?

✔ Do I have the time to cook separate meals for myself or must my diet fit in with my family?

✔ Do I usually eat healthily?

✔ Do I prefer convenience foods over regular food?

✔ Do I realize that I eat way too much garbage?

Outside Influences/Lifestyle

✔ Have I just had a baby?

✔ Do I have time to take care of myself in my current situation? (If not, don't start now. A false start is worse than no start. See page 54).

A World of Choice (Which Diet Should I Choose? An Analysis)

Now that you know yourself a little better (and are best friends), let's find out what some of the major diets are all about, without trying them all only to find out the hard way that what works for Aunty Abigail won't necessarily work for you. Let's analyze a few of the most popular diets in the Jewish world (**note that we are *analyzing, not promoting* any one diet**).

Weight Watchers

The Diet

You can eat whatever you want and still lose weight if you keep within the prescribed range of points suitable for your current weight. Each food is attributed a point value — basically the higher the calorific value, the higher the points. It's your job to keep track of how many points you are spending as you go through your day. No food is banned. No one food is compulsory.

In addition, Weight Watchers is based on group meetings encouraging support and contact (see "Troop to Group," page 133, for the benefits of group support).

The Evaluation

This diet is based on restricting the number of calories and saturated fat (the bad fat[9]) in your diet. In order to get "value for money" in terms of spending your points, you are automatically encouraged to eat foods that have low point values. These are typically your vegetables, fruit, carbohydrates, and lean proteins.

The Verdict

Although the diet can encourage healthy eating, it can also be abused. If you want to eat potato chips and chocolate all day, you can. You might get hungry, but if you stay within the boundary of your points allocation, you will still lose weight. If you continue subsisting only on the goody-gumdrops type of foods, you will not be providing your body with the necessary nutrients to ensure long-term good health.

---

[9] See "Fighting Fats," page 99.

Pros	Cons
• You can eat whatever types of food you want. This provides natural variety.	• You MUST write everything down — a few points out can make the difference between losing or staying the same (even though you think you've been good).
• You can eat whatever combination of foods you want.	• Fruit also costs you points. (This might deter you from snacking on fruit.)
• Proven weight loss method with a strong track record.	• Not everyone enjoys the social side of dieting — especially if you haven't lost weight that week.
• You can indulge in often-forbidden foods (like chocolate and potato chips).	• Although weighing food is not compulsory, it is important in the beginning until you get an idea of what they mean by a small/medium/large portion. This can be a big-time pain in the neck.
• You can save up points for Shabbos/ Yom Tov/Celebrations.	• Portion sizes must be controlled (i.e., small really is small, not just your version of small).
• Convenience foods can fit into this diet.	• You are more likely to have food on the brain all day because you must account for everything that goes into your mouth.
• No waiting between foods.	• You might feel like you are on a diet because you have to be so conscious throughout the day.
• Diet is safe and promotes good eating habits.	• The food you eat does not have to be healthy.
• Exercise is promoted.	
• Since there are no off-limits foods, it is flexible and can be adapted for Shabbos and Yom Tov.	
• Educates the participant about nutritional values.	
• Promotes group support.	
• It works.	

The Complete Scarsdale Medical Diet

(Herman Tarnower, MD and Samm Sinclair Baker)

The Diet

The diet is based on a high-protein, low-carbohydrate consumption ratio. Protein is unlimited. Very little fruit is included. Milk is excluded, as are all chocolates and treats. There is a day-by-day set menu to follow, i.e., Monday is cold cuts, Tuesday is hamburgers, etc.

After you have completed the two-week diet program, you embark on the maintenance plan for two weeks. This is basically the same except you can have milk, more fruit, and an alcoholic drink.

The diet expects a rapid weight loss. A pound a day is not unusual.

The Evaluation

You will lose a lot of weight on this diet (proportionate to the amount you have to lose).

Due to the high protein content (taken in conjunction with unlimited specified vegetables), together with low carbohydrate and fat levels, you are automatically creating a calorie deficit that will result in weight loss. (The diet provides roughly 1,000 calories a day compared to a regular weight loss program of 1,500–1,700 calories.)

Not many of the healthy eating guidelines are being met here. The basis of the diet is protein, not carbohydrates, and you don't get a full five portions of fruit and vegetables every day. The regime is strict and must be followed to the letter. This means that there is very little freedom of choice in terms of menu-planning. So tough-cookies if you have fish leftover from Shabbos that needs to be eaten.

Actually, you can forget about the cookies entirely — even tough ones. The diet leaves no leeway for Shabbos/Yom Tov treats.

When it comes to the crunch, The Scarsdale Diet does not promote a variety of foods and is basically boring. Chances are you'll get fed up of the strict regime before you lose all your weight anyway.

The Verdict

Not all the weight you lose is coming from your stores of fat. You are also losing water, which is making up the downward spiralling number on the scales. If you like protein, you'll enjoy it. If you like carbohydrates, you're going to be miserable. If you like variety and having whatever is around, don't bother starting the Scarsdale Diet.

Although this diet works in reducing weight, your long-term health benefits may be compromised. As a direct result of this high-protein diet, ketones are produced in the urine (which basically alter the acid/alkaline balance in your blood) and may produce one or several of the following undesirable effects:

- Make the urine smell like acetone (nail polish remover);
- Result in bad breath/body odor;
- Cause nausea;
- Increase your loss of sodium and potassium, which raises your risk of an irregular heartbeat;
- Increase your loss of calcium in the bones, raising your risk of osteoporosis.

Great stuff, eh?

In short: At best, this diet works short-term; at worst, it does not conform to the guidelines for long-term healthy eating and can lead to ill health.

Pros	Cons
• Follow the plan and you will lose — lots.	• You lose water, not just fat.
• You will also lose quickly.	• You might get bored.
• You don't have to wrack your brain thinking about what you are going to have for lunch.	• You might feel frustrated at not being able to eat what you want because it's not on that day's plan.
• You'll save money by not buying nosh.	• It's expensive because of the quantities of meat and fish.
• If you like meat and fish, you might like this diet.	• You can't indulge in any tempting treats.
• Very little measuring.	• No milk, only little fruit.
• No writing down/keeping track of what you eat.	• Convenience foods are out.
• Good for someone who has only a small amount to lose and a short time to lose it in.	• It could be unhealthy (and restrictive) if continued long-term.
	• Low in many vitamins and minerals.
	• Does not conform to healthy eating guidelines.

Remember, I am not advocating any one diet over another — I am simply presenting you with a menu from which you might want to make your selection.

Dr. Atkins' New Diet Revolution

(Robert C. Atkins, MD)

The Diet

You can eat as much protein and fat as you like. While this might sound like a dieter's utopia (ahh, steak…full-fat cream…butter…), there are rigid restrictions on your intake of all and any carbohydrates. Just for the record, carbohydrates are not only found in breads, pastas, and potatoes. They are also found in fruits, vegetables (the kind you cook), and raw salad veggies.

There are four basic phases to the diet. The first phase is "induction" and is the most restrictive — allowing a miniscule 4g serving of carbs a day. In real "what do I put on my plate" terms, this comes out to the equivalent of three loosely packed cups of salad.

During the second phase, there is a gradual weekly increase in carbohydrate consumption until there is no further weight loss. Then, a small amount of carbohydrates is subtracted from the daily intake for continued weight loss.

The third and fourth stages are pre-maintenance and maintenance, and involve increasing carbohydrate consumption to avoid further weight loss without gaining.

The Atkins diet is less restrictive than The Scarsdale Diet in terms of not binding you to a pre-set menu plan. You can decide what and when you will eat, as long as you follow the guidelines.

The Evaluation

This diet slaps a hard fist into the face of all that health professionals espouse in terms of good nutrition advice (i.e., eat lots of high-fiber whole-grains, at least five portions of fruits and veggies a day, etc…). The final, least restrictive phase of the diet still falls short of the nutritionists' recommended allowance[10] of over 200g of carbohydrates a day (on a 1,700 low-calorie diet), and recommends a maximum of only 60g per day.

Although rapid weight loss inevitably results, its long-term success is hampered by the fact that the diet is so restrictive and automatically will involve lots of cooking (snacking on fish or chicken anyone?). In addition, eating such high-fat foods on a long-term basis is one sure way to increase your risks of heart disease and cancer (remember, we're supposed to be living *longer*, healthier lives…).

---

[10] That fifty-five to sixty percent of your calories come from carbs.

The Verdict

The good news is that the unlimited consumption of fat will result in making you feel full longer. This means you will automatically eat less. You therefore eat fewer calories — which results in, hey presto, weight loss.

The bad news is that although following the diet may well result in speedy weight loss, much of that weight is due to excess water loss. This is because when the body needs energy, it turns to its supplies of glucose. Glucose is usually a product of breaking down carbohydrates. In the absence of carbs, the body goes looking elsewhere. On this diet, it finds fats and proteins — but will have a hard job breaking them down. This results in the production of water as a byproduct of breaking down the fats and proteins. (That's why people who follow a low-carb diet visit the bathroom more often.) This weight loss is temporary. As soon as you begin eating normally again (i.e., more carbs), the weight is regained.

In addition, low-carb diets such as this one may cause the body to quite literally "eat itself up" (ugh) by seeking energy from the body's own muscle fibers (which are protein).

As we mentioned before in The Scarsdale Diet (see page 23), a particularly unpleasant effect of following such a low-carb regime is the production of excess ketones, resulting in bad breath, perspiration, potential nausea, increased risk of loss of sodium and potassium (thereby raising the risk of an irregular heartbeat), excess uric acid[11] (potentially causing kidney stones), and loss of calcium (increasing the risk of osteoporosis).

Lack of fiber will also result in an increased likelihood of constipation — plus, because the diet is so restrictive in terms of fruits and veggies, vitamin and mineral requirements will not be met without supplements.

On the non-medical side, beefburgers without the bun, steak without the potatoes, and melted cheese without the toast might leave you craving their counterpart.

The Atkins diet is effective in the short term, but its success depends largely on how much you enjoy eggs, meat, and high-protein food.

---

[11] Produced during the breakdown of protein for energy.

Pros	Cons
• Rapid weight loss.	• Limited bread, crackers, rice, potatoes, carrots, etc. (i.e., carbs).
• Unlimited fat permitted.	• Nutritionally unbalanced.
• No calorie counting or measuring.	• Very limited fruit and vegetable intake.
• Easy menu-planning.	• You still have to count carbohydrate grams.
• Likelihood of reduced hunger.	• Lots of cooking (unless you like sushi,[12] sushi, sushi).
• Less restrictive than Scarsdale in terms of planning meals.	• Deficient in essential vitamins and minerals.
• Unlimited protein foods allowed (if you are a meat/fish lover, this might work well for you).	• Constipation likely.
	• Increased likelihood of certain undesirable health conditions (and bad breath).
	• Expensive.
	• Does not conform to healthy eating guidelines.
	• Weight loss is temporary.

The Zone

(Barry Sears, PhD with Bill Lawren)

The Diet

The Zone diet claims to put you into your personal optimal state of well-being — both physically and mentally. It is also a low-carb, high-protein plan that is based on a daily calorie distribution of 40-30-30[13] ratio of carbs-to-protein-to-fat. In this respect (increased carbohydrate allowance), the Zone is not as restrictive as Atkins or Scarsdale. The diet suggests you eat three meals a day and two snacks, but only allows you approximately 1,200 calories per day. (As we mentioned earlier on page 23 this is compared to a regular weight-loss allowance of 1,500–1,700 calories.)

---

[12] Raw fish.
[13] Most nutritionists recommend about fifty-five percent of our daily calories come from carbs, fifteen percent from protein, and up to thirty percent from fat.

The big evil in today's weight loss world, it claims (as with all high-protein diets, including Atkins and Scarsdale), is our diets' excessive amounts of carbohydrates that create too much insulin, which adversely affects the way our bodies break down fat. The diet therefore limits carbs, and, at the same time, recommends that the amount of carbohydrates in any meal or snack be matched by proteins (to ensure a good balance of eicosanoids[14]).

The diet recommends low-fat meats (versus salami, red meats, etc.), most raw/cooked vegetables (except carrots, corn, peas, potatoes), and fruit. It seriously limits bread and pasta, preferring to ensure a carbohydrate source from fruits and vegetables.

The fats recommended are the "good guy" type of fats, namely, monounsaturated. (See "Fighting Fats," page 100.)

The Evaluation

The Zone is one of the less restrictive high-protein diets. However, your weight loss is ensured, not because the pseudo-scientific research is earthshattering, but because your calorie intake has been significantly reduced.

Due to its more generous allowance of carbohydrates, the common unpleasant side effects of a high-protein diet, such as consuming an unhealthily high level of saturated fat, or forcing the body into ketosis, are not a problem on this diet.

Beware; the diet in its original form, *Enter the Zone: A Dietary Road Map*, does not make for gripping reading. Best read when you want to go to sleep anyway. It's complicated, boring, and very technical. If you are interested in this diet, it's easier on the brain cells to read the sequel *A Week in the Zone*, which was obviously written to clarify the original version.

The Verdict

The Zone is a healthy diet if you want to try out a high protein diet (it *is* fashionable, after all…). Take care not to consume more than the thirty percent of calories from fat, which may easily occur due to the diet's focus on protein.

The diet can potentially thwart hunger quite effectively due to the combination of fats, proteins, and carbohydrates at every sitting. But the portions are tiny, and the time spent in the kitchen may just be too overwhelming for many people.

---

[14] There's a lot of talk in the Zone about eicosanoids (eye-koh-suh-noids). Basically, the author defines them as "superhormones, that control virtually every vital physiological function."

Pros	Cons
• Good weight loss.	• Weight loss is also from water, not just fat.
• One of the more generous high-protein diets in terms of carbs.	• Expensive.
• Generous allowance of protein (good for meat and fish lovers).	• Very limited bread and pasta.
• Generous allowance of most fruits and vegetables.	• Not enjoyable to read (and that's an understatement).
• Easy palm-sized portioning for proteins.	• Complicated to follow and overly scientific.
• No calorie counting.	• Restrictive due to the small amounts recommended.
• Low in saturated fats.	• Recommends eating when not hungry as the best time to eat. This is not good dieting practice.
• Easy menu-planning.	• The diet insists on eating breakfast within one hour of waking (some people can't face food before they're fully awake…).
• Likelihood of reduced hunger.	• Eliminates some highly nutritious foods and is low in whole grains and calcium.
• One of the healthier high-protein diets.	• Time consuming, as you should have five meals a day.
• Steady weight loss if followed exactly.	• No room for convenience foods and treats.
	• Lots of time spent preparing meals (protein foods need cooking).
	• Low fiber intake may result in digestive problems.

The "Eat More, Weigh Less" Diet

(Dean Ornish, MD)

The Diet

The "Ornish diet" (as it's known to its friends), is a low-fat vegetarian diet. You might ask what there is to eat if you can't eat meat and fat, and the answer is…complex carbohydrates (bread, etc.), fiber-rich foods (Bran Flakes, etc.), plenty of fruits and veggies, and moderate amounts of nonfat dairy products. Of course, all the usual no-nos apply — such as no alcohol, refined sugars, oils, and nuts.

The Evaluation

The diet's downside has to be the *extreeeemely* low fat content. The diet is based on only ten percent of your daily calories coming from fat, and this is mega-restrictive as well as contravening the medical world's recommended thirty percent score. It may also be unhealthy in the long term — see "Fighting Fats," page 100.

The Verdict

This diet will work to help rid oodles of weight because, even if the quantities of allowed food are unlimited, your daily calorie intake will still be very low due to the absence of any meaningful fats. Watch out for boredom setting in or for desperate cravings for cheese, chicken, meat, chocolate.…

This one doesn't work for Shabbos or Yom Tov (no chicken or meat).

Pros	Cons
• Unlimited high-fiber carbs (wheat, rice, barley, oats, etc.) — a bread-lover's delight.	• Very little fat allowed.
• Tons of most fruits and vegetables.	• Lack of fat may reduce appeal of food.
• Baby-simple to understand and follow through.	• Lack of fat may affect health adversely in the long term.
• No calorie counting.	• Can become boring.
• Easy menu-planning.	• Zero animal products may conflict with Shabbos/Yom Tov menu.
• There's always something to eat, so hunger is relegated to memories of yesteryear.	• No leeway for sheer pleasurable naughty bits.
• The diet book is easy to read.	• Vegetarianism isn't everyone's cup of legumes (peas 'n' beans).
• Solid weight loss (if you accept vegetarianism as a lifestyle).	• Excessive high fiber may result in gas, diarrhea, or constipation.
• Effective as a diet to counteract the ills of heart disease.	• Multivitamins recommended.

Slimming World

(Possibly the second most popular diet in England — the first being Weight Watchers.)

The Diet

The first thing you have to do each day (after turning off the snooze button) is to decide whether you are feeling in a carbohydrate (Green) mood or a protein (Red) mood. Whichever one you choose will dictate the unlimited consumption of that type of food for that day. For example, on a Green Day you will be allowed to graze freely on pasta, rice, potatoes, barley, spaghetti, etc.; on a Red Day you will be allowed a free hand on (lean) meat, fish, (skinless) chicken, turkey, etc.

The diet does not promote strict food combining, where absolutely no protein may be eaten with carbohydrates and vice versa. There *are* ways to combine the two food groups on either day.

In addition to whichever day's plan you choose to follow, you are allowed a limited amount of fiber-rich, complex carbohydrate-type foods (pasta, whole-wheat bread, etc.) plus a milk/cheese selection. Eggs are also "egg-xempt" from restriction (although the diet suggests not more than ten per week). Plus, you can have your naughty-but-nice snacks too with a "Sins allocation" of fifteen points per day.

Whichever day you choose, you may consume fruits and vegetables with wild abandon.

The Evaluation

Even though you are not formally counting calories, the natural byproduct of filling your plate with a majority of veggies accompanying either your carbs or proteins is that you will automatically be partaking of a low-calorie diet.

The diet's most powerful claim is that you never go hungry. This is true. Only you might not want another baked potato when your husband is having chicken casserole, or another turkey breast when he is having french fries. But it's best not to look at his plate anyway.

The Verdict

This diet promotes some of the guidelines to healthy living. It promotes high consumption of fruits and vegetables but it falls short in its allowance of bread (remember, only whole-wheat) and cereals. All cooking must be low-fat; all meat and poultry must have all visible fat removed (say goodbye to that crispy chicken skin).

The high number of eggs allowed might raise the eyebrows of a health professional or two, but recent research is showing that eggs are not all about cholesterol and heart disease — they do have some very healthy nutritional benefits as well. However, heart patients should proceed with care.

Pros	Cons
• There is always something to eat. You don't run out of points to spend.	• Although you don't have to keep track of what you eat during the day, you do have to watch how you spend your Sins.
• The nature of being allowed to eat unlimited quantities of either Green or Red Day foods makes the diet uncomplicated.	• Fifteen Sins isn't a great deal of sinning. When you want an extra chocolate bar, you're stuck.
• The diet does not "sit on your head" all day because you don't have to keep track of what you have eaten.	• If you are a bread-lover, this one's a nightmare.
• Tons of bananas, kiwis, nectarines, peaches, strawberries, etc., make this diet a real winner.	• It can be hard to vary the types of food you are having.
• Egg-cellent if you like eggs.	• Convenience foods are very costly in terms of Sins.
• Veggies are freeeeeeeeee.	• The things that are measured, must be (you guessed it) measured. We are talking *exactly*.
• Limited weighing.	
• No waiting between foods.	
• Can combine proteins and carbs if you want (to a degree).	
• It works — if you stick to it.	

The Original Hay Diet/Food Combining for Health

(Dorris Grant & Jean Joice)

The Diet

Don't eat starchy foods at the same meal as protein foods (this one is the diet's Cardinal Rule). It is based on the idea that the body cannot cope with proteins and carbohydrates at the same time because of the way they are digested. Proteins, starches, and fats should only be consumed in small quantities. Use whole-wheat products for your starches. Skip sugar. And, get your stopwatch out: You may only eat a protein meal four and a half hours after a starchy one, or vice versa. In addition to all this, you can have oodles and oodles of salad, vegetables, and fruit.

The diet claims to reduce/cure many diseases/medical conditions and general digestive discomforts. It also claims that those who undertake this diet feel healthier/lighter/better all around.

The Evaluation

When checking the ingredients for a generally healthy diet against The Hay Diet, we find that all the rules promote good health in eating.

It is true that some people feel better when embarking upon a food combining program such as Hay. This may well be because they are forced to fill their plate with healthy salads and veggies together with their baked potato or grilled fish as much as it is due to not combining proteins with starches.

The diet works as a weight-reducing diet because your overall calorie intake is reduced — especially when you consider that you are supposed to be consuming only twenty percent starch/protein and eighty percent fruits and veggies, minimal fats (butter, no margarine), and no sugar.

The Verdict

The Hay Diet is a healthy diet that works. Whereas some might find food combining an abnormal way to eat, some swear by it. The principles of separating starch and proteins, together with the diet's encouragement to eat foods in their raw state (e.g., apples whole versus pureed/stewed) might well improve energy levels, medical conditions, and general feelings of well-being — but the same could also be said for adopting a general healthy diet as well.

Pros	Cons
• Easy to follow and understand.	• There is no scope for the wicked stuff (chocolate, potato chips, etc.).
• Less cooking required because of emphasis on raw fruits and vegetables.	• You can forget about convenience foods (since when should life be convenient?).
• You may well feel lighter and healthier.	• In between meal times you are stuck with fruit (no nibbly-bits on this one), plus if you want to snack on crackers you'll have to wait hours to have your chicken for supper.
• Can easily select from whatever you are making for the family.	• You might miss ole favorites like spaghetti Bolognaise or hamburgers with the buns.
• May improve certain medical conditions.	• May not improve your particular ailment.
• Encourages a general awareness of healthy eating (even if you don't want to stay on it for life).	• It can get boring to always eat "rabbit food."
• Fruit and vegetable lovers will love it.	• You might feel different to friends and family (unless you are living in a Hay-loving home).
• No calorie counting.	• Baked beans not advocated.
• No weighing/measuring.	
• Bread-lover's delight.	
• It works.	

Fit for Life

(Harvey and Marilyn Diamond)

The Diet

The philosophy behind this diet lies in the premise that the body has three different digestive periods.

4am–12pm (morning) is the best time for "elimination" — whereby the body is encouraged to eliminate unwanted matter;

12pm–8pm (day) is the best time for "appropriation" — whereby the body is encouraged to ingest whatever foods it needs;

8pm–4am (night) is the best time for "assimilation" — whereby the body is encouraged to break down the food necessary to its well-being.

Added to this is the Hay's principle of not combining proteins with starches and you basically have the Hay Diet with some additional restrictions. For example, this diet advocates eating only fruit or fruit juices all morning till lunch. You must wait thirty minutes after fruit before you can eat anything else. In addition, look at your watch again — you must wait three hours after a starch or protein meal before consuming any fruit. Better make sure your watch works.

The diet also strongly advocates juices — both fruit and vegetable juices. Milk is a no-no. Fruit must be raw and butter can only be eaten with your carbs.

The Evaluation

This diet was designed before 1985 (the first publication date). More recent research says that the premise of three digestive time periods is nonsense at worst and "imaginative" at best. This diet bears the same principles of food combining as the Hay Diet, but with a different book cover. It seems to be stricter in its adherence of eating what with what, and at which times.

The Verdict

Fit for Life is a healthy if cumbersome diet. (Who can be bothered to look at the clock after an apple?) Again, it works because it's based on a consumption of seventy percent fruits and vegetables and thirty percent other.

Pros	Cons
• As above (see Hay Diet).	• Only fruit to be consumed till lunch.
	• You must wait three hours after lunch or supper before eating fruit.
	• All this waiting and refraining might drive you a bit up the wall.
	• No scientific basis to some of its claims.

Meal Replacements

(Liquids, Cookies, Formulas, Etc.)

There are different categories of meal replacements. Liquids, cookies, formulas, etc., all offer the typical "fast-slim" claim and can easily be bought over the counter.

Their plan of action requires you to substitute two of your three daily meals with a supplemental beverage. This is calculated to bring your overall daily calorie intake to under 1,500 calories, which will cause you to lose weight. These types of convenient "don't have to think about what to have for supper" quick-fixes sell because they take away the "dieting is a pain in the neck" headache.

These diets might work well in the short run, but long-term, they may prove inadequate. They often backfire because they provide too few calories for your body to successfully zap away the fat. Once you don't get enough calories, your body slows down and hoards the few calories it does get. In addition, you are likely to feel weak, tired, and irritable on these plans because your body is not getting enough fuel. Plus, the sheer monotony can easily drive you off the plan before you get anywhere near your target weight.

And, of course, they have no connection to a healthy eating regime (remember the five food categories?).

These plans do not work on a long-term basis, nor do they promote learning how to eat healthily or sensibly for life. And watch out — some of them can be downright dangerous.

Diet Pills

Diet pills, such as Phentermine, should never be used unless under a doctor's instructions. A doctor might prescribe medication in instances where he determines that the medical risks of obesity outweigh the pill's risks.

Diet pills work by suppressing the appetite via a central mechanism in the brain. It's worth noting that after a few weeks, the body starts to build up a resistance to the drugs. Therefore, diet pills, even when recommended by a doctor, can only be effectively used as a short-term measure to boost a patient's weight loss while simultaneously encouraging permanent long-term changes in attitude to food and exercise.

Some of the less desirable side effects associated with diet pills are: blurred vision, dry mouth, insomnia, irritability, stomach upset, chest pain, racing heart, difficulty urinating, breathing difficulties, and swelling.

Understandably, doctors are not fond of administering these pills unless the patient is at significant medical risk as a result of being overweight. Diet pills are potentially dangerous and should not be abused. They do not treat obesity; they only suppress the appetite while deeper, more long-lasting psychological counselling can take effect.

Pills of any description, whether diuretics, amphetamines, or laxatives, etc., should never be used to lose weight. The effects are short-term, detrimental to good health, and poor substitutes for healthy eating habits.

Fad Diets (Quick-Fix Diets)

Go to any bookstore and the number of diet books you'll find there is simply staggering: celebrity diets, low-carbohydrate diets, three-day diets, diets designed to fit your blood type, astrological sign, age, gender, nature... These diet books are as appealing to us as Eve's apple was to Adam (and look where he ended up...). Through their glitz and screaming titles, they promise us quick, easy, painless — even miraculous — weight loss. Who can refuse? Indeed, who wants to refuse?

The truth is, we are creatures with both brains and hearts. Our hearts jump somersaults in glee when it seems that one of our strongest desires can be so easily satisfied. Our brains, however, are skeptical. As well they should be. They realize that it all sounds rather fishy, but on what grounds?

Why are there so many diet books published? And why are there new ones coming out all the time? Didn't the old ones work? How do we know that a diet is safe, healthy, or effective?

Rabbi Dr. Abraham J. Twerski writes in *Hamodia*:[15]

Let us realize that every month there are about ten new, "guaranteed-to-work" miracle diets and regimens that promise to reduce weight dramatically. Over the years, there must have been hundreds of such "guaranteed-to-work" techniques. If even a single one of them would have lasting results, why would there be a place for new ones every month?

But hope lives eternal, and people believe what they would like to be true, that there can be a diet or a magic pill that will control their weight. Obesity is the nation's number one health problem. Millions of people are overweight, and the "guaranteed-to-work" diets just do not work over the long run. Most of them can indeed produce a rapid weight loss, but almost invariably, the person regains the weight and then some.

"Hope lives eternal." And so it should. The crying shame about all of these quick-fix diets is that they so callously, thoroughly, and reliably dash all our hopes to smithereens. Although they promise maximum results with minimum investment, they just don't work in the long term, no matter how much we might want them to. **If it's fast, it won't last**.

Obesity has become such a pressing national health concern that all sorts of reputable organizations (such as the American Heart Association, the American Diabetes Association, the American Dietetic Association, not to mention all the relevant government agencies), are doling out sensible weight loss advice. Strangely enough, they're all saying the same thing: *Eat less, eat a variety of foods, get the nutrients you need, exercise, and take the time to lose pounds safely.*

---

[15] November 21, 2003

Is this what we want to hear? No, not really. Would we rather it were easier and quicker? Yes please. Is this quick way going to guarantee a long-term, healthy, effective, safe, enjoyable weight loss? No way.

What Exactly Is A "Fad" Diet?

OK, we get the picture. We want long-term successful weight loss. But how can you tell which diet is healthy and which is just a scam?

In true Sherlock Holmes style, you have to don peak cap and pipe and remain ever vigilant against those infamous "fad" diets.

Fad diets come and go, which is one of the reasons why they are called fads. But all fad diets have several factors in common:

- **Quick-fix**: They claim you can lose lots of weight — fast, faster, and even faster than that;
- **Special**: They promote "special" foods or promote a diet restricted to specific foods;
- **Low Calorie**: They often fail to provide even the minimum number of calories necessary for good health;[16]
- **Nutrient-Deficient**: They often fail to provide the necessary RDA amounts of essential nutrients;
- **No Exercise**: They claim to help you lose weight without the huff 'n' puff of exercise 'n' stuff;
- **Dubious Research**: They quote unheard-of sources or rely on case studies with before-and-after pictures/testimonials;
- **Scientific Evidence**: They have no long-term scientific backing;
- **Dodgy Endorsement**s: They come with approbations from uninformed/unqualified persons;
- **Contradict Health Professionals:** They contradict the currently accepted advice of established health and nutrition bodies.

Words Of Wisdom

Here's what the Food and Drug Administration and Federal Trade Commission advise:

Be skeptical about any weight-loss scheme that claims to be:

- ✔ Easy
- ✔ Effortless
- ✔ Guaranteed

---

[16] i.e. 1,200 calories a day for a woman.

✔ Magical

✔ Miraculous

✔ Exclusive

✔ A new discovery

✔ Mysterious

✔ Exotic

✔ Secret

✔ A breakthrough

✔ Ancient

Conclusion: The Same Old Story...

If you take a close look at many of these fad diets, you'll see that, in actual fact, almost every book is a rehash of a previous one. (There ain't much new under the sun...). But these diets are written and promoted in such a way that we are led to believe they are all "new" or "revolutionary." Each author, in his own way, will promote his heretofore unheard-of formula that assures weight loss once and for all. **Despite all these tempting claims, the bottom line still is (and always will be...) a matter of calories in versus calories out. Period.**

Yo-Yo Dieting

Most likely, you've dieted before. You might have lost a few pounds. Or even many pounds. But the reason you are reading this book is because you gained them back again. This is the familiar yo-yo diet pattern (also known in the medical field as "weight cycling"). You try this new diet for a while and then you get bored and try a different diet, and then you try this other, even newer diet, and then...(you get the message).

I have even seen this yo-yo pattern of dieting on conventional, healthy diet plans. The dieter becomes impatient and whoops, off course they go.

Yo-Yo Dieting: Fact Versus Fiction

There has been much written on the effects of going on and going off diets, so let's separate fact from fiction:

Yo-yo dieting:

✔ Does *not* mess up your metabolism;

✔ Does *not* do long-lasting harm to your health;

✔ Does *not* have a permanent effect on your metabolic rate;

✔ Does *not* increase the amount of your fat tissue;

✔ Does *not* turn you into an "apple," causing you to regain lost weight as fat deposits in your abdominal area (for more on apples and pears, see page 382).

So, what *does* it do (that's so bad)?

The worst thing about yo-yo dieting is that it is discouraging. Even worse-than-worst is that it doesn't work.

Who wants to end up back where they started after all that hard work?

The "I'm Just Being Careful" Diet ("IJBC" Diet)

The Diet

This one is not published, but it could be — by everyone who has ever laid claim to wanting to lose weight, but can't be bothered to follow a diet plan. Instead, they follow what in their own, individual mindset is a weight loss campaign of having less of what they think is bad for them, and more of what they consider the good stuff.

The Evaluation

Although it is unfair to overgeneralize and say that this diet *never* works, it is true to say that this one is not a guarantee for weight loss.

If you've been eating like an elephant let out of starvation zoo prior to embarking on a healthy eating regime, you might well shift the pounds. But I have had so many people come to me complaining about how they are stuck at a dieting plateau — when they've only just begun — that my first question is a well-justified, "Which diet are you on?" Of course, they are on the "I'm-just-being-careful-diet" (IJBCD for short). To which my invariable answer is: "Being generally careful generally means generally not losing weight." Generals like to stick together (just like in the army).

Why? Well, there are a number of contributing factors.

✔ Formal diets are designed and researched to help people lose weight. The calorie values have been calculated to ensure a deficit significant enough to result in weight loss. Not that I'm casting aspersions or anything, but when was the last time you had your IJBCD checked out for its calorie content? The "careful" person often does not understand the basics of how many calories she is consuming and how many she needs to consume to lose (a sensible diet plan usually does);

✔ The "careful" person might not understand all healthy eating guidelines fully (I had one "careful" lady who was noshing on almonds instead of potato chips, thinking it was healthier — nuts have ceiling-high fat content *and* more calories than the chips);

✔ The "careful" person might be eating simply too much — even of the right types of food (e.g., six slices of whole-wheat bread spread with…);

✔ The "careful" person cannot fully quantify how much of the forbidden stuff she is consuming ("I'll just have a little piece of cake/a taste of that kugel, etc.").

The Verdict

The most frustrating part about the IJBCD is that you will probably feel quite deprived (of your favorites) and will feel that you are exerting terrific effort for little dividends. If you are already psyched to lose weight and are prepared to invest in yourself to this end, do yourself a favor and go on a diet instead of relying on mis-judged guesswork. Sounds obvious, maybe, but it's true nonetheless.

Pros	Cons
• No diet book to read.	• You are never quite sure if what you are doing is going to work.
• No limit to indulging in whatever you think is OK.	• You might forget (conveniently?) whatever indulgences you have had.
• Flexible.	• You cannot guarantee that you are following a healthy eating plan (or getting the correct nutritional requirements).
• No food combining.	• It might take you longer to lose the weight you want to lose.
• Not restrictive/no rules to follow.	• It might not work.
• Plenty of variety.	
• No weighing/measuring.	
• No waiting hours between foods.	
• It's better than not embarking on a diet at all.	

Grand Summary

I am definitely *not* advocating any one diet over another. I do not get commission for increasing participants to any of the above diets (or for that matter, decreasing). I *am* trying to give you the relevant information for you to choose a plan that will best cater to your own personal preferences, rather than have you start a diet only to find out that it's not quite your cup of tea.

Additional Points To Ponder

✔ Any diet has to be thoroughly "digested" (analyzed and understood) before starting it. This means reading the brochures very carefully and following the rules. My short summary is just that — a short summary.

✔ Consider yourself a lucky ducky if you find the perfect diet. There isn't such a thing (at least I haven't found it yet! — if you find it, please send me a copy).

✔ **Every diet (that works) must limit something. If it didn't, it wouldn't be called a diet**. It's a purely personal choice which restriction of a diet is the least "painful" for you. Some might find "no milk" doesn't bother them, as they don't drink coffee anyway. Someone else might prefer to be able to eat half a chicken. No one can make the match between diet and person, except you.

✔ **Choosing a diet is not signing a life-sentence**. If you get bored on a diet, or your life circumstances change (your mother-in-law is coming to stay with you for a month), or you see it's not working for you (in terms of lifestyle/weight loss), you can always change diets. I often suggest to stale dieters that, instead of giving up completely and diving into mom's apple pie, they try a new diet instead. This way they don't sabotage all their good work till now, *and* they can continue forwards with renewed zest. See "Change Diet," page 259.

✔ Remember, I am not pushing any one diet here. I am merely presenting you with the facts and hereby wish you a sincere "Happy Diet-Hunting!"

Chapter 2

———— ◆◆◆ ————

Are You Ready?

Y ou've analyzed your lifestyle and decided which diet suits you best *and* conforms to the guidelines of promoting good health. You've done all the research and are itching to take dieting out of the realm of the theoretical, into the world of the practical. You're psyched, charged, and excited about this new, success-promising venture. You're ready to begin…but (you knew there'd be a "but"…) are you *really* ready?

Before we get to the practical side of what it means to be really ready, let's see if your attitudes are really ready. "Attitudes? What attitudes? I want to start dieting — what other attitude do I need?" I'm glad you asked. Below are seven attitudes that a successful dieter must internalize before starting out on a dieting journey. Without them, a dieter is doomed to failure before beginning. With them, well, I can almost wish you congratulations on reaching your goal weight already.

Correct Attitudes

Who's Responsible Anyway?

I was once in a park and a heavyset teenage girl came over to the swings where I was standing. When she tried to sit down on one of the swings, she found out that she was too large for it. Her reaction? She exclaimed, "They made this swing too narrow!" not, "I made me too big."

> When you've internalized the information in this chapter, you will be mentally and physically ready to start your diet.

Responsibility. **There's only one person responsible for how much you weigh, and that's *you*.** You are the only one who makes the decisions time and again throughout the day as to what exactly goes into your mouth or not. No one is forcing you. You are not a toddler being force-fed mushed-up banana in between pacifier thrusts. No one is watching you or monitoring what you consume. No one is going to slap your wrist if you go for the chocolate, or kiss you if you choose the apple instead.

It all comes from you — every decision, every step of the way.

Don't blame anyone else if *you* are overweight. Take yourself in hand and tell yourself (and mean it), "I put it all on and I am going to take it all off and keep it off." Don't bother reading the next attitude if you haven't internalized this one yet.

Willpower

Now that you have taken responsibility for your actions, you are probably saying, "But how can I succeed?" The answer (after you have digested the information in this book) will boil down to one word: willpower. What is willpower?

It is our response to motivation. It is determination. It is persistence in the face of problems, perseverance in the face of setbacks. It's strong, unyielding. It's non-negotiable, non-compromising. In other words, it means, "I really want this." It says: "I want to be in shape more than I want to stay out of shape." It's the difference between "I'd *like* to lose weight and be healthier/slimmer…" and "I *am going to* lose weight and become healthier/slimmer."

People look at successful dieters and say, "It's OK for you — you've got willpower…." This way, they automatically exempt themselves from even starting to think about dieting, because they see themselves as lacking enough of this vital ingredient to be successful.

This is not true. Willpower is not a magical elixir — a potion to which only a select few are privy. It is not in the genes ("I have brown eyes, black hair, and a willpower gene…"). It is not contingent upon receiving a degree or being particularly intelligent. It is something that anyone can develop. There is only one condition to getting willpower and that is to want it.

Check out the mind-blowing results of a five-year study of 120 of America's top performers to determine how they achieved their extraordinary success. The six fields studied included Olympic swimmers, tennis players, concert pianists, sculptors, mathematicians, and research neurologists.

The researchers analyzed the lives of the performers, their backgrounds, their home environments, etc. They interviewed the performers, their families, and their teachers. The researchers themselves admitted that they "had expected to find tales of great natural gifts" but didn't find that at all. "The mothers often said it was their other child who had the greater gift."

The most brilliant mathematicians frequently said they had trouble in school and were rarely the best in their class. Some world-class tennis players remembered that their coaches viewed them as being too short to ever be outstanding, and the Olympic swimmers said they were regularly "clobbered" in races as ten-year-olds.

So what was their secret? It was their awesome drive and determination. The researchers heard accounts of willpower and dedication through which, for example, a child would practice playing the piano several hours daily for seventeen years to attain his goal of becoming a concert pianist. A typical swimmer would tell of getting up at 5:30am every morning to swim two hours before school and then two hours after school to attain his or her goal of making the Olympic team.[1]

Pablo Saraste, the famous Spanish violinist and composer from the late nineteenth century, captured this thought when he said "A genius! For thirty-seven years I've practised fourteen hours a day, and now they call me a genius!"

Willpower. Determination. Dedication. Drive. Persistence. Perseverance. Whatever name you want to call it, it all means the same.

You see the goal before you; you want to reach its target. It's willpower that is the fuel that gets you there. Willpower will help you day by day, choice by choice. Want it, go for it, and get it.

Now that you have checked your willpower gauge and found that it reads full, it's time to go on to the next attitude.

Be Realistic

It isn't gonna happen overnight. Let's make sure we realize that right from the beginning. Unless you have only a few pounds to lose, you are in for a nice, long journey. Expecting to lose more than half to two[2] pounds per week, week after week, is not only unrealistic, it's diet-sabotage. You are going to get so frustrated that eventually you will throw the whole concept of dieting out the window, along with your self-confidence and self-esteem. So just remember who won the race (clue: It wasn't the hare!), and settle in for a long-distance excursion.

Focusing on Yourself

Once you've taken responsibility for your actions, summoned up the willpower, and internalized that you're here for a while, you can take a deep breath and brace yourself for this next attitude adjustment, 'cause this one is not so easy for us ladies.

We get caught up in focusing on other people so often that it can be a thunderbolt shock to realize that we need to focus on ourselves as well.

We do carpool for a friend, we have someone's kids over for the afternoon, we nurse the baby, we wipe the toddler's nose, we aim to please the boss, we make supper for the brood, we empathize with the teenager, we welcome our husbands from their long day…the list is as long as the day is full.

---

[1] From *Lifelines* by Avi Shulman, page 78.
[2] Except the first one or two weeks, when a higher weight loss involves the loss of water as well as fat.

With all that kindness oozing out of our hearts and souls, it can be easy to lose our sense of self amidst the busyness and demands involved in caring so selflessly for others.

That's why we have to make sure that we are ready to focus on ourselves. We have to be ready to put ourselves at the top of our list of priorities. We also need nurturing, care, and support. And we are just the right ones to give it. Without this kind of focus, it just isn't gonna work.

For example, you'll need to:

- ✔ Buy (or make) special meals that promote low-fat/low-calorie contents;
- ✔ Plan your diet menu in advance so that it will be easy to implement within the family infrastructure;
- ✔ Make sure that you eat before the kids get home;
- ✔ Make sure that you can create the time and space within your week to attend an exercise class or a diet group;
- ✔ Take the time to fill in your food diaries and monitor your successful weight loss, etc.;
- ✔ Take yourself into account at stressful times like erev Shabbos/Yom Tov or changes in routine, like summer vacation.

Another very important part of focusing on yourself is to make a written list of all that you stand to gain by succeeding in losing weight. List *all* the benefits you can think of — even if they seem petty or silly. They're not. They are the very real catalysts that will help you make very real changes in your life.

Examples of reasons might be:

- To fit into your favorite skirt again;
- To avoid the embarrassment of feeling awful in a swimsuit when you go swimming;
- To feel healthier;
- To avoid insults or sniggers behind (and in front of) your back;
- To feel better;
- To feel lighter;
- To feel in control of your eating;
- To look (and feel) good for a special occasion (like getting married);
- To make mom proud;
- To make yourself proud;
- To be able to sit crossed-legged on the floor;
- To be able to play action-type games (like ball) with the children;
- To prove to yourself that you don't have to live a life in the fat lane.

The more specific and personal you can be, the better. Take the time to do this task properly. It's an investment and will help you maintain focus throughout your diet. Plus, it'll make you feel good. So stop reading, right now, find a pen and paper, and start listing. When you are finished, read on…

In a real, yet strange sort of way, focusing on yourself will give you several positive messages. You will be telling yourself that you are important enough to focus on; that your needs are important enough to be met, and that what you are doing (dieting) matters. These are powerful messages.

In a nutshell, focusing on yourself will aid a positive sense of self-esteem and self-confidence that will spur you forward in your weight loss campaign and will help you to stay focused.

While we're talking about focusing on ourselves, it's worth mentioning that people frequently view the process of dieting as just another thing to be put on the "to do" list. Just like they have carpool and dentist appointments to schedule, now they have an extra person to take care of — themselves. This is such a shame.

One of my clients once said, at only her second weigh-in, *"I feel like I am lifting my spirits as I lift the pounds because I'm beginning to feel so much better about myself."*

To view dieting as a burden is *one* way to look at it. But why choose it when you can embark on an uplifting journey of self-nurturing instead?

Take Pride in How You Diet

Now that you have decided that focusing on yourself is a great idea, let's make it even better. Let's invest a sense of pride in your diet and diet-related areas.

Because you are a worthwhile person, what you do is also worthwhile. Giving yourself this message breeds healthy confidence. And **confidence breeds action**.

Slap-dash, corner-cutting, *haimishe*[3] dieting just doesn't achieve the same results as carefully calculated, self-prioritizing dieting does. The more you put into an investment, the more you stand to gain in dividends. How much more so when it is yourself that you are investing in.

Let's go through some of the areas that could help you take pride in yourself by taking pride in them.

Papers

You've been given the diet book. You've collected leaflets on healthy eating. You've cut out inspiring magazine articles. You've exchanged diet recipes with friends or fellow group members. Now what do you do? Do you leave these papers scattered around the house, under coffee cups, crumpled and susceptible to children's "creativity?" Let's not mince words. These papers are going to look torn, dog-eared, and dirty by the time you complete week three.

---

[3] Home-brew.

Is this really how you want to perceive your diet? Isn't a diet more appealing if the papers are all collated, hole-punched, and filed in a pretty binder? Apart from the positive practical aspect of actually being able to find what you want easily, you will also be showing yourself that this project is worthwhile and that you care about it succeeding.

Scales

OK, you got married ten years ago and you still have the same kitchen scale. It still works (you think), even if the corners are a bit chipped and the beet coloring never did come clean.

This is a new venture and new ventures require new tools. Not only will buying a new kitchen scale add to the buzz and excitement of your new diet, but the improved accuracy will help you too.

Electronic scales allow you to weigh each food item individually, directly onto the plate you are going to use to eat. No scale bowls to wash up — and no excuses (when you see the pointer fluctuate between two numbers and choose the lower one so you can add another ounce of cheese…).

Even a non-digital, regular, cheap scale will give you a heightened sense of new-venture. Just be sure to look for a wide margin between numbers so that you have a clear definition of how much the food weighs.

Speaking of weighing…if you share the bathroom with mini-demolition-men-toddlers, it might be an idea to treat yourself to a personal, brand new, "Mommy-only" bathroom scale.

Be Prompt

Diet group today? Squeezing in a lunchtime exercise class?

Give yourself the message that it's important, and try to be there on time. Treating your chosen appointment with respect breeds respect on both sides of the fence, from the people around you and from you, yourself.

Clothes

When you see your skirt swish around your hips and you need a safety pin to keep it up, then it's time to take a trip — either to the seamstress to take the skirt in, or to the shopping mall for a new skirt.

It's not time to downplay this huge accomplishment. We're women. And women like to look and feel good. If we don't look good, we won't be likely to feel good.

Just like we buy Shnocky a new coat because he grew out of last year's, so too, we should just as quickly buy ourselves a new outfit when needed.

Apart from the practical side of fixing up old clothes so that they fit well or buying new ones, there is also the psychological side. We experience an inherent dieter's boost when we take care with the way we dress.

Money Matters

Dieting costs money: the book, the group, the diet foods. Exercise costs money: the classes, the equipment, the sneakers… Agreed, if money is tight it's very difficult (but not impossible) to diet and exercise. But often enough, we won't spend on ourselves, even if we have the money, because, "How can we, when there are so many other pressing things to do with the money?" Read: "It's all right to spend on everyone else in the family, but if it's for me, I don't really need…"

This attitude has to change right now. **You are worth spending money on.** Your good health is worth spending money on. Your sanity, your peace of mind, your happiness, your self-esteem, your self-confidence, and your looks are all worth spending money on.

Sometimes husbands may not understand why our losing weight or getting into shape is worth spending money on. But believe me, if they were pressed to tell the truth, there is no question they would rather have a thin, trim, healthy, well-dressed wife than a fat, out of breath, baggy-clothed one, even if it would cost them a few bucks to get one. And even more so, if dieting and exercise is a real health issue in your life, i.e., you suffer from high blood pressure, high cholesterol, obesity, etc., of course your husband would tell you to spend whatever you need to save your health/life.

So remember, what you spend your money on shows you what's really important in your life. It's time to realize that there is no one more important in your life than you. Take care of yourself, even if it costs money to do it. And do you know what? In the long run, all those people you care about, and would spend money on before yourself, will also benefit. What a difference good health, stamina, endurance, mental happiness, self-esteem, and self-confidence makes in a mother and a wife. When you feel good about yourself, everyone around you benefits — practically, emotionally, mentally, and spiritually. So go on, spend the money. And spend it guilt-free.

Rewards

Speaking of spending money… Do you want to know one of the most powerful tools in goal achievement? In one word: Rewards.

"Rewards? For *dieting*? Whatever next?" I can just imagine your tut tut — "We're supposed to be restricting ourselves, depriving ourselves, and there she goes and tells us to treat ourselves! What's going on here?"

And besides, since when does a busy wife, mother, or any woman for that matter *ever* reward herself for anything?

But just take a moment to consider the fact that we reward our children with all sorts of goodies when they have accomplished their various milestones — be it toilet training, memorizing math tables, or going to bed nicely. Our fathers/brothers/husbands reward themselves when they complete a *mesechta*[4] or *sefer*[5] by means of a *siyum*.[6] So why shouldn't we reward ourselves when we succeed in accomplishing the goal we set out to achieve?

But it's more than just, "Why shouldn't we reward ourselves?" Rewards are one of the best-kept secrets in Diet Land. They can be vital to success. So vital that we are going to spend a little more time (and ink) on explaining this hidden jewel of the diet world.

Rewards work in two ways, either pull-me's or push-me's.

Pull-Me's

The desire to look better, to feel good about oneself, etc., are often not powerful enough stimuli to carry us through the pockets of turbulence that occur along our chosen path. We may need something more to pull us through the hard times. That's where rewards come in. A promise of a reward at the end of a hard day of dieting may be all you need to resist that day's fare of temptation. A reward at the end of the week may help you to bounce back from a disheartening reading on the scale.

A reward should be used like a magnet, drawing you towards your desired destination. Rewards at the fifteen pound-mark all the way to a massive one at the final goal all help us struggle past the tough patches that inevitably occur on any road to success.

Push-Me's

Rewards work in another way, after we have accomplished some stage of our final goal. Whether it be a day, a week, a month, fifteen pounds, the halfway point, or complete success, we tend to belittle our accomplishments.

This usually occurs for one of two reasons, and sometimes for both. One reason is the feeling that there is so much more to go — we tell ourselves that this doesn't count as a milestone or even an achievement to acknowledge. The second reason is the feeling that if I accomplished this, it couldn't have been so difficult after all, and therefore it's not worth recognizing.

Both of these thoughts destroy one of the most powerful tools in dieting, or, for that matter, in any goal achievement: ***the energy that comes from an awareness of success***.

By rewarding yourself, you are telling yourself, "Yes, it was hard work (make that *really* hard work), and even so, I achieved what I set out to accomplish. I did it and therefore I can do it again!" In this way, a reward is not only acting as a magnet that draws you forward, but also as an energy pack — a high-powered motor that propels you onward.

---

[4] Gemara tractate.
[5] Holy book.
[6] Celebration upon completion of a holy book, or part of such a book.

By rewarding an achievement you turn it into a success. And the key to goal achievement in any area is building on small successes. So don't lose the opportunity to channel the energy of accomplishment into the challenge of the future. (Go on, read that again.) Acknowledge that you have achieved, highlight it with a reward, and tap into the awesome energy of success.

An additional side benefit of rewarding yourself is an injection of self-esteem and self-confidence (you've met these Siamese sisters before…) that will overflow into other areas of your life. A reward calls out, "Hey, I set out to accomplish a goal and I succeeded. I can succeed in other areas of my life as well!"

True Story

Rochel[7] had been coming to our Weight Loss Group for several weeks before she lost her seven pounds mini-goal. In true Group tradition, she was awarded a beautiful presentation of quality lotions-and-potions products. Following swiftly on the heels of her first success were success experiences two and three. All duly rewarded. When I asked her what these rewards did for her, she responded (and I quote), "I felt that I did something big — it wasn't easy to see that as I lost one pound at a time. I felt not only was it an accomplishment, but it's also worthwhile to keep going (because I'll get there). The reward gave it *chashivus*[8] — *it isn't just nothing*."

How Do I Reward Myself?

✔ **A reward should be commensurate with the amount of effort one puts into achieving that goal.**
It's no good buying yourself a plastic $3 watch if it's just taken you a year to lose thirty pounds. At the same time, it defeats the purpose to over-reward, i.e., a new dress for a week's resistance. It belittles the entire process.

✔ **The reward needs to be what *you* like,**
not what others like or is the "done" thing, otherwise you won't feel rewarded.

✔ **Write the reward down.**
Be specific in both the goal and the reward: "When I lose five more pounds, I will buy myself a new CD."

✔ **Refer to the written-down reward every so often**
in order to keep it fresh in your mind. This keeps the magnet's pull-me power solid and steady.

✔ **Reward *all* goals —**
whether they are short-, medium-, or long-term goals; a day, a week, a month, fifteen pounds, the halfway mark, or complete success. (Yes, you'll get there.) Remember, we are building on small successes. Any achievement skipped is an unacknowledged success and a squandered opportunity for re-energization. Basically you lose out on a big-time push-me.

---

[7] This name has been changed.
[8] Magnitude, weight.

✔ **Build up the reward as the goals get bigger.**
Don't fall into the trap of using the same value reward for each goal. I.e., the first ten-pound mark is nowhere near as major an accomplishment as the fifth ten-pound mark. The reward must say: "Look what I have accomplished since my last reward," and "WOW, look how far I have come since I started this journey."

✔ **Re-evaluate your rewards regularly**
to ensure that they are working for you, and change them if they are not. Don't let a reward get stale, i.e., the same chocolate bar every night might not work past week two. Pay attention and dare to be creative.

Example of Rewards

- A mini chocolate bar at the end of the day.
- A guilt-free morning in town to window-shop just for yourself at the end of a week.
- An evening out at the end of a month.
- An inexpensive pair of earrings, new lipstick, or mascara at the fifteen-pound mark.
- A new dress/wardrobe (!) at goal.

Be imaginative; don't be afraid to be original. All that counts is that you really feel that it is a reward commensurate with the accomplishment and that it's for *you*. Because you deserve it.

Remember the song, "The knee bone's connected to the leg bone, the leg bone's connected to the hip bone, the hip bone…"? Well, as we have proven, there's more to dieting than food. Dieting is connected to our attitudes. Once you can nod away in full agreement with each of these seven attitudes, you know you are ready. Well, nearly ready…Just like the song, if, "Dieting's connected to our attitudes, our attitudes are connected to the practical side of being ready.…"

The Practical Side of Being Ready

Avoiding False Starts (Is Now the Right Time?)

Ever seen professional athletes line up at the start of a race? They crouch forward, feet balanced on specially designed springing blocks, alert and poised, ready for the gun. Every muscle is taut, senses are heightened… aaaaaaaand they're off. Ever seen a false start? One of the competitors jumps the gun and pounces out of the blocks a split second before the gun. What's the result? When they all restart, there will be very few world records set. Some of the enthusiasm, adrenaline, and concentration will have been spent and the athletes just won't have the necessary edge the second time around.

So it is with dieting. At the beginning, we, too, are poised and eager to start. We have the enthusiasm, the energy, and the focus that will carry us into the "diet race." But if we jump the gun, i.e., if we begin before we really should, all that important initial energy and enthusiasm will go up in smoke. To get started again next time, to sum up another reserve of energy, to refocus, isn't that easy. And sometimes it's downright impossible.

For this reason, **a false start is worse than no start**. At least if we don't start at all, we still have our reserves of energy, eagerness, verve, etc., at our disposal for when we do eventually start. And that increases our chances of success.

So if you've just had a baby, no matter how fat and flabby you feel, don't start yet; it usually isn't an auspicious time to start your diet. The demands of a newborn are such that they come first, and any intention of prioritizing yourself more than you usually would (as dieting entails — at least at the beginning) will only be met with frustration. For sure, you don't *have* to eat platefuls of cake and finish off every box of chocolates your friends send in, but to begin a new project at this time will only end in frustration.

Other inauspicious times to begin a new project might be:

- Illness (your own or a family member's);
- Visitors are coming (if viewed as a pressure);
- Serious involvement with other projects (e.g., learning computers/taking a course/organizing a play);
- Emotional turbulence (such as bereavement, family tensions, postnatal depression);
- Stress (e.g., moving, making a shidduch, husband going away);
- Being away from home (not being able to whisk up a salad, not having a routine, or being dependent on your hostess);
- Making a simchah (this is because the chances are that you'll have visitors, be seriously involved, experience emotional turbulence, and might suffer from stress!).

Included in the concept of false starts could be starting your let's-get-into-shape campaign by jumping on the exercise bandwagon at the same time as entering Diet Land: You might end up in a state of overload.

Don't get me wrong, I'm the first to shout from the treetops the benefits incurred from both dieting *and* exercise. But whenever we undertake a major project, we will automatically need to channel our focus and reserves to bring it to fruition. That's why taking on two major projects at the same time might not be such a good idea. Apart from becoming tired and irritable, you might be inclined to give up both projects shortly after lift-off.

There's just so much energy (psychological and physical) involved in new beginnings that you may be spreading yourself (and your reserves) too thin. Instead, try becoming familiar and confident in one area first before taking on another self-improvement scheme.

By undertaking one project at a time, you will increase your ability to focus and your chances to succeed at both.

Study Your Chosen Diet

The next stage in getting ready to start a diet is an obvious one. Once you have chosen your diet plan, read it. This means understanding and familiarizing yourself with all its rules.

The more familiar you are with the diet, the less stress or inconvenience you will feel it is creating. If there are points that you do not understand, pick up the phone and challenge the big sister who lost twenty pounds on exactly the same diet (or speak to anyone else who has experience with that diet).

Clean-Up Time

Next, once you have digested (sorry…) the diet and all that it entails and expects from you, it's time to do some serious cupboard purging (of chocolates, chips, Shabbos party nosh, etc.). Less obvious but equally dubious items in your kitchen include packaged snack foods, cheeses, and high-fat cold cuts.

Give them to the kids, the neighbors, the dog. If you can't, then put them up high or under lock and key, or anywhere that won't be right under your nose. 'Cause let's be realistic, who wants a rice cake when a chocolate éclair is staring you in the face?

Stock Up on Staples

Finally, after you've made room in those cupboards, it's time for some "diet" shopping to fill them up again. Follow your diet book and see what you'll need: fruits, veggies, whole-wheat bread, low-fat goodies, diet drinks, etc. If you don't have your dieter's staples in the house, you might just turn all that resolve into the familiar procrastination of "starting tomorrow." Or worse still, you'll get started and suddenly find (when you are hungry) that there are no whole-wheat crackers left in the pantry, there's only chocolate fudge brownies and…there goes the willpower, the initial enthusiasm, and, quite possibly, the diet. Don't be lazy: this stage is well worth the investment before you officially start.

To Conclude

✔ Have you internalized all the right attitudes?

✔ Do you feel that you have the emotional space in your life right now to start?

✔ Have you read and understood the diet?

✔ Have you cleared the temptations away (or at least put them up high so that you'll need a chair to get them)?

✔ Have you stocked up on all the food items you are going to need?

If you can check off these five questions, then you won't just think you're ready, you'll be really and truly ready…

For those of you who are so anxious to start your diet that you already want practical dieting tips, you can skip this section and go to "Section 3: Go! — Tips To Keep You On Track," page 89 (Do not pass "Go" and do not collect $200…).

However, be warned. You will be skipping an amazing chapter that is also very relevant to weight loss. After all, don't you want to know why you are eating even when you are not hungry and what you can do to change it?

SECTION

2

Get Set – Taking Charge Of Your Eating Habits

*B*efore you start your diet, it's a good idea to understand why you're really eating (even when you are not hungry) and what you can do to change.

Ask any person in the street why she eats and she'll look at you in surprise and reply, "Why? Because I'm hungry..." This is a true statement, but by no means is hunger the only reason we eat. Probe the very same person and she'll eventually admit that actually there are other, albeit less obvious, reasons why she will choose to lift up her fork and knife.

In this section we are going to analyze over twenty reasons why people eat. Then we'll try to help you analyze why *you* eat. After that we'll give you some practical suggestions and thoughts on how to take charge of your eating habits, so that you end up eating only when you really want and need to eat.

Chapter 3

—— ◆ ◆ ◆ ——

Twenty-Four Reasons Why We Eat And What We Can Do About Them

Why Do We Eat?

Hunger

What Is Hunger?

You may think that hunger is all in your mind and dieting is all about your body. The truth is that hunger is regulated by the body's chemical reactions. The body has a well-honed feedback system that connects the brain, the organs (stomach, salivary glands, etc.), the body's cells, and the senses (smell, taste, sight, etc.).

The body's cells send messages to the brain to tell it that fuel is needed and it's time for lunch. This is the body's signal to eat — not to be confused with the signals of the mind, also known as *tayvahs*,[1] which we will discuss next.

---

[1] Desires for the physical.

> This chapter should empower you to eat only when you really want to be eating.

When the body really needs food, it produces physical symptoms such as:

- Difficulty concentrating
- "Growling" tummy
- Gnawing, crunching sensation in the stomach
- Headache
- Feeling faint/light-headed
- Irritability

These are the body's warning signs. The key is to learn to differentiate between the signals of the body and the temptations of the mind. To listen to one will make you fat, to ignore the other will make you disappear…

In a nutshell, hunger is your body's signal that it needs refuelling.

Tayvah/Desires

Perhaps the most compelling reason we eat when we are not hungry is for the pure pleasure it gives us. Let's face it — food is yummy. However, even this reason is not so simple. There are two main stimuli for desires:

Externally Triggered Desires

The sensory appeal of food (i.e., what it looks like, how it smells, or how it sounds) can stimulate chemicals in the brain to trigger an eating desire.

Examples of these triggers are:

Sight: You see an ice cream sundae with chocolate syrup running down the edges, cherry perched on top;

Smell: The waft of barbecued smoked steaks or freshly baked apple pie coming out of the oven;

Sound: The crackling/munching of potato chips, the crack-fizz of a can of cola…

These stimuli can be either real (you are in the bakery and smell the rugelach) or artificial, via advertisements (pictures in a magazine or a poster on a wall, or you hear someone drinking on the radio).

Internally Triggered Desires

An internally triggered desire is a craving triggered off by either a mental stimulus or a physical stimulus.

A mental stimulus includes your memory (you remember how something tasted or how an ice pop cooled you on a hot day) or an association (i.e., whenever you fell your mom gave you a candy, so now when you fall…).

Physical stimuli include hormone-induced desires (when you are pregnant[2] you just *have* to have pickled cucumbers, or strawberry and banana ice cream), or tastebud-induced desires (after your spaghetti Bolognaise you want something sweet, or after your afternoon nap your body craves a cup of tea/fruit/ice cream).

What differentiates these physical, internally triggered desires from everything else we've mentioned is that when you eat because of these triggers, you are not eating because you are hungry; there are no external stimuli enticing you; and you are not even mentally picturing what something tastes like. Rather, your body is craving something driven by its own inner chemistry.

According to a survey conducted by H. P. Weingarten, PhD at McMaster's University in Ontario, Canada (published in the December 1991 issue of *Appetite*), *ninety-seven percent of women and sixty-eight percent of men experience food cravings.* Researchers believe that older people are generally less driven by cravings than younger people. Food cravings may also be dictated by the time of day — late afternoon or early evening is the prime time when cravings tend to occur. ***But dieters, especially those who frequently go on and off diets, tend to experience cravings more often than non-dieters, and their cravings tend to be strongest at the beginning of their diets.***

Eating By the Clock

We are all creatures of habit. We tend to eat because the clock says it's mealtime. We might have been doing this for years without actually paying attention to it.

We might have had coffee and cake with a friend at 11am and then picked at whatever we were making for lunch for the family. But when lunchtime comes, whether we are hungry or not, we will sit down to a hearty fork-and-knife lunch.

What about the classic scenario of giving the kids supper at 6pm and then finding yourself overcome by hunger and not being able to resist having generous nibbles of their egg and fries? Yet when it comes to your official suppertime with your husband, do you hesitate for even one second before plunging headfirst into a steaming steak and potatoes meal? Or what about going to a kiddush on Shabbos morning and, after all those cream cakes and delectables, coming home and having lunch — why? 'Cause it's lunchtime, that's why.

---

[2] It is also common to have cravings when premenstrual hormones are high.

Stress

Many people turn to food to relieve their feelings of stress. The demands being made on them seem to exceed their capabilities. They have a deadline to meet, or they have three kids under three with chickenpox, etc. Knowing that the stress will still be there (together with a few added pounds on their hips) after they try to calm it down with food still doesn't stop them from eating.

Comfort

People also turn to food for comfort from an unpleasant situation that might not necessarily be stress-related. For example, when people are upset, or facing bereavement, or suffering from an insulting remark…they may find themselves turning to food to help them feel better emotionally.

Lonely

Hubby is out of town, the kids are all in bed, the seminary girls have left, and suddenly the house seems strangely quiet and you are feeling quite alone. Especially if you are a "people-person," you may feel slightly uncomfortable with this sense of loneliness. In some way it unnerves you. You seek comfort and reach out for some of that leftover apple pie…. Here, too, the pounds go on and yet the loneliness doesn't go away.

Nerves/Worry

Dale Carnegie, in his book *How To Stop Worrying and Start Living*,[3] says that "…one person out of ten…will have a nervous breakdown — induced in the vast majority of cases by worry and emotional conflicts." (Today's statistics are even higher.) He quotes the Nobel Prize winner in medicine, Dr. Alexis Carrel, as saying, "Businessmen who do not know how to fight worry die young." Carnegie adds, "And so do housewives, horse doctors, and bricklayers." He points out that, apart from all the reasons in the world why we should not worry, worry also brings on all sorts of physical ailments, which he then lists.

I am adding one ailment to his long list of worry-induced conditions: overeating. When we are anxious, when we are unsettled, when we are distracted, it is oh, so common to turn our attention to food. Watch out!

Boredom

I met someone who was trying to lose weight with little success. From one week to the next she started doing really well. What was the reason? She had found a job. Now, she was "too busy to eat." If you are hanging around the house with nothing much to do, beware of boredom propelling you towards the fridge.

---

[3] Pages 40–42, 1998, Vermilion.

Social Pressures

Since the beginning, eating has incorporated social pressures. Just think of Eve enjoying her juicy fruit with Mr. Snake egging her on, and then Adam being coerced by Eve to indulge just a little and to also take a bite.

A more updated version of societal pressures would be going to a wedding and facing unrelenting friends encouraging you to join them in their food pleasures. Everyone at your table (and quite probably from the surrounding tables as well) will ask why you're on a diet, or will urge you to tuck in because "just a little bit won't matter."

Sometimes they'll ask you whether the reason you are refraining from eating (everything) is because you don't trust the kashrus. (You might feel pressure to eat just to show them that you intend no slight to the hechsher.[4]) Or what happens when the host walks by, or actually tells you, "Please eat…have some more…have you tried this dish?"

All this doesn't include our own self-induced pressures like, "How can I not indulge when everyone else around me is enjoying themselves?" and "I don't want to look different so I'll fill my plate up as well."

Whatever the scenario, social pressure is a major force in eating even when we are not hungry.

Socializing

People like people. One of man's most potent means of drawing people together is through food. Since ancient times, we have "broken bread" together to foster kinship. Let's face it, who's ever been to a no-food party? Sharing food brings with it an inherent deepening of friendships, forum for increased communication, and encouragement of intimacy.

Sisterhood functions and food are often inseparable. Would you ever invite a new neighbor over for a shmooze[5] without offering her a drink and a piece of cake?

Celebrating

Not only can food provide a forum for socializing, but it can also provide the backdrop to celebrating an occasion. Food, in all its lavish glory, helps to mark the occasion and make it one of substance and importance. Food can also render an atmosphere of festivity and joy. So why are you eating? 'Cause it's Grandpa and Grandma's sixtieth anniversary — why else?

---

[4] Kosher certification.
[5] Chat.

Procrastination

You've got a boring report to write, or Pesach cleaning to get on with. What do you do? You prowl the kitchen, fling open the cupboard doors, raid the pantry, and peruse the fridge…all for the third time. Anything to put off the inevitable.

Procrastination and eating are often synonymous.

Boring Job

Research on dieters and non-dieters alike shows that everyone tends to eat more when engaged in a boring task. Stimulation and creativity just don't seem to leave as much room for eating as a boring, monotonous job does.

Unawares

You are on the phone and the kids' leftover supper is on the counter in front of you; by the end of the call the plate will be clean without the use of the dishwasher. Or you are lying on the couch reading a great book, and the pistachios next to you will suddenly disappear before you even reach chapter three. You're in the car driving from A to B, large bag of corn chips in hand — on "automatic pilot," — you can guess the rest.

The examples may be endless, but eating unawares is perhaps the most pathetic reason to eat. You can't even remember enjoying the taste of the food, nor the sense of satisfaction that it gave you, yet the food's all gone. It's a shame really, considering it's the same number of calories as if you'd sat down and truly enjoyed yourself.

Tired

The baby kept you up half the night, and the toddler kept you up the other half. You have forgotten the definition of a full night's sleep. Your brain feels like a cross between marshmallow and cotton candy. Your eyes feel dry. It's hard to smile. Yep, you are tired.

One of the hardest situations to handle is chronic fatigue. Our tempers run high, and our tolerance levels run low. Stress, comfort, boredom, etc., are all exacerbated and therefore we reach for the cake.

Another byproduct of tiredness is that we cannot find the mental or physical energy to withstand temptation. The slightest internal or external stimuli to our *tayvah* sends us on the food rampage. There goes the last of the ice cream.

Trying to stay awake is a third reason why we may eat when we are tired. Food provides energy. Especially any of the "ose" products (e.g., fructose, glucose, etc.), which provide energy that is easily and quickly available to the body after ingestion. The benefits may be felt immediately: we get a sudden "high" or "rush," so we find ourselves turning to the chocolate bar, the fizzy (non-diet) sodas, and the cookies. We rationalize that being awake is more important now than our diet — after all "it's only one chocolate bar!"

Conditioned Response

Many of our automatic responses are the result of having been conditioned into our behavioral patterns from a young age.

So it is with many aspects of our eating habits. Why do you always finish off whatever food was placed on your plate? 'Cause Mommy always told you to. Why do you always serve dessert at the end of a meal? Because your parents did. These practices become less of a conscious decision, and more like ingrained habits.

Mitzvos[6]

There are many occasions when it becomes a mitzvah to eat. Matzah and morror and two full sedarim on Pesach, three meals on Shabbos, two on Yom Tov, all day erev Yom Kippur. Let's face it: Food plays a major part in our religious observance.

But no one ever said overeating is a passport to heaven.

Making a Transition

We live in such rushed, busy, frantic times. The pace of our lives sometimes pushes us to continue without pause. When we do finally allow ourselves a break it can be difficult to make that transition between harried housewife/rushed businesswoman into a more relaxed, calm, and centered person.

Food helps people switch gears. The businessman comes home, kicks off his shoes, and makes a dive for the sofa — with a package of cookies in one hand and a newspaper in the other. The housewife comes home from shopping with her two tiny tots and automatically makes herself a cup of coffee, with cake on the side.

Food smoothes the transition.

Thirsty

Some people would rather eat than drink. They often fall into the trap of eating — not when they are hungry, but when they are thirsty.

Studies show that when you think you are hungry, often you are not — you are just thirsty instead.

Medicine

Certain medications may have the side effect of either increasing or decreasing the appetite. Your doctor may neglect to inform you that this can be a potential side effect, because it is not life-threatening and the effect will stop when the medication is stopped.

---

[6] Commandments.

Here is a list of some medicines, from "The Essential Guide to Prescription Drugs,"[7] that may increase your appetite:

✔ Antidepressants (mood elevators)

✔ Antihistamines (allergy pills)

✔ Diuretics (chemicals that make your kidneys work harder and cause you to urinate more)

✔ Tranquilizers (calming drugs)

The correlation between an increased appetite and certain medications does not necessarily mean that the medication should be avoided. However, knowing that such a correlation exists is helpful in realizing where our eating drives are coming from.

Weather

Did you know that a person feels hungrier in cooler weather than in warmer weather? Just think about it. What do you naturally want when it's cold? Stews and thick soups. What do you want in the summer? Salads, open sandwiches, chilled fruit salad, etc. And when it's very hot outside, you might not even want to eat anything.

Amazingly enough, our bodies even process food faster when it's cold out. The stomach is emptied more often, and food travels down the digestive tract more quickly. All this means that you'll be hungrier, more often, in the winter.

Conclusion

It may be surprising to discover that there are many reasons why people eat even when they are not hungry. The more honest you are with yourself, the more reasons you will find why *you* eat. And just because I'm a nice lady, I'm going to help you make that discovery. So let's begin a little self-analysis.

Why Do You Eat?

On a scale of 1 to 10, where 1 = Never and 10 = Every day/very often, assess yourself in the following areas.

✔ Do you *ever* eat when you are not hungry (i.e., when you are not experiencing physical symptoms of hunger such as growling tummy, light-headedness, etc.)?

✔ Do you eat because you see/smell something delicious and can't resist it? (Externally triggered desire)

✔ Do you eat because it seems that your body is craving a certain spicy food/sweet food/sensation? (Internally triggered desire)

[7] New York: Harper Collins, 1995, James W. Long and James J. Rybacki.

✔ Do you always eat breakfast at breakfast time, lunch at lunchtime, and supper at suppertime, even if you are not hungry? (Eating by the clock) ☐

✔ Do you eat when the demands being made upon you outweigh your ability to cope? (e.g., the mother-in-law is coming to stay, your baby's teething, and the car's broken down. Stress) ☐

✔ Do you eat when someone has upset you or you are feeling sad? (Comfort) ☐

✔ Do you eat when no one is around and you are feeling lonely? (Lonely) ☐

✔ Do you eat when you have a big meeting coming up/your daughter is on a shidduch date/your bank overdraft is worse than expected? (Worry/Nerves) ☐

✔ Do you eat because you have too much time on your hands? (If yes, come to me and I'll find you something to do…) (Boredom) ☐

✔ Do you eat at a kiddush or wedding because everyone keeps offering you cake and insisting that you take it and you can't summon up the courage to refuse? (External/real pressure) ☐

✔ Do you eat at a wedding/Sheva Brochos because you are embarrassed to leave food on the plate (and look different) or because you are scared to insult the hostess? (Internal/self-induced pressure) ☐

✔ Do you find yourself eating more at a social event, e.g., N'shei/Bar Mitzvah seudah? (Socializing) ☐

✔ Do you eat more than usual at simchos/special occasions? (Celebrating) ☐

✔ When faced with an unpleasant task, work, project, paperwork, etc., do you find yourself in the kitchen nibbling rather than doing the work? (Procrastination) ☐

✔ Do you eat because you are involved in a mindless, monotonous task? (Boring job) ☐

✔ Do you ever find yourself surprised at finding an empty bowl of nosh next to you that was full an hour ago? (Unawares) ☐

✔ Do you eat more when you've had a bad night's sleep? (Tired) ☐

✔ Do you find yourself polishing off your plate automatically, regardless of the portion size or how full you are feeling? (Conditioned response) ☐

✔ Do you eat more on Shabbos or Yom Tov? (Hey, that's like asking, "Who's normal?") (Mitzvah)

✔ Do you eat when changing pace or project? For example, do you come home from shopping and make yourself a cup of coffee with a piece of cake before the next job? (Making a transition)

✔ Do you eat because you are thirsty? (Disguised thirst)

✔ Do you eat as a side effect to medication you are taking? (Medication)

✔ Do you eat more when you are feeling cold, or when it's cold, dark, and wet outside? (Weather)

✔ Are there any more reasons you can think of why you eat? Please insert.

_____

_____

_____

_____

_____

Now look back at the numbers in the boxes. Which ones scored 8's, 9's, and 10's?[8] Those are your main Achilles' heels, but don't ignore the 5's, 6's, and 7's either. They also deserve some attention. So, let's give it to them…

What We Can Do About the Reasons We Eat?

Hunger

If we all only ate because of hunger, I wouldn't have bothered to write this book.

It's worth mentioning, at the risk of stating the obvious, that our goal is to eat in response to our physical sense of hunger and not as a reaction to our emotions. Once we are more in tune with eating to assuage hunger (as opposed to assuaging boredom, loneliness, etc.), we will be a long way towards a healthier (and lighter) existence.

---

[8] Just for the record, I gave this test to my Diet Group and the overwhelming reason why they ate, when they weren't hungry (ninety percent of the group gave it a ten), was Shabbos.

Tayvah/Desire

(Internally and Externally Triggered Desires)

This is perhaps the most common and most compelling reason why we eat other than when we are hungry. It is also the hardest one to break, so instead of suggesting ways to eliminate *tayvahs*, we will concentrate on limiting their damage to our diets.

Try Substituting

Take a few moments to consider whether a low-fat alternative might scratch the itch just as well. Try skim milk and cocoa or a low-fat sorbet if you crave chocolate or ice cream.

If you find yourself craving something sweet and nibbly, try keeping fresh or dried fruit at hand. Raisins, dried mango, cherries, and grapes make good hand-to-mouth substitutions for cookies, cake, or candy. Dried fruits (apple, apricot, and banana) can be just as chewy and will provide more nutrition than the empty calories of a sugary chewy candy.

Use Portion Control

Nothing is going to happen to you if you do give in to temptation every once in a while — it's OK to have your potato chips or corn chips — so long as (and this is the keyword…) it's *controlled*. A handful is not the same as a bagful. Help yourself overcome your craving and opt for the small pack of potato chips instead of diving headfirst into the jumbo family pack. Try an ice cream cone rather than digging into a half-gallon ice cream tub, spoon at the ready, and see if that does the trick.

Eating By the Clock

Let's face it, it's just plain convenient to eat at conventional mealtimes. We have schedules. We have routines. It just doesn't seem efficient to start making lunch for ourselves now, two hours after clearing up the family's lunch, because *now* we're hungry.

There are, however, a couple of effective ways around this.

Eat Often

When you experience real stomach-crunching hunger, it means you've let yourself go too long without food.

A little food, often, helps to raise the metabolic rate, keeps energy levels high and optimal, and keeps the discomfort of excessive hunger at bay. That's not to mention it might help you avoid shouting at the good ole husband who doesn't know what hit him.

So, yes, eat at mealtimes, but make sure you're not overloading yourself. Rethink your definition of "mealtime." Maybe it's more constructive to view it as "snack-time."

Substitute Heavy Foods for Lighter Ones

If you are not *really* hungry, but it's convenient for you to eat now, try substituting heavy, calorie-laden foods with lighter alternatives.

For example, the family's having roast chicken, roast potatoes, and green beans. Try skipping the potatoes, or substitute them with a salad. This way you'll feel lighter while still warding off the tummy-grumbles. Alternatively, try skipping dessert at a mealtime and save it for your snack when you start to get hungry again.

Stress

Food may *feel* like the ultimate answer to a stressful situation, but in effect, eating when stressed will add pounds and may even create stresses of its own. (For example, "I feel so upset, I blew my diet again!" or, "I feel so guilty, I've just polished off a whole package of cookies!" or, "I hate myself when I'm fat." That's besides the stress of ill health, which can be induced by being overweight.)

More healthful alternatives to make you feel de-stressed would be:

Focus

Perhaps the most obvious answer to alleviate stress-induced eating is to focus on the problem that is causing you to look for comfort. Use your sense of agitation to mobilize you into looking for solutions to the problem you are facing.

A Trouble Halved

If a practical solution is beyond you right now, turn to a friend to download your frustrations. A trouble shared is a trouble halved. It's always surprising how much better we feel when we get things off our chests. True, you might not be nearer a solution by the end of the call, but you might be clearer on the issues involved. Even if she listens patiently and only makes you feel fifty percent better, you'll be fifty percent more in control.

Exercise

No, I'm not suggesting you pay your whole month's salary to a posh, rubber-plants-in-the-corner gym. Brisk, energetic (free!) walking does just as good a job. Exercise stimulates endorphins, the "feel good" hormones. Plus, it enhances feelings of self-control and self-esteem. (See "The Feel-Good Factor", page 275.)

Or try getting out to an exercise class. It will take your mind off the stressful situation and refresh your body so that you will be able to face the stress with a better attitude and more positive perspective.

Do Chew

Although we don't want our mouths to resemble Gertrude the Cow, chewing gum can occupy your mouth so that it's too busy to take in other food. Calorie-wise, it's better to chew aggressively on gum than it is to allay our aggressions via food.

Tehillim (Psalms)

We're not in charge of our lives. A Higher Power Who knows and understands more than we do is. Relax and ease the burden of your stress onto His broad shoulders.

Asking Him to help is half the answer.

Laugh

Keep something handy that makes you laugh. It could be a collection of jokes, funny emails, hysterical photographs, or cute things that the kids have said.

Laughter is one of the most effective stress busters there is. And there's no chance of an overdose.

Do a Mitzvah

We can become very self-orientated when we are stressed. Stepping back from our own problems by thinking of someone else can help us regain a more realistic perspective on our problems. ("This is not life-threatening, just life-aggravating.")

Try calling someone who is more stressed than you and watch your own problems begin to shrink.

Music

Any soothing music can have a positive effect on your blood pressure, heart rate, and general stress levels.

Keep CDs handy next to the computer when you work, or tune into your Walkman headset for a five-minute haven of harmony.

Dance

Put the music on loud and go for it — you get all the benefits listed above for exercising, plus you get to have fun. Don't worry, no one's watching.

Stretch

Stress contracts our muscles, especially the neck, shoulders, and spine. This can lead to a whacking throb of a headache. Try de-stressing by lying down (floor or sofa), lights low, and slooooooowly stretching each muscle in the body one by one. Ahh. Doesn't that feel much better?

Play Hairdresser

Take the extra time to braid your daughter's hair, or brush it for those extra few minutes. She'll be the envy of her whole class, and you might feel surprisingly soothed. The calming nature of continuous slow stroking has been proven to lower the heart rate and promote feelings of tranquillity.

If you (or your neighbor) have a pet dog or cat handy, stroking it in a slow, methodical manner works wonders too.

Get a Pedicure/Manicure/Facial

Forcing yourself to undergo a slow, methodical, pampering process just might take the frenzy out of your stress levels. If nothing else, it'll force you to sit still for half an hour and your body could probably do with the relaxation after all the muscle clenching it has had to put up with while being under stress. As an added bonus, it just might provide a timely pick-me-up, since stress usually gets us down and depressed.

Try Alternatives

If lotions and potions are your thing, how about the following:

Relaxation: Techniques such as Yoga, deep massage, meditation, and visualization may help;

Acupuncture: People use it to overcome energy blockages and improve fatigue;

Herbs: Some herbs, such as valerian, cava cava, and lemon balm, promote feelings of calm;

Flower Essences: Bach Rescue Remedy is the most useful — place a few drops under your tongue when feelings of stress or panic start to rise.

Bubble, Bubble, Boil, and Scrubble

Skip the functional "in-and-out" approach of the power shower and opt for a relaxing bubble bath instead. Feel pampered and soothed from the skin to the soul.

Do Nothing

At least once during the day, sit quietly and do precisely nothing.

It can be one of the hardest things to do because we are so used to thinking of our worth in terms of what we get done. But try it out anyway — it works.

Breathe

For five minutes, slow your breathing down to about six deep belly breaths a minute. In other words, inhale for about five seconds, exhale for about five.

Making a conscious effort to breathe deeply and correctly can be a simple and very effective way to de-stress. Just being conscious of your breathing patterns can have a very powerful relaxing effect. It's best done lying down (because then you are forcing your body to rest), but you can do it anyplace, anytime. So, go on, as you read this, take a breath — or five!

Tip: Put a dot of correction fluid on your wristwatch or desk clock. Every time you see the white dot, take two or three long, deep breaths. You'll be amazed how quickly it calms you down.

A cute aside: Just because STRESSED spelled backwards is DESSERTS, don't fall into the trap of making them synonymous.

Comfort

Maybe someone made a comment that hurt. We want to be soothed. We want to feel calmed. It might well be an automatic, unconscious habit to turn to food for comfort. But it doesn't need to be. Check out these non-food coping skills first.

Phone Someone Who Cares

She cares, she listens, and she makes all the right "ahh" noises. A listening ear is so therapeutic and can be a real pick-me-up. If mom's line is busy, try sis, big brother, best friend, neighbor, or cleaning lady. Besides making you feel better, you'll have to control yourself from downing those chocolate chip cookies until you get off the phone (it's rude to munch in someone's ear). Once you have controlled yourself for those few minutes, it'll be easier to continue to exert control.

Get Out

Being surrounded by those familiar kitchen counters and cupboards, complete with dish-laden sinks, for hours at a shot can be stagnating. Getting out and about for a walk, stroll, or saunter can be refreshing and invigorating. If it's raining, go for a drive or go window-shopping. Chances are you'll feel better and will have changed the tone for the rest of the day.

Confront the Source

We tend to bottle up our emotions. They fester and grow until we bear a full-scale grudge. But it doesn't have to be that way. If someone made a cutting remark, maybe she didn't mean the comment that way. Maybe you misinterpreted it. How about picking up the phone and (nicely) asking her what exactly she meant by it. This way you might end up with a good night's sleep, and you won't lose a friend at the same time.

Cry

My husband is always amazed at me when I curl up with a good book and box of tissues and sob away. He controls his urge to tear the book away from me only when I explain how much I am enjoying a good cry.

Sometimes it feels so good to have a luxurious wallow in self-pity and release the waterworks. We somehow feel refreshed. So, go on, ready, steady…. Cry! (Doesn't work the same when someone tells you to, does it?)

Create

Being involved in a creative project can take your mind off your upset and give you a lift. It doesn't have to be anything major, but it should be pleasant. How about arranging some flowers, or trying out a new dinner recipe? Even rearranging a room can be creative and provide you with a much-deserved boost.

Be Busy

Like you're not already? But seriously, instead of moping around, propel yourself forward — weed the garden, make a meal for a new mom, feed the birds, wash the car. The physical activity will do you good and may provide a therapeutic release. I know someone who feverishly cleans out all her cupboards every time one of her children is on a date. Saves on the nail-biting and you also end up with a spic-and-span kitchen (and hopefully an extra in-law or two).

Get a Massage

These days, massage therapists are almost like doctors. They can detect knots in the muscles that are built up over time, and can succeed in pummelling them away. Just having someone kneading your back like a challah dough forces you to focus on your body and the sensations it is going through versus focusing on those awful misery-me's. You will feel relaxed afterwards — somewhere between feeling like a double-decker bus ran over you and going through a car wash. (It's actually supposed to be rather nice.) If you are thinking of hiring a therapist, make sure she is fully qualified (you want to be able to walk away afterwards...).

Hug

Give or get a hug. (That sounds good, doesn't it?) Enjoy the warmth of body against body. Enjoy the close proximity to another's vitality. Try it out on a child who's giving you problems, your sister, your best friend…Feel yourself giving and receiving love. What better pick-me-up?

Lonely

Whereas some people revel in the luxury of their own company, some find it disconcerting and a potential source of discomfort. If you fall into this category and feel yourself unsettled by the quiet, before you fill the void with crunching noises, try these first instead.

Background Noise

In a quiet house it can feel reassuring to have the radio or music playing in the background. Music or talking sounds can fill the void and give a sense of company. You will feel less isolated and part of society.

Listen To Tapes

Maybe now is a good time to listen to those lectures you have been meaning to get around to. If this quietness is going to last for some time, or happens often, join a tape library and turn lonely time into "growing time."

Pick Up the Phone

Having a good shmooze on the phone soon blows away the cobwebs of loneliness. You get to share feelings and thoughts, and have a laugh together. Why not use the opportunity to call someone you've lost touch with — an elderly aunt or an old seminary friend? Or take the opportunity to cheer up a fellow lonely person and solve the problem of loneliness for both of you.

Invite Someone Over

If your lonely-time is planned, maybe now is the time to do some entertaining. Tea for two is great; and what about inviting a few extras over for a board game (Pictionary?) and a giggle?

Time-Out

Sometimes our lives just never seem to be quiet — the phone, the doorbell, the street traffic, the household machines, the children, the neighbors… maybe now is a good time to capitalize on a little "Time-Out" for yourself. Try having a long relaxing soak in your favorite bubble bath, or curling up in bed with the latest bestseller. Or go for a walk and take the time to smell the flowers.

Hobbies

Sometimes long-term loneliness can be coupled with boredom. If you are experiencing a life-change or transition, maybe now is a good time to pursue that hobby or interest you have put on hold for the last ten years. Shake off the dust, pull it out from under the bed, and go for it.

This could be your perfect opportunity to take a new course, develop latent skills, or broaden your horizons. You might develop parts of yourself you didn't know existed, you might make some new friends, and yes, you might even master your loneliness.

Nerves/Worry

Problems, bills, illness, aggravations, and uncertainties can snowball out of control into one huge mass of gnawing worry. Not only does worry adversely affect both our mental and physical conditions, but it does us no good either. When was the last time that worrying got you out of your pickle? That's right — it doesn't. But it sure can get you into one.

Those of us who overeat because we are nervous, aggravated, or worried stand to lose so much — not in pounds, but in peace of mind, good health, and happiness.

Let's go through some proven methods[9] for overcoming one of the all-time biggest, self-induced deterrents to successful living — worry.

---

[9] Adapted from Dale Carnegie, *How To Stop Worrying and Start Living,* Vermilion.

Live in "Day-Tight" Compartments

It's no good dwelling on past mistakes or future tribulations. Today is our only real possession. We can *do* something with today, but we can't change the past and we don't get very far by worrying about the future. Live in the present and live for what you can do with today.

Accept the Worst Imaginable Scenario

Accept the bleakest picture, relax, and then try to improve upon it. Accepting the worst-case scenario, instead of fighting or dreading it, can liberate you from the incapacitating clutch of worry. Once you accept what could be the very worst thing that could happen, whatever improvements you can make to alleviate the situation will then be conceived as a cause for celebration — not worry.

Try Problem Solving Techniques

Try out this handy little formula to help those gargantuan worries shrink into manageable pieces:

✔ Clarify the facts (without the emotions, the reservations, or the probabilities — just plain, cold, hard facts);

✔ Analyze the facts;

✔ Arrive at a decision and then act on that decision.

Is this obvious stuff? Yes. But it works. It takes away the fog of confusion that surrounds us in our worried state and helps us lift ourselves up, above, and beyond it.

Keep Busy

Since most of us can only think about one thing at a time, try filling your time with another activity. If you crowd your mind with something else, there won't be any space left for worrying.

Don't Sweat the Small Stuff

Don't spend your time and energy exaggerating the importance of minor aggravations.

Don't brood over grievances that in a month, a year, or ten years will be forgotten and insignificant. Ask yourself the question, "Will this be important to me in ten years' time?"

Balance Your Worries Against the Law of Averages

I'd bet that nine tenths of your worries would easily disappear if you would consider that *by the law of averages, whatever you're worrying about probably won't even happen anyway.*

Insurance companies bet that the disasters people are worrying about will never occur. They get rich on this philosophy. And so can we: with lives void of worry and rich in peace of mind.

Accept What Can't Be Changed

If there is nothing you can do about the disturbing problem facing you (illness, being fired, a relative's death, etc.), then do the one thing you *can* do: cooperate with the inevitable. The sooner you can accept your situation and move forward, the sooner you will be able to live life worry-free.

Put a "Stop-Loss" Order on Your Worries

A stock market broker will decide exactly when he will cut his losses on a share and sell it. He will control his margin of loss so that he is not left with huge debts.

We can do the same. Let's take control of our difficult situations by deciding just how much anxiety a thing may be worth — and then let's refuse to give it any more than that.

Think Positive

Choose to fill your mind with thoughts of gratitude, peace, courage, health, and hope, instead of drowning your sense of joy in worry. Our life is what our thoughts make it.

Act Positive

You don't have to be a trained actor to act as though you are unworried even when you are worried. Acting and thinking cheerfully will help you become cheerful. External actions always influence internal emotions.

Prayer and Faith

Why pray? Well, although there are many more answers to this question, I have listed a few reasons in terms of its role in significantly reducing worry.

- Prayer helps us clarify our problem. It is almost impossible to solve a problem when we are confused and the problem appears overwhelming and vague. Rather like putting pen to paper, prayer helps you put into words exactly what it is that is worrying you. Once you have clarified your problem, you are likely to feel more able to "view it from above" instead of suffering from a sense of oppression.

- Prayer gives us the sense of sharing and unloading our burdens. When we can't tell anyone else, we can always tell G-d.

- Prayer can empower us with a sense of *doing*. It may be your first step towards action.

- We can trust G-d. He knows it is in our best interests to be going through our present situation exactly the way it is. When we release our judgement in favor of His, our sense of calm returns.

- G-d listens to our prayers. He cares. And He answers.

Prevent Fatigue

As we mentioned earlier in this chapter (page 66), fatigue can make a mountain out of a molehill. It exacerbates and exaggerates any little stress or worry that we already have.

The answer is to rest. And in the future, to learn to rest even before you get tired. Rest is repair. It's not a waste of time. You're not doing nothing — you're positively doing something. You are re-energizing your body, your mind, and your emotions.

Boredom

This one's easy. If boredom is the culprit in sabotaging your weight loss, then a two-word answer is in order: get busy. If you have come this far in being able to analyze that boredom is the criminal, you should be able to send him to jail and get on with life. Maybe it's time to start thinking about getting a part-time job, taking a course, developing new hobbies (see "Hobbies," page 77), catching up on news with an old friend, making new friends, preparing a special dish for Shabbos, finding a good book to read...the list is as long as the imagination is short.

If you can't think of anything you'd like to do, why not volunteer your services to an organization that caters to helping others? Time is our most precious possession. Giving some of it to others doesn't just help them, it can also help you.

Social Pressures

While puttering around your own kitchen your resolve may be as steadfast as Fort Knox, but when facing society, the pressures to conform may override your better judgement. Yet it is still possible to surmount these hurdles with a little foresight.

No-no's

You are at a kiddush and the hostess is going around offering quadruple-layered oozing cream cakes. She is insisting that you have "just one." You don't want to insult her but you were really on target so far this week. What do you do? *Just say no*. This can be a tall order for those of us who like to please people and take the line of least resistance. But it is one of the most important words in the English language for a dieter to learn, no matter how giving or softhearted she may be. And here's where the foresight comes into play. Before you ever get to the kiddush/wedding/party, practice your lines — i.e., practice saying no.

If you're caught off-guard, without having practiced your answer, you will offer your most automatic response ("Thank you, yes, I will have one"). If you can anticipate the scenario, you can be well-equipped to handle it. You need to practice saying, "No," politely, firmly, and convincingly. Try practicing these lines:

✔ "No, thank you, I'm under doctor's orders" (most doctors would recommend NOT eating cream cakes, especially when you are on a diet);

✔ "No, thank you. They look delicious — did you bake them yourself?" (Changing the subject);

✔ "No, thank you, I'm full. It was all absolutely delicious."

✔ "No, thank you; they don't agree with me." (Interestingly enough, most people can handle your abstinence much better if they think you are refusing because of pain rather than because of gain!)

See also "Peer Pressure," page 229.

A Bird in the Hand...

Is worth two in the bush, and a glass in the hand is worth two cream cakes on the table.

If you walk around with something in your hand you are less likely to be offered platters of cake; you will have something to do with your hand (other than holding the aforementioned); and can look, for all intents and purposes, as though you are also indulging — just like everyone else. Our discomfort often stems from feeling different from the crowd and this simple yet effective tip can go a long way to overcoming this.

We mentioned earlier that sometimes the social pressure that we feel is self-induced. We don't want to look different from everyone else. To counteract the risk of overindulging because of this reason, try the following:

Pile Up Your Plate

If you prefer not to look different from the crowd by having an empty plate — then fill it up. Of course, we are talking about filling it with the salads and veggies and only taking a controlled portion of the roasties and schnitzel. Full is full and will usually fool most people (including yourself).

Socializing and Celebrating

Sometimes the whole joy and/or importance of the occasion is so greatly enhanced by the wonderful food backdrop that it can be irresistible to even the most self-controlled dieter. See if any of these tips can help:

See "Planning Ahead," page 240;

Split It Up

Most Sheva Brochos/weddings have several courses. Why not start your meal at home (having in mind to *bentsh*[10] at the hall) and have bread and the first hors d'oeuvre (soup/fresh fruit/chilled melon-type foods) before you go. This way your hunger won't get the better of you as you step towards your table and dive into the challah.

---

[10] Say Grace After Meals.

Waist-not, Want-not

Wear a well-fitted suit/skirt/waistband. It will be a marvellous reminder of your progress as the evening develops. Need I say more?

Don't Pollute — Just Dilute

And if you are surrounded by high-calorie drinks at a simchah, don't sit back and drown your sorrows. Try asking a waitress for a pitcher of cold water. If she tells you she doesn't have any spare pitchers, wait for one of the soda bottles to empty and present her with your own makeshift version.

See "Clink a Drink," page 243;

Enjoy Your Surroundings

If you find yourself three arm-lengths away from anything remotely low-cal, try organizing yourself so that the low-cal drinks, salads, fresh fruit, pickles, etc., are all near you, and the nuts and croutons are on the other side of the world. Even just pushing them to beyond your reach serves as a deterrent. This way if the speeches go on (and on and on) you will have plenty of opportunity to choose the right kinds of nibbles.

STOP!

No, I'm not telling you to stop enjoying yourself, I'm suggesting that when the speeches start, or there is some other break in the festivities, stop eating. Taking a few minutes' break from eating will give your stomach the chance to catch up with you and send signals to your brain that you are full (or getting fuller). See "Practice Feeling Full," page 122.

Devilish Desserts

OK, you have been an angel all night, but when they bring out the triple-decker choco-whopper cake, the devil in you takes over. Before you sprout horns and pronged fork, how about trying the following:

✔ Go halves with a neighbor. Ask the waitress (she'll be your friend by now) for an extra empty plate, and what d'ya know, you've halved the calories immediately;

✔ Ask your neighbor for just one bite of hers (yes, she would have to be your close friend);

✔ Skip the dessert and choose fresh fruit instead;

✔ Say, "No, thank you," straight away. It'll only take a second to say no and you can rest assured that your resolve will continue because they don't usually offer dessert more than once;

✔ Schedule your trip to the ladies' room for dessert time. By the time you come back, they will probably have cleared the tables for *bentshing* already.

And Lastly…

Aim to be the last one at your table to finish. This will ensure that you chew your food properly, taste it, and enjoy it to the fullest. It will also mean that you will eat quantitatively less food and will feel more in tune with your body's signs of satiety. Plus, people won't have the chance to offer you seconds.

Procrastination

Instead of eating when you don't want to do the job at hand, try any of the following:

Carrot Dangle

Heard about the donkey that didn't want to walk? His master dangled a carrot in front of his eyes so that he would move towards it. Not that I'm calling you a donkey…but do yourself a favor and find an incentive to encourage you to move beyond the inertia.

Stovetop needs cleaning? Promise yourself a relaxed long distance phone call with an old seminary friend. Putting off that Pap test (don't!)? Reward yourself with a cheap pair of earrings on your way home. Unpleasant jobs will be around for a while; our job is to find our own personal carrots to overcome our resistance to them.

"Help!"

Let's say this donkey was really stubborn and the carrot just didn't seem to get him to budge. Another way to get him up and running (we'll settle for walking at this stage) would be to get hold of his collar and start yanking — hard. We might need the same treatment. Enlisting external support will help us attack what we have to do with renewed vigor. Try asking mom to nag you (she'll be delighted). Try asking your husband for helpful reminders (maybe he can call you from the office between clients/during coffee breaks).

Subjecting yourself to this type of accountability can be a new and effective technique in motivating you to do/move/go.

Reward and…

Well, not quite punishment, that's a little severe. Let's just call it "consequences."

If this infuriating, stubborn donkey is still sitting on his haughty haunches, another way to get him up is to start hitting him with a stick (don't tell the ASPCA). I'm not suggesting self-flagellation, but a little promise to yourself coupled with ensuing consequences might do the trick to help you get up and running.

Depending on how prevalent procrastination is in your life, you might want to write your promise down, or you can tell someone else about it to strengthen its enforcement.

Examples:

✔ If I don't take out the garbage and clean out the garbage cans before lunchtime, I'll put all the cans in the kitchen until I do.

✔ If I don't write that report by next Monday, I give my husband permission to hide my cell phone until I do.

Unawares

When we live in Diet Land we want to make every calorie enjoyable. If we're not even conscious of eating, we're also not even conscious of the enjoyment that food can give us. Considering that, by definition, dieting entails curbing our natural craving for excess calories, we should be aiming to highlight our appreciation of food — not diminishing it by eating unawares.

How can we make ourselves more conscious that we're eating?

Eat Only at the Table

Make it a rule that you'll only put something into your mouth if you are sitting at the table. Let's add another rule: Only eat with a plate and a fork or spoon in front of you.

Clear the Decks

Remove all distractions to eating. Don't answer the phone (that's what answering machines are for); put the book next to your bed instead of next to the table; put the Sony Walkman next to the exercise bike… Only eat when you eat.

Purge Those Places

Remove food from all those places where it's easy to eat without noticing. Clean out the car of crackers (fewer crumbs too); clear out the computer desk, coffee table…anywhere where you may find yourself with fingers with a mind of their own.

Tired

See earlier in this chapter, "Prevent Fatigue," page 80. And get some sleep. It doesn't matter if it comes as an afternoon nap, an early night, a late morning snooze, or by catching up on the weekend. But it might mean bringing in a night nurse if your baby is depriving you of sleep, or rearranging your schedule so you can sleep when everyone's out of the house. Alternatively, you can try sweet-talking your husband into relieving you of at least one shift in the night.

If your tiredness becomes long-term, either quit your job or check with your doctor to confirm that you don't have an iron-deficiency, a thyroid imbalance, sleep apnea (see "Respiratory Problems," page 367), or clinical depression — all of which can cause feelings of exhaustion.

Conditioned Response

If you always finish what's on your plate even though you stopped feeling hungry halfway through, you might be suffering from an ingrained conditioned response.

This habit may have been instilled in you from early childhood. ("You'll only get dessert if you finish off your plate… There are people starving in Ethiopia, you should be grateful you have food, so eat!")

Realizing this can be half the battle. When you are three quarters of the way through your plate, stop, put the fork and knife down, pause for a minute, and ask yourself, "Am I hungry anymore, or is Mommy back again?" After you do this for a while you'll find that you've broken the habit. If you can't yet manage that, try using a smaller plate and finishing that off. If you go for another serving it'll be because you are hungry and not because that "voice" is back again.

Mitzvos

If you're the type of gal who finds herself tucking in when there's a mitzvah at hand, flip to the "Shabbos" and "Yom Tov" sections of this book (Chapters 6–9) to find ways to counteract such tendencies.

Making a Transition

Facing a changeover from one job to the next might send us on the food rampage. But it's not our bodies that are craving the sustenance, it's our minds that are craving a respite.

Try relaxing on the couch with your eyes shut for a moment, or listening to some soothing music for five minutes. Read the paper or a magazine for a ten-minute break. Take a short walk. Listen to a story by Rabbi Paysach Krohn on a tape. Be imaginative, be creative. I know of wealthy businessmen who play with mini putting ranges in their offices to relax between clients. Sometimes a fast 'n' beaty CD with a five-minute dance or aerobic workout will do the trick. Give it a try. Anything's better than those extra pounds.

Thirsty

The body realizes that it needs something, but that something may be hard to pinpoint. We need to fine-tune our senses to differentiate between the need for food, and the need for water.

The signals may get confused because dehydration contributes to fatigue, and when you are tired your body is more likely to look to food for energy instead of the water that it really needs.

So Rule Number One is: Pause for a second to try and see if you really want food or if it's drink you're after. Rule Number Two is: Make it a habit to always drink before you eat and you'll be less likely to confuse the signals. Rule Number Three is: Make sure you drink enough throughout the day.[11] You won't end up with any more confusion because you'll be well-watered.

Feeling thirsty? You are already experiencing mild symptoms of dehydration. As soon as the symptoms of thirst occur, it usually means you've left it too long — that cup of coffee on the counter that you made half an hour ago is now cold. (What else is new?)

Medicine

You're on medication. Your symptoms are improving. But one of the unwanted side effects is an increase in appetite. What can you do?

Communicate with Doc

Sometimes a doctor will prescribe a medication and will automatically assume the patient is a happy camper on it. Unless you communicate your unhappiness to your doctor, he will have no idea that you're not happy with your situation. He may very well be able to alter your medication with a different brand that will still give you the treatment you need but without the negative "extras." Don't underestimate your doc — he's there to help you in *all* areas of your health — from your medical complaint right through to your weight loss.

Combine Your Combinations

Let's say that doc says you're stuck with your medication (for now). All is not lost…

If you've been merrily sailing along on a reduced-calorie diet prior to taking your medication, you may feel that the amount of food you want to consume now exceeds the recommendations. If this is the case, maybe it's a good time to try out a "Food Combining Diet."

There are many different Food Combining Diets on the market these days.[12] Basically, they promote separating carbohydrate foods from protein foods. The advantage is that quantities are unlimited even if combinations are not. Hence, you never have to feel hungry.

I once had a client who was dieting beautifully until she began her antidepressant medication. It wasn't possible to change her prescription, so, instead, she changed her diet. Bingo, she continued to lose — without feeling hungry.

---

[11] The rule of thumb is: drink eight 8oz glasses every day to keep the demon of dehydration away. (You will need to drink even more in hot weather — or if you exercise. This is because you need to replace lost liquids.)

[12] See "A World of Choice," page 21.

Weather

There's not a lot you can do about the weather, except move to a different climate. Short of that, the main test we face is in the cold climates ('cause *not* eating too much in the summer is a blessing, not a test). So let's see if there are other ways to stay warm that won't show up on the scale on weigh-day.

Lay On Layers

Help your body along by dressing in layers of clothing. Put them on when you are still warmish and let them act as your own personal insulation. If you let yourself get cold before you layer-up, your body will need extra energy (read: calories) to warm up again. Plus, sometimes, when the body temperature has dropped, it's harder to get warm again.

Neat Heat

Feeling the chill might have a really simple solution — turning up the heat. If you've set your thermostat on the same reading for years, and you have been losing weight (and the insulation that body fat provides), don't be surprised to discover that you are feeling the cold more. Just turn the dial up.

Move It

Our bodies produce heat when we exercise — so a quick jig or some jumping jacks just might do the trick.

Hot Liquid

When you're writing at the table or talking on the phone, or when you are tapping away at your computer, stay warm with a good, old fashioned hot water bottle and/or a piping hot cup of coffee. Neither have very many calories, although the coffee probably tastes better…

Conclusion

Try to remember that food should not be used as a coping device. Rather it is there to be enjoyed and to help us survive.

When we are not slaves to our food, nor to our eating habits, we become free to truly enjoy our food. **The aim of the game is to become in control of what you are eating, when you are eating it, and why you are eating it**. And with that control will come an awesome sense of freedom and power to live the kind of life that you really want to live.

3

GO! — Tips To Keep You On Track

*N*ow you are ready to start your diet. But there is a big difference between bearing the yoke of diethood and actively enjoying it. This section is designed to give you practical tips — not just to help the effectiveness of whichever diet you have chosen, but also to help you enjoy being on it. And the more you enjoy your chosen diet plan, the longer you'll stick with it. So here are some of the bits and pieces I wish I'd known ten years ago, learned the hard way, and would like to share with you.

Some of the tips might be obvious to you (and you have been doing them automatically for years); some you might find useful yourself; some you can tell your best friend to try; some might be useful now; some only useful at a different stage in your dieting journey. Whichever way, these tips should be helpful to anyone currently on any type of formal diet, or anyone who generally wants to improve her healthy eating habits.

These tips cover the spectrum of: Everyday Living; Shabbos; Jewish Festivals; External Support; Vacationing; and Eating Out.

Chapter 4

———— ◆ ◆ ◆ ————

Practical Tips

I have split this mountain of information into four parts:

- Food, Glorious Food;
- Non-Food Advice;
- Out and About; and
- Day-to-Day Advice

Food, Glorious Food

Fill Up on Plant Food

No, you can leave the flowers in the garden. We're talking fruits, vegetables, and whole-wheat/high-fiber food.

From a purely dietetic point of view, plant foods take up more space in the stomach than calorie-dense foods, making you feel fuller faster, on fewer calories.

Putting this into real-food terms: one tiny dollop of butter has as many calories as three cups of broccoli; a matchbox-size slice of cheddar cheese (1oz) has the same number of calories as one cup (8oz) of Bran Flakes. Food for thought.

Plant food also takes more jaw-work in terms of chewing and swallowing (just imagine crunching a carrot versus licking a cream cake). More jaw-work means it takes longer to eat. The longer it takes to eat, the more we feel we are eating.

From a health perspective, plant food also has some hidden benefits. Not only does it have a whole range of essential vitamins and minerals, but recent research has shown that it may help reduce the risk of heart disease, certain cancers, and other chronic diseases. The high levels of folate (B vitamin) in plant food also seem to reduce the risk of certain serious birth defects. (And you thought it was only for rabbits…).

Dressing Down Salad

Speaking of rabbits… You've finally buckled down to getting onto that diet, so out comes Bonny Bunny's food supply — lettuce, tomatoes, carrots, celery, etc. Even if you add a few raisins, nuts, or croutons for texture, you should still be getting the benefits due a good bunny, namely, a high-fiber, high-nutrition, low-calorie fill-me-up.

But the dressing can undo all your good intentions (plus the waistband). Let's do some math (groan). One tablespoon of normal fat mayonnaise is 100 calories. One tablespoon of low-fat mayonnaise is 50 (some even boast only 25 calories). Making this simple substitution would mean that you cut your calories in half. And all you had to do was open the other jar.

Using a low-fat or fat-free salad dressing works even better (plus, they've done all the hard work of choosing which spices to add). One tablespoon of Haddar's Italian Fat-Free Dressing only costs you 2.5 calories. This means that if you open the bottle instead of the high-fat mayo jar (one tablespoon per day for five weeks), you are saving yourself a whopping 3,412.5 calories.

While we are on the subject of mayonnaise, if you customarily baste your chicken with it before roasting, try spray oil instead. Every tablespoon of fat you don't use means 100 calories cut from the "cost" of the dish.

If you're the type who likes to make her own salad dressing instead of opening the bottle or, more realistically, forgot to buy it last time you were out shopping, how about trying this economical recipe — tried and tested, it's a real winner.

Low-Fat Vinaigrette Salad Dressing

    2 Tbsp. sugar
    2½ Tbsp. vinegar
    1 tsp. salt
    1 tsp. mustard
    spices (I use Italian seasoning, garlic, and pepper)

You can even make double and store it in the fridge for when you are next in a rush (and when are we *not* in a rush?).

For more adventurous dressing alternatives, try raspberry puree and wine vinegar; non-fat yogurt or fromage frais, vinegar and dry mustard; or vinegar, soy sauce, garlic, and ginger. And don't forget that you can always make dressings from cider vinegar; regular vinegar and olive oil; lemon juice; tomato juice; spices; and herbs, etc. It's not too difficult to turn a boring plate of salad into an exotically delicious one. All it takes is a little initiative and a bit of experimenting (after all, that can be half the fun).

Extra tip: If experimenting is your thing, just make sure to taste your concoction *before* pouring it over the salad. This way, if it didn't turn out quite as you expected, you don't have to throw the salad out at the same time.

Slurp Soup

OK, you can skip the slurp (when you are in company), but soup can be a real winner when you need a wholesome filler. What better way to warm up on a cold, snowy, winter's day than with a big mug of steaming hot, wholesome veggie soup?

It's nutritious. It's low-calorie (sometimes even free). It's delicious. And it takes the edge off your hunger.

Going Out...

Going on an outing? Remember, you can heat soup up and keep it warm for hours in an insulated container — or have it ready at a moment's notice when you come home.

Batch It

Why not make a big batch at the beginning of the week, pop it into the fridge, and then portion out bowlfuls — from-fridge-to-microwave style? This is one of my daughter's favorite motzei Shabbos jobs — i.e., to try out a new soup recipe and make enough for the week ahead. (See also, "Souper Suggetion," page 216).

Recipe Hunting

Sick of all your old standard recipes? Try a new one — call a friend you've let slide and exchange news and recipes, or ask to borrow some of her favorite recipe books if you've dog-eared yours from using the same recipes over and over.

On the Go

Can't be bothered to sit down to a bowl-and-spoon serving? Try serving it in a mug — it's portable and convenient (have it with your friend and slurp together in harmony).

Keeping It Hot

Nothing is more comforting than a hot bowl of soup. The trick is to keep it that way. When serving hot soup, warm the bowls. One way is to heat them in a preheated oven at a low temperature (200 to 250 degrees Fahrenheit) for a few minutes. If your oven is being used for something else, pour boiling water from a kettle into the bowls and let them stand for several minutes. Pour out the water, dry the bowls, and ladle in the piping hot soup immediately.

New-Size French Fries

If you want to resize your old body, you have to be especially careful when it comes to fat (see later in this chapter, "Fighting Fats," page 99). As french fries have a potentially high track record of the stuff, let's look at a few ways we can still indulge without the bulge.

- ✔ Forget the pretty zig-zag edges type and go for straight-edged soldiers instead. Fat has this habit of creeping into *all* nooks and crannies.
- ✔ Make them (not you) fat. Cut them big and chunky. Avoid the thin and delicate type.
- ✔ Try using oil that is high in unsaturates (usually your sunflower and vegetable oils, but check the bottle. See later, page 100).
- ✔ Change the oil often and make sure it's really hot before you start frying. Hot oil sears the food and traps in the goodness (whatever's left after frying, of course). Warm oil is absorbed by the food (yet more calories!), and results in slimy, greasy, stomach-churning soggy fries.
- ✔ Drain them well once they are golden brown (salivating already?) with plenty of good quality paper towels.
- ✔ Best tip: Skip the smell (and calories, and fat…) of frying and go for oven-baked or microwaved french fries instead. Less fat, fewer calories, less mess.
- ✔ Even better than best tip: Wash potatoes, leave skin on (you can justify your laziness by saying you are providing the family with extra fiber[1]), cut into thin slices, and spread out over a baking tray. Squirt spray oil all over, sprinkle generously with paprika, garlic (optional), and a touch of salt, bake in a medium-high oven for about forty minutes. The kids'll love them, they're healthy, they're easy, and you'll still be right on track.

---

[1] For more on fiber, see "Appendix 5: Fiber."

Milk Your Milk for What it's Worth

Either you are a milk person or you are not. If you are, milk is an excellent source of calcium, which keeps bones strong and contributes to counteracting that much-mentioned, bone-breaking disease, osteoporosis[2] (see page 272 and "You Will Keep Your Bones Healthy," page 294 for more information on osteoporosis). Milk is nutritious without being dense, and can also be a thirst quencher.

However, due to its high level of nutrients, it would help us to think of it in terms of being a food even though we all know that it's really a liquid. For this reason, it is important to note that **milk, unlike water, is not free in terms of calories, cholesterol,[3] or saturated fat.**[4] Of course, whole milk is higher in these evil critters than skim milk. There are 150 calories in one cup of whole milk versus 86 in a cup of skim.

I am not trying to put you off having your cozy-time hot chocolate. Quite the contrary — I want you to be able to indulge without having to pay for it in terms of pounds or health.

Obviously, the least painful adjustment to improve your diet is to swap over from whole milk to skim (see later, page 105). If you just can't face the changeover, try this tip instead. In order to reduce the calories while still enjoying yourself, try diluting the milk with cold water. It is best to do this gradually, bit by bit, until you get used to it. If skim milk is limited on your diet, this tip also works to stretch out your allowance.

People mistakenly pour milk like water. Therefore, if your throat resembles a parched Sahara desert, when it comes to coffees, teas, milkshakes, etc., watch out for those seemingly invisible calories.

Snack Attack

Contrary to the old school of thought, snacking is a good habit. We generally need to eat every three to four hours. Research has shown that people who snack often are less likely to overindulge in comparison to those who restrict their eating. Snacking stops hunger dead in its tracks and prevents overeating the next time you see food. An added benefit to snacking: The body can better absorb the nutrients when it's supplied with food at regular short intervals than it can when presented with the feast-or-famine pattern of three meals a day. So go on, put the kettle on and take a guilt-free coffee break. Don't have time? On the go? Grab a low-fat yogurt, a piece of fruit, or a rice cake. They all make good "can't stop now" snacks.

---

[2] Brittle bone disease.
[3] See later, "Clarifying Cholesterol," page 102.
[4] See later, "Fighting Fats," page 99.

Prepare for Snack Attacks

For good weight control, snacking is not a vice, it's a necessity. Keep low-fat snacks handy. Try pretzels or fruit. Snacks should be substantial enough to feel filling, but not so filling that you feel full.

Another low-fat snack is popcorn. Watch out though — many microwave brands are high in fat, so make popcorn in a hot-air popper that doesn't use oil. Dusting it with an artificial sweetener works well to provide a sweet treat. Or you can sprinkle it with paprika and a shake of Parmesan cheese. Or use soy sauce, pepper, or powdered ginger (and dust off those old chop sticks…).

Take Cereal Seriously

(Try saying that one fast)

Not only is cereal a potentially high-fiber, high-complex carbohydrate filler, but it is also quick, easy, and relatively inexpensive (both in terms of calories and money). It often scratches the itch of not knowing quite what to have without leaving you too overfull after you've finished off the last spoon of milk. It also makes an excellent meal in itself or as an in-between mealtime snack (see above).

Obviously, the high-fiber cereals are better choices health-wise — cereals such as Fruit 'n Fiber, Cheerios, and oatmeal versus Corn Flakes and Rice Krispies. In addition, the high fiber varieties fill you up more and for longer, on less — but hey, you knew that already, didn't you? (Look for cereals that have 3–6 grams of fiber per serving.)

Try making the cereal go further for fewer calories and more nutrition by cutting fresh fruit into your bowl first and then adding the cereal. By "diluting" the cereal this way, it looks like more, for fewer calories. This works especially well for potentially calorie-high cereals like Muesli.

Another tip: Add dry fruits to the cereal instead of sugar — the calorie difference might be negligible, but you are providing your body with better "value-for-money" in terms of nutrients.

Halt Salt

Although health professionals will tell you to go easy on pouring teaspoons of salt onto your steaming chicken and broccoli, it's processed and prepared foods — not the salt shaker — that are the greatest source of salt (and therefore sodium) in people's diets.

Too much sodium has been connected with increasing the risks of osteoporosis.[5] Dieters, especially, have to be careful to avoid too much sodium, as they generally tend to fall short in their consumption of calcium (which helps to counteract the disease). Other lovely side effects of excess salt are high blood pressure and an increased risk of strokes.

---

[5] See page 294 for more about this disease.

Salt itself does not make you gain weight, but it does cause water retention, which will show up on the tell-all love/hate scale, albeit temporarily (see later on in this chapter, "The Weighing Way", page 106). Therefore, if it's the day before weigh-day, go easy on the salt unless you don't mind crying buckets into a tissue as you step off the scale.

Spice Up Your Life with Spices

Open your cupboard doors and I bet you've got the same selection of spices you had when you first got married. While revamping your own body image, maybe you should take the time to "spice up" your stale staples as well.

Not only do spices add terrific flavor, but they also help mask the blandness that can ensue from reducing fat in all your favorite recipes.

Ever tried cumin? Makes a great curry. How about coriander? Can be used in beef, chicken, and lamb meals, soups, stews, cakes, and cookies. Don't know where to start? There are some great books out explaining which spices to use for which type of dish. Why not treat yourself to a bookstore spree, or drop brick-like subtle hints to your husband?

Substituting spices for salt will help lower your intake of sodium (see above) as well as add an extra pizzazz of flavor to your meal.

So go on, give it a zap!

Banish Booze

At 7 calories per gram, alcohol is almost as fattening as fat (9 calories per gram). And the higher the proof, the more calories it has. Worse, after a drink or two, nutritional judgement falters. After a few drinks and a plateful of hors d'oeuvres, you have consumed the equivalent of an extra meal's worth of calories, without even noticing.

Tipsy Tips:

- ✔ Choose seltzer or mineral water with a twist of lime or lemon for your first drink or two, as the first drink goes down so quickly anyway. Only then move on to your glass of wine.
- ✔ Order a bottle of mineral water or a pitcher of iced water to come to the table when the bottle of wine is ordered. After that, alternate your glasses: first water, then wine. You'll pace your drinking and limit your calorie intake.
- ✔ Instead of alcohol, try adding your favorite fruit juices to sparkling water — you'll still be able to clink your drink — and retain your smile beyond the party.

Sweet Treats

Subject: Sugar

Pure in its sweetness, pretty in its sprinkles, sugar can be seductive. But just consider that sugar contains only calories with no other nutrients. It's what health professionals call "empty calories" — i.e., the calories do not provide the body with any wholesome nutrition, nor do they fill you up.

Contrary to the tired, chocolate-bar-in-hand housewife's cry of needing it for more energy, you do not need sugar for energy. You can get energy from all the other food you eat.

The Problem with Sugar

Sugar is a classic case of "more for less." You get more calories for a tiny, itsy-bitsy amount.

Coffees, teas, herbal teas, etc., have no calories. One teaspoon of sugar contains a sneaky 20 calories. Multiply this by five (five cups of coffee/tea a day [I do like my tea-breaks…] with one teaspoon of sugar in each) and your no-calorie winner of a drink shoots up to 100 calories. 100 calories a day, times 7 days a week, and you've got an eyebrow-raising 700 calories. That's the equivalent of twenty rice cakes or fifteen fresh pears. Is this the time and place to mention that artificial sweeteners offer sweetness without the calories? Mmm…

Sugar's Favorite Hiding Places

Of course, the most obvious place he's likely to hide is inside the kitchen cupboards, somewhere between the flour and the teas and coffees.

But sugar is also a master of disguises. All good food manufacturers know that if the food labels always said, "fattening, empty-calorie-sugar" as an ingredient, we'd all run a mile. But they don't all list sugar as sugar. Beware its many less-familiar disguises. Watch out for the following: sucrose, glucose, dextrose, fructose, lactose, and maltose. They are all sugar — just wearing different hats and glasses. Honey, molasses, syrup, raw sugar, brown sugar, cane sugar, muscovado, corn syrup, and concentrated fruit juice are also worth avoiding — they are sugar's first cousins and you don't want to fall into bad company.

Tips for Reducing Sugar:

- ✔ Try drinking teas and coffees without sugar. Do it in stages if you find this one difficult.
- ✔ Try substituting some or all of the sugar with an artificial sweetener.
- ✔ When buying soft drinks, opt for the low-calorie ones. Try unsweetened fruit juices diluted with water, soda water, or even diet lemonade. If your kids pull faces at the changeover, challenge their tastebuds by taking off the bottle wrappers — see if they can *really* tell the difference!

✔ An easy substitution: Buy canned fruit in natural juice versus syrup. You can hardly tell the difference if you're using it for a fruit salad or drowning it with ice cream.

✔ Try halving the sugar you use in your favorite recipes. It works for most things except jam, meringues, and ice cream.

✔ Choose whole-wheat cereals rather than those coated in sugar/honey. If you need extra sweetness, you can always add your zero-calorie sweetener or bite-size pieces of fresh fruit.

✔ Seriously limit all those really obviously fattening goodies. You know the ones I mean…candies, chocolate, cakes, cookies, jam. (I knew you wouldn't like this one so I saved it for last.)

Don't Choke on Chocolate

Although I said we should limit chocolate, note that I never said to abandon it altogether. Chocolate belongs on every diet. It's the ultimate sweet tooth-lover's delight. It's the "I've been good all day and I deserve this" treat at the end of the day. But, read on…

Opening a big bar of milk chocolate and sitting down with a cup of tea could be the beginning of the end (of the chocolate, and your resolve). So try one of these chocolatey tips:

✔ Help yourself resist the temptation by breaking off whatever portion you are permitting yourself for that day — ***before*** you sit down. The hassle of having to get up again once you've plopped onto the sofa will keep you from overindulging.

✔ Alternatively, try putting the chocolate somewhere not-so-accessible. If you have to stand on a chair to reach it, for example, chances are that you won't be doing it every five minutes (unless you like to feel like a human yo-yo). They call this Behavioral Modification. I call it using laziness to overcome cravings.

✔ Buy fun-size bars instead of jumbo bars. They're portable, easily grab-able and…fun.

✔ Keep your chocolate in the fridge or freezer for a longer lasting chewwwww.

Fighting Fats

To oversimplify a very unsimple subject…

There are three basic types of fats:

Saturated Fats: Found in butter, ice cream, whole milk, other dairy foods, hard margarines, some soft margarines, meat (the white stuff visibly surrounding the meat), palm oil, coconut oil, hydrogenated vegetable oil, cakes, cookies, puddings, sausage rolls, etc.

Monounsaturated Fats: Found in olive oil, peanut (and other nut) oils, canola oil, peanuts, hazelnuts, almonds, Brazil nuts, olives, avocados, and margarines made from olive oil or labeled "high in monounsaturated fat."

Polyunsaturated Fats: Found in corn oil, fish oils, cottonseed oil, safflower oil, sesame oil, soybean oil, sunflower oil, oily fish (such as trout, sardines, mackerel, and salmon), and margarines labeled "high in polyunsaturates."

According to the U.S. Department of Agriculture's Dietary Guidelines, no more than thirty percent of our total daily calories should come from fat. For example, someone on a diet of 2,000 calories per day would be permitted up to 600 calories from fat each day.

However, since the real bad guys of the fat "family" are the saturated fats (they're the ones with curly mustaches, beady-eyes, and fat cigars…) the USDA recommends that no more than one third of our fat intake comes from saturated fats. In our example, that would mean limiting your saturated fats to 200 calories.[6]

Besides the world-famous health problems of digesting too much fat, like an increased risk of coronary heart disease,[7] diabetes, some forms of cancer, etc., it's worth noting that gram for gram, fats have more than twice as many calories as protein or carbohydrates. I.e., there are 9 calories in every gram of fat as opposed to 4 calories in a similar gram of protein or carbohydrate. (As we said earlier, even alcohol has less calories than fat, at 7 calories per gram). With that type of math, you can see why limiting fat plays an important role in weight reduction.

But, as you have probably guessed by now, nothing's as black and white as it looks at first glance. So you won't be surprised to know that fat is mighty important to your good health as well. Just to mention a couple of its positive contributions…

- Fat helps to make body tissue and hormones, and it helps to grease the wheels of our gallbladders and brains.

Here's a useful tip in dieting terms:

- By adding a bit of fat to your meal, you will feel fuller for longer. Fat has staying power. This way you will get hungrier less often — and just might end up eating fewer calories in the long run.

So if you were thinking of removing fat completely from your diet, think again, and don't. Just try to limit it to the above-mentioned percentages. I know, I know, easier said than done. But don't worry, I'm not abandoning you yet. Here are some tried and tested tips for controlling your fat intake. Try them and test them yourself.

---

[6] These numbers are for adults. Infants, toddlers, and children need more fat to aid their physical and mental growth.

[7] As we mention in Appendix 1, page 364 — coronary heart disease is the number one killer in the Western world.

HVO: "How Very Oily" or Hydrogenated Vegetable Oils and Margarine

✔ If you must have your toast and margarine and eat it too, then try to look for margarines labeled "high in polyunsaturates."

✔ If you are used to cooking with margarine or HVO, try switching to sunflower oil, soybean oil, sesame oil, etc. (See the Polyunsaturated Fats list.)

✔ For baking alternatives, see later table on "Full-Fat Favorites," page 105.

Butter Made Better

✔ When it comes to butter, measure out your permitted tablespoon(s) before you sit down at the table. This way you'll be less tempted to just cover up those "bare" edges.

✔ If you're the type who really lays things on thick, and religiously has butter with jam, butter with…try replacing the butter with honey, or pear and apple spread — or just about anything else other than a high sat-fat little devil like butter.

✔ For baking alternatives, see later table on "Full-Fat Favorites," page 105.

Milk

See earlier, "Milk Your Milk for What It's Worth," page 95.

Nice Cream Ice Cream

✔ Creamy dairy ice cream may taste like heaven, but that's one place you're not in a hurry to visit just now. Try substituting low-fat ice cream or sorbet. Tofutti can also be a great low-fat substitute (it's best to check the label to be sure). Just compare forty-five low-calorie frozen fudge bars (at 30 calories each) to the equivalent number of calories in one pint of rich real-stuff ice cream.

✔ Instead of an ice cream bar, why not choose a fruity popsicle (same hand, less fat) — or make your own concoctions using fruit juice?

Yummy Yogurt

At the risk of writing the obvious, try the low-fat and fat-free versions, or fromage frais. You might like them. If you don't, try adding a sugar substitute, vanilla essence, or low-sugar jam. Putting creativity and fruit into them might just turn a high-fat snack into a low-fat fruit-pack.

Say "Cheese"

These days the cheese manufacturers are getting the message and are producing low-fat versions of many different types of cheeses. There's low-fat Mozzarella, Cheddar, soft cheeses, creamy cheeses, cottage cheeses…even a mouse looking to lower his fat intake can have a field day.

Salad Dressings

See earlier, "Dressing Down Salad," page 92.

Business Meating

✔ Go for lean cuts of meat. Take the few extra seconds to trim off excess fat. If you can see white bits, chop 'em off.

✔ If you've got a choice of different types of meat, it's best to go for less of the "organ" types of meat (as in body parts, not as in music…e.g., liver, kidney, etc.). These are very high in cholesterol. Same goes for processed meats (e.g. salami, hot dogs, etc.): Avoid them when you can.

✔ Because red meat generally has a high saturated fat content, it's wise to use your eyes when it comes to portion size. Try eating smaller portions than you usually do. One small portion would be the equivalent size of a deck of cards; a large portion would be double.

✔ If you can't manage to acquire a low-fat chopped meat, try this trick to reduce the fattiness. Heat the chopped meat in a pan with a little water, and when it's cooled (it's best if it's left in the fridge overnight), pour off the fat with the water. Then cook the meat as desired. This also works for fatty sausages or beef burgers.

✔ Before cooking chicken, take the skin off (or save yourself a job and buy it ready-skinned). Most of the chicken's fat is just under the skin (to keep the little darling warm). As a side benefit, you will automatically be reducing calories as well.[8] (A fried chicken breast with the skin on has 217 calories; without its skin, 160.) So it's off with his skin to keep ourselves trim.

✔ If you are roasting a fatty joint of meat, try "dry roasting" it by using a trivet so that the fat can pour off. (See later section on "Cooking Methods that Start with 'B,'" page 119).

Clarifying Cholesterol

Since we've just spoken about fats, let's move over for a brief look at one of fat's closest relatives — cholesterol.

Unlike fat, cholesterol has no calories. That's the good news. The bad news is, if you have too much cholesterol it can kill you. High levels of cholesterol in the average Amercian are why Coronary Heart Disease is the leading killer disease in the western world. But surprisingly enough, eighty percent of our cholesterol is produced by our own bodies (this is called "blood cholesterol") and only twenty percent comes from eating foods high in cholesterol (this is called "dietary cholesterol"). This means if we are going to control our cholesterol levels (and we better…), then we will have to lower the levels of cholesterol our body produces as well as limit our intake of dietary cholesterol.

---

[8] Similarly, cook your chicken soup the day before you need it, refrigerate it overnight, and skim off any visible signs of fat. What you see is the saturated fat happily doing the breaststroke.

Here is where those bad guys, saturated fats, come into the picture again. They are the nasty critters that increase our levels of blood cholesterol and they are the ones we have to severely limit, just like we discussed earlier. On the other hand, research has found that foods high in polyunsaturated or monounsaturated fats actually help to lower our levels of blood cholesterol. So out come the sardines, mackerel (polyunsaturated), and olive oil (monounsaturated) and away goes the butter, margarine, and full-fat cheeses (saturated fats).

But, as usual, there is always the other side of the coin to take into account. Even dreaded cholesterol has some endearing qualities. Cholesterol helps our cells, aids in the production of vitamin D and certain hormones, and helps our gall bladder do its job properly. That's why the USDA suggests that we don't completely cut dietary cholesterol from our lives, but that we just make sure we don't take in more than 300 milligrams of it per day.

Just to give you a rough idea of what this means in terms of what's on your plate:

A 3oz serving of Cheddar cheese = 90 milligrams of cholesterol

A 3oz serving of beef stew = 87 mg

A 3oz serving of roast chicken breast = 73 mg

A 3oz serving of tuna in water = 48 mg

3oz of whole milk = 13 mg

One large egg = 213 mg

Now that we realize fats and cholesterol are not the flavor of the month for several reasons, try these substitutes…

Subject Yourself to Substitution

Full-Fat Favorites	Substitute With
Potato Chips	Low-Fat Pretzels
Full-Fat Soft Cream Cheese	Reduced-Fat Soft Cheese
Sugar	Artificial Sweetener
Candies	Sugar-Free Candies/Raisins
Cream Cheese	Low-Fat Cottage Cheese
Oil	Spray Oil
Cookies	Low-Fat Crackers with Jam
Full Fat Fromage Frais	Low-Fat Fromage Frais
Full-Fat Yogurt	Low-Fat Yogurt
Salad Dressing	Low-Fat Salad Dressing
Tortilla Chips/Potato Chips	Vegetable Sticks with Dips (made with low-fat yogurt)
Heavy Puddings	Fruit Salad
Cheesecake	Meringues/Raspberry Coulis
Ice Cream	Sorbet/Non-Fat Frozen Yogurt
Ice Cream Bar	Tofutti Fudge Popsicle
Strawberry Ice Cream	Sliced Strawberries with generous dollops of Fromage Frais or Sorbet
Apple Pie	Baked Apple with Raisins and Artificial Sweetener
Chocolate Bars	Low-Fat Crackers with a scraping of Chocolate Spread
Fruit Flans/Cakes/Cookies	Fruit Salad/Fruit Platters/Compotes

In addition, if you are baking and want to reduce the calories without compromising on taste, how about trying the following substitutions:

Full-Fat Favorites	Substitute With	You Save
½ cup butter in frosting	½ cup Marshmallow Fluff	574 calories; 92g fat
½ cup vegetable oil	½ cup unsweetened applesauce	910 calories; 109g fat
2 Tbsp. butter or oil when sautéing	2–4 Tbsp. Wine	Up to 200 calories; 25g fat
1 cup heavy cream for soups	1 cup 1% milk plus 1 Tbsp. cornstarch	688 calories; 85g fat

Just for the record, I once had a client who had never been on a diet before. She made only two changes to her diet: she substituted low-fat mayonnaise for full-fat, and switched whole milk to skim. She lost four pounds in the first week.

Making substitutions enables us to enjoy our favorite types of food without having to pay the penalty of eating something unhealthy and fattening.

BLT: Bites, Licks, and Tastes

Also known as "The Invisibles," all those bites, licks, and tastes mount up when you are not looking. Just straightening up the cakes' side and, almost unawares, swallowing the slither can add real calories to an otherwise careful day. Don't be caught off guard: each bite, morsel, nibble, mouthful, or crunch adds up (and up, and up…).

I once attended a lecture on our little friends B, L, and Ts. The lecturer had amassed quite a collection of food. She had half sausages; leftover, soggy french fries; bits of cookies, chips, pretzels, nuts, croutons, raisins, chocolate, and oven latkes; and an array of children's suppertime leftovers. When all the food was displayed she announced that each food was what she had eaten either on the go, unawares, or while clearing up. Though most of it hardly looked remotely tempting anymore, the message was powerful. Calories are being consumed and we are not even conscious of them.

Far be it from me to suggest permanent muzzling in between mealtimes. But, being truly conscious of these facts and your tendencies can help you overcome them.

Extra tip: It's often irresistible to have a nibble when you find yourself carrying platters or plates of goodies to and from the table. Try putting something in your mouth (carrot stick) so you can't nibble on what's in your hand — or make sure both of your hands are utilized (on both journeys) to stop you from being able to pick from the plate that you are carrying. (For more advice on this topic, see "Eat from a Plate," page 119).

Non-Food Advice

Until now we have focused on food-related issues. Let's turn our attention to some non-food areas. As we leave the kitchen, turning our backs to the mess, we turn left towards the living room, grab a five-minute time-out, and close the door. Now we can hear ourselves think.

The Weighing Way (At the Scale)

Yes, I know, the numbers going down mean you're doing something right, and well, the rest we'll talk about someday. This principle is true whether you weigh yourself in the bathroom (door bolted, padlocked, and barricaded), at the gym, at your Diet Group, or in the supermarket. The bottom-line question is really: How often should you weigh yourself?

The ideal is to weigh yourself once a week at the same time of day, with the same weight of clothing, same denier tights, same eyeliner — you get the picture. You want to create circumstances as similar as possible from week to week, so that you can feel assured that the scale is showing you a real weight loss. Incidentally, if you think it's ridiculous to wear the same outfit from week to week, know that I had one client who lost three pounds in about three seconds flat when she took off her sweater! (Ahh, if it were only that easy...)

"Can't I weigh myself every day?" I hear you ask. Far be it from me to stop an obsessive, compulsive, overall discouraging habit, but...because there are so many day-to-day variables that will *not* show an accurate picture of your weight loss (like the weather — yes, I'm serious — and whether you ate a food that results in water retention,[9] the "time of the month," and things like *barometric pressure* [the earth's pressure against your body]), maybe it's an idea to reconsider.

Seeing the numbers fluctuate daily can be discouraging (you don't see a steady downward trend) and can make your weight loss feel like it's taking forever. So weigh yourself only once a week if you can manage to hang on that long. I've tried both ways, and believe me, it's just more motivating to go for the once-a-week trip.

While we are on the subject, have you checked out those ten-year-old bathroom scales recently? Try weighing sacks of potatoes/flour/etc. to check the accuracy of an old scale. Hey, you never know, maybe you're really five pounds lighter than you thought! Remember, a scale should lie on a hard, even surface. So if you've got yours at the foot of the bed, all ready to be jumped on after Modeh Ani,[10] try placing them on a hard board instead of the carpet for a more accurate reading.

---

[9] Like pickles, canned soup, tomato juice, rice, or salty foods (see earlier, "Halt Salt," page 96).
[10] Prayer of gratitude for seeing a new day, said upon waking.

Monitor and Motivate

Whenever you begin a weight loss program, it's always a great idea to monitor yourself properly. We've spoken about body weight and weighing, but there are other ways to monitor your success. Obviously, the more areas you see yourself succeed in, the more successful, motivated, and happy you'll feel. Success breeds success and therefore it's important to capitalize on the achievements you make in all areas of your body's changes.

Below is a list of ways to monitor your success:

✔ **Accurate Weighing** (See above)

✔ **"Smile, Please!"**

Taking a photograph right at the start of your campaign may feel awkward and embarrassing, but it's a wonderful motivator.

You see yourself in the mirror every day. You are accustomed to the way you look. You can't see the changes, but changes are there. After you have lost fifteen to twenty pounds or so, people may begin to compliment you. You might not see the changes they see. But if you take a photo after you have lost weight and compare the two…Wow! You, yourself, will see the difference.

It's the realization that you are succeeding that will motivate you forward. Everyone who didn't take photos before successfully losing weight regrets it. Even though you might have to force yourself to do it, it's worthwhile in the long run. So get the camera out and start clicking.

Practically speaking, the photos should include: one full-length, front-facing; one full-length, side-facing (try to resist the temptation to pull in the tummy — we are being relaxed and natural here); one close up, head-and-shoulders front-facing; and one head-and-shoulders side-facing. Oh, and don't forget to smile!

Make sure you take photos right at the start of your program, and at each subsequent fifteen-pound-loss interval. Ready, steady…cheeeese.

✔ **Pinch an Inch**

Another wonderful way to watch the body metamorphize into a butterfly is to measure the circumference of certain body parts. Sometimes you'll lose inches even if you don't lose pounds. This may seem discouraging when you are standing on the scale, but if you keep track of your measurements, you can, quite literally, watch the numbers drop and drop. Plippety plop.

Make a chart listing the following body parts to measure: Around the Arm (halfway between your elbow and your shoulder); Neck; Bust; Waist; Hips; Thigh; and Calf. Plot these in a column going down the left hand side of your paper, and a row going across the top of the page that lists Week 1, Week 4, Week 8, etc. It should look something like this:

Body Part	Week			
	1	4	8	12
Arm (Top)				
Neck				
Bust				
Waist				
Hips				
Thigh				
Calf				

It is advisable to only measure yourself once a month (at the same time of the month, etc.), because the body's fat supplies take time to be mobilized and zap — disappear.

These measurements should be taken directly onto the skin, without the bulk of clothing or a padded bra (although a bra that provides good support *should* be worn) to hinder the reading. You should aim to measure the widest part and be relaxed as you do so. (Tense, contracted muscles differ in size to relaxed muscles.) Take a deep breath in, then out, then start.

✔ Try It On

Weight loss can feel very slow at times. The changes in your body are gradual, hardly noticeable on a daily basis, and may require a motivation-boosting aid. So, after several weeks of successful dieting, try on something that used to be too tight. If you are really eager, you can try on your snug outfit every fourteen days to see how it fits you better and better. Watch how the zipper starts to glide up instead of snagging and jerking against the strain.

When presented with this concrete proof of now-fitting clothes, the realization comes that yes, your body has actually changed shape in a very real and tangible way. All that hard work has been worth it. The clothing doesn't change size, so any difference in the way it fits is an indication that you are really and truly changing shape.

Dear Diary

No, not the, "Dear Diary, I feel just terrible. Chani thought I was due next week and I had the baby a month ago!" variety — we are talking about one of the best, most effective, absolutely foolproof ways to ensure self-control. A Food Diary.

Basically, a Food Diary is a table, chart, or grid that requires you to fill in all the food you eat every day. Yes, down to the last lick and spoonful. I can just hear the non-fastidious types explode at this point, "Everything I eat? Every day? *I just can't!*" Don't worry, even if the thought of being meticulous in detailing such information sends you to bed with a migraine, know that a Food Diary is not a life sentence. Even if you can only manage to fill it in for a few days, or every other day, or when your weight loss is slow, it's still a highly effective method of maintaining hand-to-mouth control.

Why?

✔ It forces you to be conscious (note, not phobic) about what exactly is going into your mouth;

✔ It forces you to be honest ("Mommy M'eiser"[11] from Shnocky's Shabbos Party: five M&Ms, handful of Bissli, pretzels, and lemonade-soaked chips. OK, skip the chips and just picture the mess instead);

✔ A written record of what you ate will help you gauge more accurately if you really *are* following the diet plan's guidelines correctly (if not, go back to the sofa, do not collect $200, and read the diet plan's book — again!);

✔ It works! With this kind of "Big Brother Is Watching You" consciousness, you stick to your plan and really lose.

If you are going to any type of formal Diet Group, any consultant worth her salt should be able to analyze your Food Diary to see where you are going wrong. Without it, she can't help you — there's no way you're going to remember whether you had two extra cookies at 11am last Thursday or not.

When filling in your Food Diary, in addition to all of the above, take extra care with the following:

✔ Write down *everything* that gains entrance into that sanctum of tastebuds;

✔ Be specific when noting portion sizes. Write "One massive bowl of pasta" versus "Pasta;"

✔ If it's Shabbos/Yom Tov, write down before Shabbos what you expect to have, and right after Shabbos note the differences;

✔ Write clearly — taking care in writing it all down makes your Food Diary and diet plan more pleasant and pleasing (not just for you, but also for your consultant). Shmatte writing, shmatte diet. Lovely writing…

Extra Tip: An alternative method of using your Food Diary would be to use it as a menu-planner for the week and then add any extras as you go through your week. This way you can organize yourself and can shop in advance for any special dishes or ingredients.

[11] Tithe

Just to give you an idea of the look of a typical Food Diary, here's a one-day version.

Monday	
	Points/Sins/Treats
Breakfast	
Lunch	
Supper	
Snacks	
Points used today	
Points saved today	

Multiply by seven (days) and…you're up and running.

Out and About

Now we're not just getting out of the kitchen, we're getting out of the house alto-gether. Where are we going? Let's go shopping. Have you taken everything you'll need? Money, lipstick, keys, willpower… Good. Now pack the following bits of advice into your pocketbook as well, and you'll be ready to go.

Shopping When Hungry

I've tried it both ways. Empty tummy, full cart. Full tummy…well, not-so-full cart. The truth is, shopping on an empty tummy fills up the shopping wagon beyond our wildest dreams. Subconsciously we fill our carts with what we would really like to be eating (that is, eating right then and there in the middle of the supermarket). When you are hungry you are more likely to choose the cakes and cookies, as they seem even more appealing than usual. You will also be more prone to plonk them into the cart because you understand intuitively that they give more immediate satisfaction than the baked beans, which need preparation (heating up). We also tend to choose much more of whatever we are selecting because we are hungry. (The physical symptoms of hunger trigger a reaction in the brain that says: Get food).

As a byproduct, what ends up in your house has a lot to do with how hungry you were when you were shopping. Having cakes and goodies surround us on a constant basis will provide us with numerous occasions for temptation, versus not having them in the house at all and therefore having to summon up the energy to go out and buy them. I know which one I'd rather.

Conclusion? Save yourself the temptation of all those calories, have pity on your credit card, and fill up your own "tank" before setting out. Also, try to write a shopping list — and stick to it.

Shopping When in a Rush

If you go shopping in a rush, you won't have time to check out low-fat alternatives (reading the labels), new products, or cheaper items. You'll end up with all the regular staples and wonder why you forgot what you went shopping for in the first place. This will necessitate yet another trip into the lion's den of temptation — plus it's a waste of time.

Although it might be unrealistic to always shop with serenity (who is she, anyway?), giving yourself an extra few minutes when facing all those choices can help to keep you on track. Sometimes a new product will add a whole new dimension to your healthy eating program. Variety is not only the spice of life, it's the spice of your diet as well. So slow down, enjoy the choosing, and you might end up enjoying your diet as well.

If you find yourself perpetually in a rush, try making your store-specific shopping list in aisle order. It's faster to collect all like-foods at one time instead of zigzagging all over the store, plus you're less likely to forget anything.

Food Labels

During the course of our Diet Group sessions, I encourage the Group participants to bring in any new product they have found on their travels. I analyze the product's claims ("low-fat," "no cholesterol"), work out the points/treats/sins values, and either recommend they buy it in bulk and live off it for the next year, or I disparage it and risk getting sued for libel. What surprises the group (and me) repeatedly is that in the world of advertising, all that glitters is definitely *not* gold. A package of cookies can claim to be "sugar-free," a yogurt can call itself "low-fat," a pretzel emblazons "no cholesterol," a salad dressing cries out "Light" or "Reduced." Does this automatically mean we should fill our carts with these dieter's jewels? Unfortunately not.

Upon taking a closer look at the you-can't-hide-anything-from-me Nutrition Facts, we get the true, objective, and sometimes disappointing facts. First of all, advertising terms such as "Light" or "Reduced" are all relative terms compared to normal standards. It *is* light or reduced — but it may not be dietetic and certainly may not be "free." Secondly, yes, a product may be low in cholesterol, but it doesn't automatically follow that it's low in fat or calories.

What claims should we mistrust? "Lite," "Light," "Low Sugar," "Sugar-Free," "Reduced-Fat," "Low Cholesterol," "High Fiber," etc. Let's just clarify that: Mistrust *every* claim. All are guilty until proven innocent.

Coming from the school of thought that education in such matters will provide the correct tools to counteract the misleading presentations of the marketing and advertising world, let's explain what that confusing little box at the back of the package really means. Here are some useful rules of tum, I mean thumb.

Sample Label for Macaroni & Cheese

Nutrition Facts

(1) Serving Size 1 Cup (228g)
Servings Per Container 2

Amount Per Serving		
(2) Calories 250	**(3)** Calories from Fat 110	
	(5) **%Daily Value***	
(4) Total Fat 12g		18%
Saturated Fat 3g		15%
Cholesterol 30mg		10%
Sodium 470mg		20%
Total Carbohydrate 31g		10%
Dietary Fiber 0g		0%
Sugars 5g		
Protein 5g		
Vitamin A		4%
Vitamin C		2%
Calcium		20%
Iron		4%

(6) *Percent Daily Values are based on a 2,000 calorie diet. Your daily values may be higher or lower depending on your calorie needs:

	Calories	2,000	2,500
Total Fat	Less than	65g	80g
Sat Fat	Less than	20g	25g
Cholesterol	Less than	300mg	300mg
Sodium	Less than	2,400mg	2,400mg
Total Carbohydrate		300g	375g
Fiber		25g	30g

(1)

| Serving Size 1 Cup (228g) |
| Servings Per Container 2 |

(1) Serving Size

It is worth noting the portion size that you usually eat in relation to the serving size suggested. If you know that you never level the tablespoon (yes, this means getting out a knife and scraping its surface) or you always eat half a box of cookies at a time as opposed to the serving size of two, you might be underestimating your calorie intake. If you eat more than the serving size stated, you need to get the calculator out.

In this example, one serving of macaroni and cheese equals one cup. If you ate the whole package, you would be ingesting *two* cups. That doubles the calories and other nutrient values.

(2)

| **Amount Per Serving** | |
| **Calories** 250   **(3)** | Calories from Fat 110 |

(2) Calories

Calories quantify the amount of energy you get from a particular food serving. We want "value for money" from our foods when we are on a weight-reducing program, because excess calories turn into fat. Therefore we need to choose foods low in calories, so that we can eat more food, feel less hungry, and still lose weight.

(3) Calories From Fat

The "Calories from Fat" gives us the amount of calories per serving that add up from the fat in the food. Usually the two (fat and calories) go hand in hand (from mouth to tummy), i.e., where there's fat, there are calories.

In this example, the amount of *calories from fat* is 110 calories. This means that almost half of the food's calories come from fat. As we mentioned earlier in the "Fighting Fats" section, page 100, since nutrition experts recommend that we consume no more than thirty percent of our daily calories from fat (or 600 calories from fat on a 2,000 calorie diet), this spells trouble.

A handy (don't-have-a-calculator-with-me-in-the-supermarket) method to arrive at a rough idea of whether a food has a high/low fat content, is to multiply by ten the number of grams of fat as listed on the label. Then compare that "fat number" with the number of calories also included on the label. If the fat number is more than one-third of the calorie number, the item is too high in fat.

In our example, (see (4) on page 112) there are 12g fat listed. Multiply this by 10 and we're at 120. Compared to the 250 calories provided by this macaroni, we can see that 120 is almost half of 250, which means it's way too high in fat.

Total Fat 12g	
Saturated Fat 3g	
Cholesterol 30mg	
Sodium 470mg	
Total Carbohydrate 31g	
Dietary Fiber 0g	
Sugars 5g	
Protein 5g	
Vitamin A	
Vitamin C	
Calcium	
Iron	

(4) The Nutrients

The list of nutrients (Total Fat, Saturated Fat, Cholesterol, Sodium, Total Carbohydrate, Dietary Fiber, Sugars, Protein, Vitamins, Calcium, and Iron) is all-important for our health. They can be separated into two main groups: nutrients to be limited and those we need.

Total Fat 12g		18%
Saturated Fat 3g		15%
Cholesterol 30mg		10%
Sodium 470mg		20%

Limit These Nutrients: Fat, Cholesterol, and Sodium.

Most of us don't have a problem with getting enough of these — rather, we tend to overdo our consumption of them. These "baddies" are highlighted in grey 'cause grey makes them look really mean.[12]

Dietary Fiber 0g
Vitamin A
Vitamin C
Calcium
Iron

Get Enough of These: Fiber, Protein, Vitamins A and C, Calcium, and Iron.

Most of us don't consume adequate amounts of dietary fiber[13] or these essential vitamins. Eating enough of these nutrients can improve your health and help reduce the risk of some diseases and health conditions. These are the "good guys," but often get ignored because they are surrounded by all those ugly numbers and percentages.

For example, in real terms, a food is considered to be high in fiber if it has at least 5g of fiber per serving. We should try to have those cereals with *at least* 3g of fiber per serving. So goodbye Corn Flakes, hello Bran Flakes.

---

[12] For further elaboration on these, see earlier, "Clarifying Cholesterol," page 102.
[13] Dietary fiber does not mean that only those people on a diet should eat it. It is referring to the fiber we eat, not the fiber we wear (like cotton, wool, etc.).

⑤

	%Daily Value*
Total Fat 12g	18%
Saturated Fat 3g	15%
Cholesterol 30mg	10%
Sodium 470mg	20%

⑤ **The Percent Daily Value (%DV)**

I know, it looks really unappetizing. But, believe me, it's worthwhile familiarizing yourself with this little column of numbers. It's a simple yet effective method of knowing what and how much you are eating in relation to your day. The Government has done much research to determine how much of which nutrients we should aim to consume each day to ensure we eat a healthy diet (not necessarily a weight reducing diet). The %DV (Daily Value)[14] shows us the percent (or how much) of the recommended daily amount of a nutrient is in a serving of food. By using the %DV, we can tell if this amount is high or low. Without a %DV, we may be told that a food has 12g of Total Fat, but this information is meaningless without a greater context of how much we are supposed to be having. Here, we are told that 12g Total Fat, in this product, contributes to eighteen percent of the total amount we should consume each day. In other words, after eating this macaroni and cheese we will be left with eighty-two percent of our fat allowance to spend throughout the rest of the day.

⑥

*Percent Daily Values are based on a 2,000 calorie diet. Your daily values may be higher or lower depending on your calorie needs:

		Calories	2,000	2,500
Total Fat	Less than		65g	80g
Sat Fat	Less than		20g	25g
Cholesterol	Less than		300mg	300mg
Sodium	Less than		2,400mg	2,400mg
Total Carbohydrate			300g	375g
Fiber			25g	30g

⑥ **%DV Based on a 2,000 Calorie Diet**

For labeling purposes, the Government set 2,000 calories as the reference amount for calculating %DVs. Even though most people don't have a clue about how many calories they consume each day, you can still use the %DV as a rough frame of reference, regardless of whether you eat more or less than 2,000 calories[15] each day.

Still with me? Just a few more numbers…hang in there. Look at the Total Fat information in this box. It tells you that if you eat a 2,000-calorie diet, you should eat *less than 65g of fat in **all** the foods* you eat in a day.[16] This means that if you eat 65g of fat, then you are eating 100% of your %DV for fat.

---

[14] Just to confuse us, the DV (Daily Value) is sometimes referred to as the RDA (Recommended Daily Allowance).

[15] As we've said before (see "The Equation," page 17), each person has a different level of calorie consumption necessary to lose weight. Factors such as present weight, build, age, and activity levels influence the number of calories you need.

[16] Incidentally, the recommended values for the consumption of Sodium and Cholesterol stay the same, regardless of the number of calories you eat.

What All This Means For Us

As a guiding quick-fix rule, when it comes to %DVs, know that 5% or less is low for all those nutrients we want to limit (e.g., fat, saturated fat, cholesterol, and sodium), and is also low for those nutrients that we want to consume in greater amounts (e.g., fiber, calcium, etc). On the other hand, a DV of 20% is considered a high reading for all nutrients.

Let's look at our macaroni and cheese again. Is 18%DV Total Fat contributing a lot or a little to our maximum fat limit of 100% each day? You see that 18%DV is not quite 20%DV, (i.e., considered high), but if you went ahead and polished off the whole package (two servings), you would double that amount and be way over your twenty percent. This amount, coming from just one food, would leave you with sixty-four percent of your fat allowance for *all* of the other foods you eat that day, snacks and drinks included. (Now you see why it's a good idea to get a handle on all this math.)

What This Information Means For Us When We Go Shopping

✔ Comparisons

The %DV makes it easy for us to make comparisons. We can compare one product or brand to a similar product. It's easy to see which one is higher or lower in a nutrient, because the serving sizes are generally consistent for similar food types (for example, a 30g serving when comparing two cereals).

✔ Nutrient Content Claims: No More Tricks

We can quickly distinguish one claim from another, such as "reduced-fat" versus "light" or "nonfat." Just compare the %DVs for Total Fat in each food product to see which one is higher or lower in that nutrient. No need to trust the advertisers or Cousin Shuli — you can go right ahead and trust the label.

For example, let's take a look at two salad dressings. Pfeiffer Italian "Light" Dressing has 8%DV of fat, in comparison to Pfeiffer Italian "Fat Free" Dressing, which has 0%DV of fat. Notice that the 8%DV of fat is called "Light." As we are going to "label" ourselves discerning consumers after we have read this chapter, it's worth taking a closer look at the calorie content of these enticing looking bottles. As we mentioned earlier, fat and calories are buddies and go through life hand in hand. We shouldn't be surprised to see that the Light Dressing has 60 calories per its two tablespoon serving, whereas the Fat Free Dressing has only 20 for the same two tablespoon serving. And they thought they could fool us. Ha.

✔ Dietary Trade-Offs

We can also use the %DV to help us make dietary trade-offs with other foods throughout the day. We don't have to give up a favorite food to eat a healthy diet. For instance, when a food you like is high in fat, you can balance it with foods that are low in fat at other times of the day. Also, you need to pay attention to how much you eat, so that the total amount of fat for the day stays below 100%DV.

"Fats" it for now, enough of the brain-strain number crunching. Math never was my strong point anyway, so don't feel bad if all those numbers make you as nervous as a schoolgirl facing an algebra exam paper. Just make sure to go shopping not only with list in hand, but also with your reading glasses perched on your nose for peering closely at the Nutrition Facts label — your new friend.

On the Town

If you are planning to spend a morning in town, taking the extra second or two to think ahead may be a real bonus. Imagine the scene: you've just visited hosiery store number five, which has also just run out of Shnocky's won't-wear-anything-else-except Levante tights. Your feet hurt, your patience levels are getting dangerously low, and yep, you are hungry. Do you dive into the nearest kosher deli and drown your sorrows? Do you make a half-crazed beeline for the kosher nosh corner in the supermarket? Why, no. You have come prepared with your inseparable nosh bag: crispy Granny Smith apple, just-ripe pear, rice cakes, low-fat yogurt, and ahhhhh, a refreshing drink. Now doesn't that make you feel better?

Not only will you save time (and money) by taking food with you, but you will also be avoiding the temptations of a deli when at your lowest willpower ebb. You even get to rest your weary bones and rub your feet for a spell.

Day-To-Day Advice

Dieting doesn't just involve mealtimes or the ten minutes before mealtimes. It's a mindset. Let's look at some tips to help us out on a day-to-day basis.

Weigh To Go (Weighing Food)

The definition of dieting means limiting something. You can pick and choose which ingredient you can most easily live without (hence 101 different diets on the market), but whatever that ingredient is, you'd better blast it out of your kitchen.

If the diet calls for x number of fat grams per day, get out the calculator and throw out the mayonnaise. If the diet calls for zero carbohydrates, "Pesach clean" the cupboards and freezer. If the diet calls for no milk, sell the cow, etc., etc.

Most diets work. They might not entice you, excite you, invigorate you, or inspire you, but they sell because, if you follow their rules, the pounds will probably drop.

See that sneaky little phrase snuck in there…"if you follow their rules…"? That's because without cutting out what needs to be cut; or weighing out what needs to be weighed; or measuring what needs to be measured, it ain't gonna work.

I've seen the same scenario replay itself time and again in our Weight Loss Group meetings. The first client will swear that she did exactly what the second (successful) client did and yet she (the first client) didn't lose an ounce. When quizzing her on her in-depth familiarity with her digital kitchen scale (or even on its existence), she looks at me blankly, as though questioning, "Are you for real?" If you want a real weight loss, you need real measuring.

Showing the Group a set of measuring spoons is another tactic I have tried using to bring about a heightened awareness of exactitude. Everyone who's ever browsed around a kitchen store will know the sort I mean — usually four different sized spoons, grouped together, family style, in one bunch. There's Daddy spoon: the tablespoon; Mommy spoon: the teaspoon; Sister spoon: the half-teaspoon; and even cutie-pie Baby spoon: quarter of a teaspoon. These spoons are so often relegated to the back of some junk-infested drawer that we tend to "guesstimate" the amounts we are using.

Just to prove my point, let me ask you a question. When you last made coleslaw, did you use a measuring spoon for the mayonnaise, or did you free-pour? (Hmm, no wonder it was so delicious.)

There's also a world of difference between a level tablespoon and a heaped table-spoon. We can add invisible calories to a dish depending on how high the heap. Even if it means dirtying a knife to level the mayonnaise, go for it. Exactitude is a sure-fire dieting policy (consider it akin to dotting the "i"s and crossing the "t"s).

Tip: If you don't want to face the bother of measuring out one cup of cereal every day, try marking your cereal bowl with nail polish to mark the permitted level.

Serving: Here and There

Often it's the small changes in our behavior that will reap the greatest dividends.

Try serving the food onto plates in the kitchen (i.e., skipping the serving bowls stage) and bringing them directly to the dining room or kitchen table. This way, you won't be tempted to pick from the serving bowls in front of you or be tempted to help your-self to seconds when firsts sufficed. You will also be forcing yourself to leave the com-fort of sitting to go and get more food. This provides you with a few seconds of intro-spection. You may either change your mind ("No, I'm gonna stick to this diet…"), or know for sure that you require more food ("I really am still hungry").

Extra bonus: because you are not using serving bowls, there's less washing up.

Cooking Methods That Start with "B"

Cooking meat with any of the following methods saves lots of calories over frying, stewing, or sautéing. That's because the fat inside the meat has a chance to drip, drop, drip away from the roast (and away from your plate).

- ✔ Broil;
- ✔ Barbecue;
- ✔ Bake (on a rack);
- ✔ Braise.

Be clear
It's a winner
To cook with "B"
For your dinner.

Although technically not methods beginning with "B," you can also try just about any other alternative to frying, such as steaming, grilling, poaching, and microwaving.

Downsize Portions

Often a heavy person's food choices are the same as a thin person's. What's different is portion size. To exercise quantity control, you need to think *quality control*. If you're after the real stuff and low-fat substitutions just won't meet the grade, then concentrate on its essence, not its volume. Try a tiny smear of real cream cheese rather than a massive blob of the low-fat version. This way, cravings are satisfied without piling on calories.

Small is Beautiful

Instead of serving your meal onto a dinner plate, which is typically ten to twelve inches in diameter, try using a side plate (about eight inches across). By automatically reducing the surface area available for food, you automatically reduce your calorie intake (after all, we don't want to start scooping mashed potato onto the tablecloth...). All the taste, no waste.

Same idea applies to swapping the dessert spoon for a teaspoon at dessert time. More time to savor the flavor.

Eat From a Plate

Just in case you thought I was going to accuse you of eating from the dog bowl, I'm not. But making a ground rule that you'll only eat from a plate or bowl will help to curb nibbling from packages, straightening cake edges, or picking at leftovers (see earlier in this chapter, "BLT," page 105). When you have portioned out your food onto the plate, put the package/serving bowl/container back into the cupboard/fridge/freezer/etc. and then sit down and dine like a (conscience-clear) queen.

Short-Circuit Binges

Hint: Mint

Everybody overeats sometimes. But thin-thinkers have tricks to help them cut short a binge. For example, try brushing your teeth. The toothpaste (or any strong mint flavor) breaks the stranglehold that high-calorie snacks might have on those tastebuds.

Handy Activity

Another tip is to adopt an activity, such as knitting or painting, that can't be done while you are eating. After ten minutes of distraction, you stand to dissipate those cravings more effectively than looking longingly at the cookie jar for the same ten minutes.

Procrastin-eat

When you feel the urge to grab at those leftover chocolates, pause and ask yourself these two simple questions: Am I really hungry? Can I wait until my next meal to eat?

If the answers are a loud "Yes!" and "No!" help yourself to something quick and nutritious first, before pouncing on the goodies. But if your answer is, "Well, maybe," take five and drink a glass of water, read a magazine, go for a walk, or make a phone call.

With any luck, you'll be distracted enough that — if you weren't hungry — you'll forget about bingeing.

How To Eat

Although you might think that you learned this within minutes of being born, let's take a quick refresher course (after all, it was a while ago…).

🍽 Eat slowly.

It takes twenty minutes for your brain to register the fact that your stomach is full. And by that time, the stomach has been overloaded and stretched past its happy limit. This means we need to take our time while eating to recognize when we've had enough.

Try putting your knife and fork down every so often and give the person you are talking to your full attention.

Try taking sips of water in between bites. Only "allow" yourself to arrange the food on the fork for the next bite after you have finished chewing and swallowing what's in your mouth.

Take the time to chew the food properly. Remember, there are digestive enzymes present in the saliva. Therefore, the more you can help to break the food down before dispatching it to the stomach, the kinder you will be to your digestive system.

These aids to help you slow down will enable you to recognize more easily when you are full.

🍽 Concentr-eat When You Eat.

Give food your full attention. If you sit nibbling while shmoozing on the phone, you're likely to eat, and eat, and…right until the end of the call (if it ever ends, that is). Do yourself, your meal, and your enjoyment of the food a favor; only eat when you know that you are eating. And then enjoy the experience by concentrating on what you are eating — i.e., its tastes, textures, smells, etc.

🍽 Redefine the Word "Meal."

Most of us grew up thinking a meal means meat, potatoes, vegetables, and dessert — more than many adults need. So try out some dinnertime sittings of just a bowl of vegetable soup with a crusty roll, or a chicken and salad sandwich. The change from routine might also perk you up (and move your weight down).

🍽 Don't Wait Until You're Ravenous Before You Eat.

If you wait too long (by skipping or skimping on meals), it'll be excess hunger, not dieting resolve, that leads the way to overeating. Eating small amounts regularly throughout the day will ensure that you are never either too hungry or too full. Bear in mind that it's the overall number of calories that counts, not how often you eat.

🍽 Tune in to How Your Body Feels.

Instead of piling the plate high with all those yummy foods (even if they *are* permitted), try piling it only half-high and take your hunger and fullness clues from your body. Actively concentrate on how hungry you are feeling (rate yourself on a 1–10 scale) and only then decide whether you *need* to take more food or not.

🍽 Don't Eat from Jumbo/Giant/Economy Size Containers.

There's eating from a single, individually wrapped ice cream cone, and then there's sitting in front of a half gallon tub of ice cream, spoon in hand, poised and ready for action. No points for guessing who's going to consume more. Go for controlled portion sizing. That way you'll know what you've had, plus, there's less temptation to overeat.

🍽️ Practice Feeling Full.

As with any skill, this might take time and practice. If you follow the above tips (eating slowly, etc.) you will become more in tune with your body's sensations of natural satiety. When you feel that fullness — stop. Yes, really. Just stop. Sometimes we don't even consider the obvious. If you are full, your body is telling you that you have had enough and you should stop. Try it out a few times. It'll become easier as you go along. (See "Listen to Your Body," page 177).

All these tips are a help-yourself smorgasbord in Diet Land. But we don't live in a vacuum (it's too dusty in there anyway). We are surrounded by friends, family, relatives, neighbors…in short, people. These people can help us in so many ways. Sometimes all it takes is to ask. Let's look at a few different ways that people can be one of our strongest dieting assets.

Chapter 5

———— ◆ ◆ ◆ ————

Enlisting External Support

*A*lthough you may well argue that *you* are doing all the hard work, not your husband, friend, or Auntie Ruthie, they and others like them are still possible sources of encouragement. And in this game, a little encouragement goes a long way.

In this chapter we will discuss the different categories of people who can support your dieting enterprise, and what kind of support to expect from each. We'll even talk about the stumbling blocks such "supportive" people can put up to impede your path in Diet Land, and how to avoid those stumbling blocks.

Why Do I Need Support?

Most of us are not born with an intense, lifelong supply of willpower. To accept ourselves as the sole generators of our own motivation is to under-utilize the power of the influence of others.

Let's put this into context. What does the project of dieting entail? Dieting is not a two-minute job waiting to be checked off the "To Do" list. It is relevant on a constant basis (i.e., not just between the hours of 9am — 5pm, but rather all day and, dare I say it, all night as well). It requires planning, preparation, focus, motivation, willpower, etc. Is it possible? Yes. But it makes the ride far more enjoyable (and successful) if we take advantage of all the positive sources of support available to us.

By the end of this chapter, you won't feel like you're dieting alone anymore.

Here's a list of reasons why getting support might be the best idea you've had all day:

✔ As the process of dieting may be new to you, you may feel strange and over-whelmed by the new information and skills required. (Contrary to popular belief, dieting isn't just about the body. It's about the mind too). Whenever we embark on a new project, it is always advantageous to enlist advice and help from others. This type of help clarifies issues and makes your goal more attainable.

✔ External support can remind you of your goal, which can help you to stay focused when other issues threaten to overwhelm you. ("Would you like one of those crunchy apples instead of that spoon of ice cream perched by your lips?")

✔ External support can offer you empathy (and tea) with lots of "Ahh"'s and "Ohhh"'s in all the right places. This will make you feel better and give you the emotional strength to continue.

✔ External support can be a source of encouragement and motivation when the going gets tough.

✔ External support can make your project easier to execute practically. (A friend can babysit your toddler while you go to your Weight Loss Group).

With all these advantages, maybe the question should read: Why *not* get support?!

Why Do I Need To Know What Type of Support I Can Get From Each Group?

Just like it's useless to go to a bookstore for Shnocky's pink frilly socks (to match the pink frilly dress), it's useless to ask for nutritional information from a diet-ignorant, already overwhelmed husband, or for emotional empathy from your skinny-from-birth sister who doesn't even know how to spell "calories," let alone wage war with them.

Knowing who can provide which type of support, will reduce that killer of all good intentions — frustration. By reducing your levels of frustration, you are creating the optimum conditions for success.

Why Do I Need To Know What Stumbling Blocks I Might Encounter?

Although as a rule I try to steer clear of any black, ugly, aggressive negativity, some-times positive can come from the negative.

Knowing what obstacles I might encounter within the confines of each support system can go a long way in overcoming or avoiding them. As my grandmother always said: "An ounce of prevention is worth more than a pound of cure". And she was some clever lady.

In addition, when embarking on any new project it is essential to have realistic expectations of who can help for what and who won't help for beans.

Now that we've got that all taken care of, let's analyze each system of support.

What Types of Support Are There?

Although you might be able to recruit support from an unexpected or unusual source, you should generally try to get support from the following groups (and ideally from all of them):

- Nearest and Dearest;
- A Dieting Partner;
- A Weight Management Group;
- A Mentor.

■ Nearest and Dearest

Parents

☺ **Support Expected**

- A listening ear;
- Encouragement (no mother wants her daughter to suffer or experience ill health from being overweight);
- Advice (often when unasked for, but that's a mother for you);
- Practical help (if she's one of these super-moms, maybe she'll make a salad for you, or pick up some good quality fruit from a superior grocery store, or buy you the latest nutrition bible — and take the kids along for the ride. Can I have her number?);
- Emotional support ("You know I love you whatever size you are, but if this is important to you, I'm right behind you.");
- Financial help (earmark this one for Dad).

☹ **Potential Stumbling Blocks**

- Insults ("You've really let yourself go, haven't you?" I know, it even hurts to read.);
- Just because she tells you what to do, the rebellious teenager inside you may come out and resist her advice, come what may;
- Nagging ("Oh, you don't want to have that cake — remember, you're supposed to be on a diet, aren't you?");
- Pressure ("How did you do this week, darling?");
- Disinterest.

Advice

Talk It Through (Insults)

Although you can't control what your parents say to you, it might be wise to explain to them, right at the start of your program, what you are doing, how you plan to succeed, why this is important to you, what support you would appreciate from them (i.e., a listening ear, encouragement, advice when asked for, etc.), and even what things you don't want to hear (i.e., no insults, no nagging, no pressure, etc.). The more specific you can be in this regard, the better. If you are not the type to speak your mind, you could always photocopy this section and pop it in their coat pockets when they're not looking, or leave the book open, strategically placed under their coffee cups — as subtle as a brick through glass.

Knowing When Not to Talk About It

Alternatively, if you lack supportive parents or are afraid they'll be too intrusive, it's probably better to keep quiet and avoid the whole subject altogether. Sometimes, in this case, it can help to get one parent on your side and have that one explain it all to the other parent (i.e., "Let's not criticize her but rather let's make an effort to only say positive things"). We are looking for support here, not confrontation.

Friends as Sounding Boards (Rebellious Teenager)

If you find yourself acting like a rebellious, pouting teenager and rejecting any advice your parents give you, don't be too hasty in casting their words into the garbage can — rehash their advice with an objective friend and then make a rational decision on whether this advice will/won't work for you. Don't worry, your friend won't think badly of you — she was also a teenager once upon a time. And if you do end up taking their advice, you can always tell yourself you are heeding the words of your friend (without lying). Emotions aside (I know, impossible), it might be a good idea to explain to mom and dad that their advice is wonderful, but you feel you can grow better from the opportunity of working things out yourself. Obviously this is better received when they haven't *just* offered their sagacious words of wisdom.

Nag, Nag, Nag, Nag… (Nagging)

Being prepared to be nagged will go a long way towards curbing your temptation to bite the nagger's head off with sharp 'n' spicy retorts. You know your nearest and dearest better than most people. If they are likely to be the nagging type, preempt them ("I'd appreciate it if you don't remind me I'm on a diet, I can cope better this way…"), and preempt yourself in case they slip ("Thanks for trying to help, but it's better for me if I choose what I'm eating myself").

Investing in Interest (Pressure)

If you are the type to buckle under the pressure of someone else's interest in what you are doing, pick and choose who you want to tell about your new venture. If they pass this screening and you really do want them to be interested (and show it), let them know under what circumstances you would like them to express it. For example, you could say something like, "If I come into the house on a Monday morning after weigh-in and I'm smiling, please ask me how I've done…if I come in frowning, please change the subject and find something nice to say to me…."

Mom's Cover-Up (Disinterest)

If mom shows disinterest, it may be a cover-up. She, herself, may be desperate to undergo a physical makeover, but she's too scared to even start. Try deliberately "forgetting" written, diet-related material in her house. Hearing advice from you may be too hard for her to swallow. If she really *is* disinterested, focus on your own enthusiasm and on its delivery. If you are excited about something, people like hearing about it, even if it's the boring stamp collection/how many times I woke in the night/what the dentist said varieties.

Kids

☺ **Support Expected**

- Sharing in your weekly success at the scales;
- Cheering you on (kids can make a great fan club);
- Reminding you not to nibble unawares (with derech eretz,[1] of course);
- Practical help (older daughter can make a fruit salad for you or babysit while you go to an exercise class).

☹ **Potential Stumbling Blocks**

- Chutzpah ("Mommy, you're not allowed to eat that!");
- Thoughtless insults ("Is there really any hope for you? — Aren't you just too fat?");
- Pressure ("Did you weigh yourself yet?");
- Jealousy ("Why are you always going out and leaving us?" or "You've always got time to make nice things for your own supper, but we just end up with soggy fries and stale bread!");
- Lack of confidence in you ("She's just on one of her diets again. By September we'll be back to normal.").

---

[1] Respect.

Advice

Kids Will Be Kids (Chutzpah)

Children sometimes lack the social graces of knowing when to say what to whom. Accept this fact first and then try to improve upon it.

"Put Yourself in My Place" (Insults)

Therefore, if you want to diminish those soul-crushing negative comments (chutzpah/insult: "Mommy, you're *so* fat!"), it is important to preempt the situation with an open, kids-put-yourself-in-my-place discussion. ("People are usually sensitive about their size, so it's always a good idea *not* to draw attention to their fatness or thinness. How do you feel when someone calls *you* a name?")

"I'll Manage Better if You…" (Pressure)

If you find their involvement too intrusive, try explaining that you like to take responsibility for your own diet, and that it helps you succeed if you are allowed to do this in your own time — just like they don't like to be nagged to do their schoolwork.

"You Are Important to Me…" (Jealousy)

Children are very prone to jealousy when it comes to their precious mommy. However, you can take the sting out of their tail by asking them for their opinion. ("What should I do? The doctor told me I had to lose weight, and going to Group helps me achieve this. Should I go to Group and increase my chances of losing weight, or stay at home and risk putting on more weight?") Reassure them that they are very important to you. Explain to them that you love them even if you have to go to a diet group one afternoon a week and won't be home to greet them from school that day.

Prove 'Em Wrong (Lack of Confidence in You)

Advice for their lack of confidence in you? Only this: Prove them wrong — go out and stick to that diet (say goodbye to yo-yo dieting). Show them you can do it. Yeah.

Best friends

 Support Expected

- Understanding ("Yes, that must be really hard…");
- Empathy ("Oh, you poor thing.");
- Support ("I've made a salad. Should I leave you some without the full-fat dressing?");
- Listening ear (No response required, she just has to be there.);
- Encouragement ("You can do it!");
- Practical Help ("Would you like me to drive you to Group?").

☹ Potential Stumbling Blocks

- No time for you ("Sorry, gotta run, I'm late!");

- Jealousy (They need to lose weight themselves but can't buckle down to it. They are jealous of you choosing to take control of your situation and your life.);

- (Unintentionally) sabotage your efforts ("C'mon, it's only a little piece, it won't hurt…!");

- Inconsiderate ("We all went out for pizza, but since you were on a diet, we didn't invite you.").

🔅 Advice

Ask Up Front (No Time for You)

As people these days lead very busy lives, it is safe to assume that most friends have schedules, appointments, and pressures to deal with on a daily basis. It is unrealistic to expect your best friend to *always* be available for you. An easy solution: Ask her up front, at the start of the conversation, if now is a good time for you to get something off your chest or have a shmooze[2]. It takes seconds to ask such a simple question and can save you much heartache and frustration. Bracing her in this way will also better prepare her for listening to you. Alternatively, find out *her* schedule and ask her when she has some spare time for you or, better yet, fix a weekly coffee break chat with her.

Juggling Jealousy (Jealousy)

If your friend is not supporting your diet, her attitude may indicate some deeper, as-yet-unresolved issues. Unless you are prepared to unearth a hornet's nest, maybe you should steer clear of seeking her support on this matter. Try other friends who have similar interests or who feel less threatened.

Mean Business (Sabotage)

Unless your friends realize that you mean business, they won't feel it is inappropriate to entice you to indulge. If you do mean business, tell them. Let them know how important this is to you and how hard you are controlling yourself in order to resist. Ask them not to make it even harder for you. If they are true friends, they'll understand and support you.

Asking for Explanations (Inconsiderate)

If you are hurting from their display of inconsideration — ask them why they didn't invite you (without the whine) and request that in the future you be included in their plans. Let them know that although you are on a diet, you are capable of facing the food-challenges of being socially active (and then you'll *have* to be capable).

---

[2] Conversation

Spouse

 Support Expected

- Emotional support ("I think you're great to take on this new project/diet");

- Encouragement ("You're doing *so* well!");

- Practical help ("I'll take the kids to school on Mondays so you can go to Group");

- Shared enthusiasm ("Wow, well done! That's fantastic!");

- Shared experience ("I care about the diet because you care about it");

- Financial incentives/rewards ("I'll buy you the new CD you want when you've lost ten pounds.");

- Support ("Of course you should spend the money to join a group/gym... you're worth it.").

 Potential Stumbling Blocks

- Offers solutions instead of empathy ("Maybe you should try a different diet" versus "Ah, yes, I realize how demoralizing it can be to stay the same weight after all that hard work.");

- Nagging ("Are you supposed to be having that?");

- Insults ("You're right, you do look fat in that outfit.");

- Insecurity ("If *I* think you look beautiful, then other men will too.");

- Financial ("We can't afford your gym membership.").

Advice

Ah...Men (Solutionizing)

Men are from Mars, women are from Venus. It sometimes really does feel like they come from a different planet. Understanding this will reduce your frustrations. A man will automatically offer solutions to any problem presented to him. This is the way he views himself as helping. If it's a solution you want, all well and good. If it's empathy you are looking for, you can either sit down for hours to explain the female/emotional perspective on life, or phone your fellow Venusian instead. Latter recommended — it's quicker. If you do find yourself getting frustrated by his inability to know when to offer his solutions versus empathy, understand that he is offering his solutions only in order to try to help you. Husbands really do care, they just have funny ways of showing it.

Logic: The Male Language (Nagging)

If your husband seems to be watching over your shoulder with conscience-style questioning ("Did you weigh that first?"), it is worthwhile explaining in clear, logical language (note: *not* exploding) why his interaction is not beneficial. He thinks he's helping, so let him — by letting him know how. Some people, however, like this type of help (maybe you actually did forget and appreciate the reminder). One woman's pleasure is another woman's poison.

Expect an Honest Answer (Insults)

If you don't want an *honest* answer to your question, don't ask your husband the question. This may sound unbelievably obvious, but just think — how many times have you asked your husband the following questions:

- "How do I look?"
- "Does this make me look old?"
- "Is this too tight?"
- "What should I wear?"
- "Can you see any wrinkles?"

Being a logical, answer-the-question-at-face-value type of guy, he may well give you an answer you did not expect (i.e., the truth). He is then surprised at your emotional outburst, which escalates into a…well, we'll close the door on that one. So steer clear of emotionally charged questions (unless you really *want* to hear that yes, you are looking fat, old, and wrinkled) and opt for the safe approach of silence instead.

Dress for Him (Insecurity)

When you succeed in losing weight, you will inevitably get compliments. You will look and feel healthy, radiant, and more attractive. All this extra attention may make your spouse feel unsettled. To counteract this, ensure that you make him feel that his opinion is important to you. Asking him which outfit he prefers (and being prepared for an honest answer) will make him feel that you are dressing in order to please him, which in fact, you are. If he expresses his preference for a particular outfit, take note of it. If he has a favorite color/style/etc., try to accommodate him when buying a new dress or suit. We all dress in order to look attractive to our husbands, so let him know this, loud and clear, in your selection of what you wear.

Financial Investments (Financial)

If money is an issue, try discussing how you view this to be a financially beneficial move (as well as a healthier move). After all, nosh is expensive; doctors' consultations and subsequent medication for weight-related conditions such as diabetes, high blood pressure, etc. are expensive; therapists are expensive, etc. Try to make him feel like he is getting a bargain: a healthier, happier, slimmer wife at a fraction of the cost of getting an unhealthy, miserable, fat one.

■ Let's Be Partners (A Dieting Partner)

What is a partner?

As supportive as our husband or best friend might be, let's face it, they don't usually share our enthusiasm for exactly what we have eaten since the last time we saw them. One of the most effective ways of avoiding such boring suppertime conversations is to find a diet partner. Ideally, she should be on the same diet, possibly attend the same Diet Group, and be (at least) as motivated as you to shed those unwanted pounds. If you are new to the delights of dieting, it's wise to choose a veteran-type partner who can give you free advice and show you the ropes.

Your partner can help you plan your day's menu, give you good ideas, share recipes, and lend her support. She will receive the same support from you. Your friendship will flourish, your husband won't be bored out of his mind at mealtimes, and you will edge ever nearer to your goal.

☺ **Support Expected**

- Listening;
- Empathy ("I know just how you feel.");
- Advice ("I tried this last week and it really worked.");
- Encouragement ("Of course you can do it! We're in this together — I'll help you.");
- Practical help ("How about sharing Shabbos salads this week?");
- Sharing and Caring (You lose, she claps; you gain, she commiserates.).

☹ **Potential Stumbling Blocks**

- Unhealthy competition ("I beat you this week!");
- Jealousy ("It's not fair! How come you lost and I gained two pounds this week?!");
- Unbalanced partnership (You give, she takes.).

Advice

You Win, I Win (Competition/Jealousy)

If you see that your partner's sense of competition is more acute than yours and you want to bop it on the head before it turns ugly, try suggesting that whoever loses the most weight that week treats the other to a snack-size treat or muffin. This way the "loser" becomes a "winner" too, and the negativity of unhealthy competition is diminished. This will also work to diminish potential jealousy.

Taking Turns (Unbalanced partnership)

In the event of being the goody-two-shoes in a partnership, where you are doing all the recipe sharing and menu-planning, try taking it in turns each week to be the supportive one. Some people need this type of structure and responsibility in order to shine. This way the guidelines are defined and are therefore easier for your partner to fulfill.

■ Troop To Group (Going To a Weight Management Group)

What is a group?

Your average Weight Loss Group takes place on a weekly basis, at the same time each week. The first half hour or so is usually spent weighing-in and sitting around chatting to like-minded people. The Group leader then gives a short talk on a variety of different topics pertaining to weight-loss: techniques, motivating factors, health issues, troublesome areas, etc.

Either before her talk or after it, she will usually praise those people who have done well that week or take recalcitrant souls to task. She then analyzes why they lost or gained and suggests advice to counteract any problems. This is an excellent opportunity for people in the same situation to benefit from her advice, even if they are shy or too embarrassed to ask questions. There is also an inherent motivation-boost from realizing that other people have the same problems that you have.

She may also bring certain food products or tips to the group's attention, and give out awards at certain milestones. The session can last anywhere from one to two hours (find out how long it lasts before you step inside), and is attended by, between ten to fifty people.

Why Group Support Works

✔ **The weekly weigh-in provides an accurate monitoring.**
There's no room for excuses: "The scale's batteries are low." There's no body-gyrobics-balancing act of leaning excessively to the left to render a lower reading (been there, done that). The scale is accurate. It's the same scale each week. Basically, the reading is indisputable (so you can leave the boxing gloves at home).

✔ **Someone else is monitoring you.**

Just having someone else witness the weekly weigh-in and keep an eye on you in general can serve as a powerful motivating factor.

✔ **The people in the Group lend their support.**

All the people who go to a Group are there for the same reason. Just being surrounded by people whose focus is the same as yours has a powerful, almost osmotic effect in motivating you. If they are motivated, you will be motivated. And since their goal is the same as yours, together, you can share worries and concerns, tips, recipes, failures, and successes. Feeling part of a larger unit reduces the feelings of isolation — it's not you against the world.

✔ **The Group leader is trained to help you.**

The Group leader is usually someone who has lost weight herself and has successfully kept it off. She is, therefore, a living role model of someone who has succeeded. This inspires you to succeed. She knows the diet like the back of her hand, can answer practical questions about the diet, and can offer suggestions to make the diet more enjoyable. She understands, commiserates, and empathizes in all the right places. If you have a good Group leader, you'll want to take her home with you for good.

✔ **An additional side benefit of going to a Group is that it helps you maintain a focus on yourself.**

We do so much for so many that sometimes it is difficult to take time to focus on ourselves. One of the benefits of going to a Group instead of "going it alone" is that you will feel psychologically pampered. This makes for happy wives, mothers, seminary, or ex-seminary girls. The happier you are, the more chance of success. The more successful you are, the happier you become. (Are we talking in circles?)

An additional word or two about groups is in order.

✔ **Groups convene at the same time each week (come rain, sun, or snow).**

This includes erev[3] Yom Tov and motzei[4] Yom Tov. Both of these are times when you might feel least like turning up, but would benefit greatly by going. They are reliable and formal. Therefore, you can make your arrangements (babysitting, etc.) accordingly.

✔ **Not all groups allow admittance of children.**

It's wise to check this out before arriving at the door with your screaming toddler in tow only to be told goodbye before you've even said hello. Although it may seem inconvenient to be unable to bring Shnocky with you, you (and everyone else there) will be able to concentrate on the lecture and gain the most from the group if you are not distracted by nudging, noises, or diapers.

---

[3] The day before.
[4] The day after.

Support Expected

- Accurate monitoring;
- Group support;
- Leader's advice and inspiration.

Potential Stumbling Blocks

- Regular commitment;
- Embarrassment in front of others;
- Financial;
- Dislike of Group participants or leader.

Advice

Reassess Your Time of Stress (Regular commitment)

If commitment makes you ballistic, maybe now is not the right time to embark on this project. Stressful times are not conducive to subjecting oneself to extra commitments. Therefore, get the calendar out and see how many celebrations/appointments you have on the horizon. Also, if you have just had a baby and can't imagine finding the time to undertake such a commitment, maybe you should give yourself a few weeks and then reconsider when things have calmed down (do they ever?). (See "Avoiding False Starts" page 54.)

If it's a question of a commitment-aversion-by-nature, maybe you could get together for a weigh-in with a few friends and enjoy the loose structure. Either way, if you are going to take this program seriously, you have to face the fact that you are going to have to be monitored somehow, sometime, someplace.

Go Private (Embarrassment)

If the thought of a cheering crowd or a booing audience (they don't really do that) sends shivers up your spine, maybe you could enlist the help of a weight consultant privately.[5] This way you get the advice, tips, and general support without the frills. (However, you will miss the extra support that a Group provides).

Paying Up (Financial)

Groups do cost money. (You usually have to pay a weekly fee — whether or not you attend every week; i.e., you pay double the following week.) The benefit of this is that you feel that you have invested (literally) in your ability to lose weight. You will want to make your investment worthwhile and you will therefore be more inspired to work hard to achieve your goal. Paying also makes your commitment to the program more concrete. You will feel it's a waste of money to gain weight. If coughing up the money each week seems

---

[5] See "Find a Mentor," page 136.

off-putting, try calculating how much money you will be saving on nosh while on such a weight-loss plan. Or, think of the money spent as a preventative measure — spending it now prevents ill health, instead of later supplying doctors with a bank balance that will take them comfortably around the world via the Bahamas.

Shop Around (Dislike of Group participants/leader)

If the people or leader in the Group are not to your liking, don't throw the baby out with the bath water and give up on your goal. That particular Group may not have clicked with you, but maybe another one will. Shop around — ask the leader if you can sit in on a session first before you commit yourself. Or ask a friend to take you along as her visitor. Most Groups allow a guest. However you do it, just make sure you do it, because Diet Groups have a proven track record of success — why pass up such a golden opportunity?

■ Find a Mentor

What is a Mentor?

The dictionary defines a mentor as a wise advisor, a trusted teacher and counselor. Avi Shulman[6] maintains that "a more complete meaning would be someone who *was* where you are, is where you would like to be, and is willing to help you get there."

If you go to a Group, your mentor will be your Group leader. If you can't manage to go to a Group, it is worth your while to try to find someone who can be your mentor to help you navigate the sea of overwhelmingness.

Ideally, your mentor should be:

✔ Someone who knows more about dieting, health matters, and weight loss than you;

✔ Someone who has also struggled with a weight problem and succeeded;

✔ Someone who has time to give you advice.

Even if your chosen mentor/wonder woman is not a Group leader, or is not used to giving advice, or is not formally involved in health issues, or is a combination of all three, it is still very worth your while to speak to her on a regular, preferably weekly, basis. Interview her; ask her questions about her own struggle, how she overcame obstacles, how she now maintains her weight, etc. Chances are she will feel flattered by your attention and you will come away with a healthy injection of motivation each week.

There aren't many Olympic gold medalists who won their medals without a coach. They needed the direction, clarity of vision, experience, understanding, and motivation that a coach can give. Do yourself a favor and find a coach so that you, too, can win your own personal gold medal.

---

[6] *Lifelines*, 1998.

To Summarize

✔ The benefits of enlisting external support are immeasurable.

✔ Being realistic in what to expect from each support system will reduce your frustration.

✔ Understanding what stumbling blocks you may encounter can help you overcome them.

If you'd be the general in charge of a team of soldiers involved in an all-important, world-saving mission, you'd try your hardest to pick the best kind of soldier. The mission depends as much upon you, the general, as it does the soldiers you have at your service. So, too, with your Battle of the Bulge: picking the right troops, whether it's enrolling mom but leaving out dad, or educating your kids how best to support you, is going to set you up for your very best chance at what you truly want — ultimate victory.

Chapter 6

————— ◆ ◆ ◆ —————

Friday a.k.a.
Erev Shabbos

*D*ieting is not a 9am to 5pm job. It's a 24/7 consciousness. If we adopt the mentality that we are only going to be vigilant Sunday through Thursday, we're reducing our total dieting potential by about a third (two days lost out of seven).

So when it comes to Shabbos and the natural break in routine, it's going to pay to stay focused. Let's look at how we can tackle each section of Shabbos.

Introduction

Devorah[1] would bemoan her weight loss at the scales every week. It was the same old story. Throughout the week she could pin on her angel's wings and follow her diet plan to the letter, then, on Shabbos…she threw caution (and her weight loss) to the winds. She realized she was sabotaging her own efforts and just couldn't seem to get herself out of her voracious (as opposed to "vicious") cycle.

She is not alone. So many women have complained to me that they manage beautifully all week with their toast and salad (there's a good idea for Monday's lunch) and baked potatoes and cottage cheese (Tuesday?), but when it comes to all that delicious challah and homemade ice cream, their resolve disappears as magically as it reappears on Sunday morning with promises of doing better the following week.

> *Erev Shabbos may be the busiest day of the week, but it doesn't mean your diet has to go out the window.*

———

[1] This name has been changed to protect privacy.

It doesn't take much to sabotage all the good work of Sunday through Thursday. Just a couple of days of over-and-above-the-allowance extras and we're either back to where we started, or (groan) pounds heavier.

Dieting over Shabbos is pivotal to our success. It can mean the make-or-break of our week's weight loss, and it can contribute to our feelings of frustration and disappointment, or to that awesome sense of accomplishment.

As we mentioned earlier, out of a potential twenty-four reasons why we eat, my Diet Group chose Shabbos as their Number One reason. So, if you fall into this category and are nodding away as you read this, know that you are not alone.

As you sit on your armchair thinking, "Oh no, she's going to tell me to eat nothing but carrot sticks and celery all of Shabbos!" rest assured that I'd never do such a wicked thing. Besides, it's not sound nutritional advice.

Shabbos is such a special day. It can create an oasis of calm and relaxation within a busy, frantic, and high-paced weekly framework. It is a day that is designed to be enjoyed. I want to help you enjoy it — without the pitfalls of frustration, broken diets, and increased pounds. I want you to achieve your goals of weight loss happily within a life that embraces Shabbos for the day of rejuvenation that it is.

Since Shabbos is such a cornerstone to our success, we have dedicated an entire chapter to it. However, in a dieter's world, Shabbos doesn't start with candle-lighting. It starts with erev Shabbos.

Erev Shabbos can either be a dieting disaster in itself, starting us on a fast downward spiral, or it can help minimize some of the potential stumbling blocks of Shabbos when it comes. So let's take a look at erev Shabbos before we tackle Shabbos.

Avoiding an Erev Shabbos Dieting Disaster

Busy Bee

Erev Shabbos's most characteristic feature lies in the huge amount of things to do within a short timespan. This makes for busy bee (should I be honest and call it *frantic*?) housewives. Don't know about you, but I think I am allergic to deadlines, especially ones that are non-negotiable. Just knowing we have a deadline kinda gets our backs up, our nerves strained, and our decibel levels higher.

And whenever that happens, our dieting guard is down. So, what can we do about potentially overeating because we are so busy?

Space Out

One of the best tips I learned the hard way was to create space for Friday. Instead of leaving things for the end of the week (even if it's a long summer Friday), build a block of "empty time" into your Friday schedule.

Practically speaking, this means doing all those annoying little errands on a different day; planning and shopping well in advance; not making appointments (dentist, doctor, chiropractor) for Friday; etc.

Creating this leeway in our busiest of days will not only enable us to handle any unforeseen event with equilibrium (Shnocky's muddy footsteps and an, "Oh no, I just washed the floor!"), but we may also choose to use this time to perform an extra task either in honor of Shabbos, or not. For example, we could try out our mother-in-law's recipe for a marble cake, or else we might find that this extra time is just what we need to sort through that messy cupboard.

The difference lies in the importance and urgency of the jobs to do. If our cupboard remains messy, we'll still have a great Shabbos. If, however, we haven't *cooked* for Shabbos…well, don't invite me over. Jobs that *have* to be done before Shabbos may well have to be done before Shabbos, but they don't *all* have to be done on *Friday* morning.

The jobs that we choose to do are not just more "things to do" on our list. If you have enough time, great, bake away. If your created space was filled with some minor calamity or suddenly remembered errand, you will be able to accommodate it calmly while executing all of the jobs still on your "To Do" list.

Of course, you can always choose to fill this slot with some shuteye (see later) or with a coffee while you finish off that book.

Look into the Future

You can put away the crystal ball, because all I am advocating is thinking things through way before you get to the stage of becoming Mrs. Highly-Vocal Stress Case.

Sunday is none too early to begin your preparations if you need to pace your workload. A job a day keeps stress at bay. Yes, there's a lot to do, but there's no reason why *everything* has to be left for erev Shabbos. Break it up. Make the ice cream (for the family, of course…) on Sunday, the Swiss Rolls on Monday, meringues on Tuesday, etc. One little job each day versus a mountain on Friday — take your pick.

Create Your Own Oasis

Doesn't that sound nice? Unfortunately, I'm not planning to take you to the Bahamas next week (do you want to take me?), but instead I am suggesting that you create your own oasis right inside your own house (I know, not quite as picturesque).

With all the rush and bustle of erev Shabbos it's easy to feel wound up. This one may not be for the faint-hearted, but it's a wonderful tip:

Try preparing your own lunch on a tray. Have everything ready and attractively laid out, complete with drinks and bentsher.[2] When there is a lull in the Shabbos preparations, take yourself out of bounds, go into an empty room for ten minutes, and have lunch. *Toute seule.* (That's French for "I vont to be alone.") Take a deep breath and enjoy being able to think again. If you have little children, enlist the support of hubby or a neighbor's big daughter. You're not asking for the world (or a cruise to the Bahamas), you're only asking to have lunch.

The benefits of relaxing in this way are multifold:

- This oasis will prevent you from getting more and more wound up;
- It will help you to actively "wind down" if you are wound up (feel like a clock yet?);
- It will refresh your perspective;
- It will re-energize you physically (you'll be eating properly instead of noshing on the go);
- It will recharge your physical, spiritual, and emotional batteries to enable you to face the rest of the day with a positive (we're talking batteries, remember?) attitude.

Try it and just see how it refreshes your nerves as well as your body.

Shuteye

Although shutting your eyes to the mess of strewn coats, Sedrah[3] quizzes, and mismatched shoes sounds like a great idea, it's not quite what I had in mind as a stress-reducer.

If the previous tip (of creating an idyllic "away-from-it-all oasis") was not for the faint-hearted, then this tip is for the very-not-faint-hearted.

Having a quick forty winks (or hundred) will take the edge off extreme exhaustion (and your temper), and will refresh you both physically and mentally. Please don't sue me for being impractical, but, tried and tested, I can testify to its benefits.

Accomplishing this might sound like a tall order, but I have spoken to people who use their Friday mornings (when the kids are in school) to peel back the sheets and taste the joys of slumber from within. This nap is especially effective if your littlest one still wakes you in the night.

Practically speaking, if you work or save Friday mornings for making Shabbos, you can still create a timeframe for clocking-off for an hour. It doesn't have to be in the morning. How about right after lunch, when everyone's been fed and watered? Or maybe early afternoon, before the tempo picks up? Or what about putting your feet up *after* you have lit the candles?

---

[2] Grace After Meals card.
[3] Weekly Torah portion.

If the children are home while you are trying to sleep, think about investing in a pair of earplugs to deaden the decibels.

Some people find it hard to allow themselves to relax. They jump from job to job, pushing themselves ever onward. Some don't even know they're doing it. Relaxing is a worthwhile investment. **Not only are you allowed to relax, but you'll also function better because you are taking care of yourself.**

Therefore, although it can be tempting to spontaneously whisk up another type of lukshen kugel[4] on erev Shabbos, we have to stay focused on exactly what we are creating.

Yes, we want a beautified Shabbos replete with tasty dishes; yes, we want the house to sparkle. But we also want *to enjoy the process* and keep our cool. Welcoming Shabbos in a truly centered, calm fashion can create new meaning to the phrase "day of rest."

More Chores for Less Work

Doing a job perfectly usually means doing it yourself — but not always. It is a worthwhile skill to learn how to develop the art of delegating. If you are going to go apoplectic if the job is not done to your own standards of perfection, then yep, add it to your own "To Do" list. If, however, it doesn't faze you if the napkins don't match, or if the shopping isn't put away with army-like precision, then utilize any and all hands on deck — large or small. Easy-peasy jobs like separating the laundry basket's darks and lights; tearing the perforations of the paper towel roll; returning a container to a neighbor; etc., can all be executed by a little child (who won't feel so little if he's allowed to help).

If you have children in the house (doesn't matter if they are your own or borrowed), encourage them to become involved in your Shabbos preparations too. They'll love it and will anticipate Shabbos even more. If your children have not yet arrived on the scene, or if they have flown the nest, "borrowing" children from a neighbor may be a two-fold blessing. Not only will you benefit from their help, but their mother will be better able to focus on her remaining brood and remaining jobs.

Because delegating comes easier to some than others, here are a few tips to ensure a "happy delegation."

✔ **Make the job age-appropriate**

It's no use asking your toddler to polish the silver or Daddy's shoes without expecting to pay the price of mess and spills. Try giving your little ones simple, tidying-up or sorting jobs. Five-year-old kids can do near-to-home errands or can supervise a younger child; seven-year-old kids can set the table (especially effective with a picture of a place-setting for them to "copy"); ten-year-olds can fold and put away laundry, etc.

Expecting too much of a child can result in a negative experience for both of you. Instead, give him a job he can handle easily and let him experience the sweet joys of success. Increase the level of difficulty gradually, allowing the child to dictate his own pace.

---

[4] Noodle-based dish.

✔ Pep Talks

Similar to the pre-football game motivation speech, a pep talk forges an atmosphere of cooperation, togetherness, and motivation. Try this:

"Kids, we're going to play a game called 'Teamwork.' I've got ten jobs on this list and I'm going to give each of you a job. This is your special job — do it to the very, very best of your ability. Any team members who need help may ask an older team member to help them. We're going to give this our best shot. Anyone who does the job properly and before the deadline gets a bonus. We're up against the clock. We've got to be finished in thirty minutes. This means if you see someone having a tough time, offer to help. We're in this together, team. I'm going to go through the list with each of you then it's 'Ready, steady, GO!'"

Want to join the team?

This pep talk is also the ideal time to specify any stickers/rewards/treats you might like to give them upon their jobs' completion. This prevents miscommunication ("That's not fair! I wanted to stay up for the whole meal instead!") and increases your workforce's desire to succeed both in their own job and as part of a team.

✔ Specify Exactly What You Want

If your five-year-old son has never tidied the toy closet before, he might think "clean up" means haphazardly inserting everything onto one shelf. You, however, meant that each toy should go into the right container. It is unrealistic to expect him to understand what you want ("Clean up the playroom") unless you explain it very clearly. State the obvious rather than give him vague instructions. ("All these train pieces go into this red box…all these jigsaws go into this yellow box…etc.")

Having a clear job description gives the child a sense of security — he knows what is expected of him and he thinks he can do it. Furthermore, he is motivated to do it because he knows it is within his ability.

It can be especially useful, particularly to a younger child, to physically demonstrate what you mean. ("See? I'm putting this book on the shelf with the spine facing me.") Not only will you end up with a more obliging helper, but you will greatly increase your chances of achieving your expected results (especially if he doesn't know what a "spine" is).

✔ Preempt any Difficulties

It is the responsibility of the delegator to ensure that his workers know what to do in case of difficulties. This is like offering the trapeze artist a safety net. Who should the helper go to with his questions or problems — you/older sibling/Daddy? Let's remember it is erev Shabbos, so maybe you would rather not be the person to answer everyone's questions as you stir the cholent. You can delegate this one too.

Preempting difficulties also means trying to imagine "what if" scenarios. This gives the helper direction. For example, "Please put this laundry away. If there's no room in your closet, put it in the hall closet; if there's no room there, try the spare room."

Alternatively, try getting your helper to come up with the answer himself. This will increase his sense of self-confidence. "When you go to put this laundry away and find your closet's full, what do you think you should do?" It will also help to create the ability to think for himself instead of always coming to you for direction.

✔ What Did I Say?

One of the most effective methods of ensuring that your message has been accurately received is to ask for a replay. After giving Shnocky his instructions, a question such as "Now you tell me, what are you going to do?" will enable you to see how fully he has (or hasn't) understood what is being asked of him. This is a great precursor to the job's execution because it can go a long way in helping to overcome both his and your frustration — and ending up with a job well done. Nip a miscommunication in the bud and the job's a breeze.

✔ Reporting Back

It is important for your helpers to know that they are required to inform you when they have finished their tasks. This is for a number of reasons:

- You will be able to affirm whether he has done the job or not — and whether it was done to your satisfaction. If he is not required to report back to you, you will presume that he has done his job — but maybe he hasn't.
- Your immediate positive response to his job is more powerful than a brief, "Thanks, son," hours after the job has been completed. (There's nothing like a child's face lighting up when they see your obvious pleasure at their success);
- You will know where he is holding, i.e., it doesn't take an hour to match up socks, so where *is* he? (Playing football, kicking his sister, waking up the baby…).
- Your helper will experience a sense of completion and satisfaction by reporting back to you. It makes him feel important and it makes him feel that his job is important. If you show that you care about his job, then he is more likely to care about his job too.

✔ Be Positive

However the job turns out, it's a wise policy to find the good in what he has done. That's because it builds the child versus breaking him, and also because we want to encourage him to help us another time. Let's say Shnocky set the table. He also scrunched all the napkins into the glasses so they look like shmattes[5], and the knives and forks are the wrong way around. Yes, I'll agree he may well need some guidance to further his career in table-setting, but we must make sure that our initial response is positive. Maybe something along the lines of: "Oh, how nice! You chose such lovely color napkins!" or, "You put the plates so neatly next to the knives — well done!" etc. It's always easy to criticize someone when he doesn't do the job the way we imagine it should be done. Taking the time and patience to find the positive in his efforts is an investment that will reap many dividends.

Hunger

If we really want to paint a picture of Mrs. Hassled on erev Shabbos, not only would we envisage her with a list of things to do longer than her daughter's Chinese Jumprope, but we'd also add a particularly effective stress-enhancer that's a sure-fire method to break the diets (and good character traits) of the most iron-willed. Hunger.

Imagine the scene. Somewhere after grating the potatoes for the kugel and getting it into the oven before it goes brown (she's got about fifty seconds), her two-year-old toddler decides to throw a tantrum for the fifth time that morning. Amidst flailing arms and loud, urgent vocalizations, the bottle of open oil goes flying across the newly washed kitchen floor. (I was going to use cocoa, but I think oil is worth more of a scream.) Maybe she is a born angel and might still keep her cool. But let's add that she hasn't had breakfast, and, whooaaa, now we've got the Wicked Witch of the West. Poor kid, let's not stick around to hear the rest…

Although I can't promise that she would coo patiently, lovingly, and calmly to her terror, I mean darling, maybe she (and her larynx) would have had an easier time if she'd only helped herself to a couple of Weetabix before clearing the brood's breakfast war-zone.

If we would have stuck around the scene, we would have witnessed Mrs. Witch flinging open fridge and freezer doors, raiding cupboards, and finishing off leftovers with wild abandon as she succumbed to her by-now-overwhelming hunger.

This takes us to our Number One tip to conquering hunger on an erev Shabbos:

Eat

This one is sooooo obvious I bet you didn't think of it. If you are hungry, that's your body's way of nagging you to pay attention and fill it up with gas before you get stranded on the highway. If you are hungry, it's healthy to eat.

---

[5] Worn-out rags.

"Breakfirst"

Having breakfast at the beginning of the day used to be quite fashionable. In this high-paced, fast-living generation, we are tempted to skip it to save time.

This trap is so easy to fall into. We prioritize everyone and everything else before ourselves. (Here I go repeating myself, here I go repeating myself, here….) After all, we justify, there's sooo much to do, I just *have* to keep going before I allow myself the *luxury* of eating. Maybe you don't feel so hungry yet. Maybe your tummy rumbled but you chose to ignore it. If you leave hunger to its own devices, it'll get even with you and will ensure that by the time you *do* listen to it, it'll overpower both you and your resolve.

Let's say you overslept and you wake up with that awful stomach-lurching sense of panic. All those jobs are waiting for you and now you've got even less time to do them. Add a few pressures and deadlines for work, for school, for buses, morning prayers, etc., and you have the beginnings of a treadmill workout set on maximum speed. Where are you heading? Onto the downward slope of overeating when you finally do manage to meet food face to face.

Do you begin the day the Bran Flake way?
"Who's got time?" you sharply say.

In Nechama Berg and Chaya Levine's book on time management, *It's About Time*, they list one of their most insightful tips to becoming better organized. If you've got lots to do, rest before you begin. This way, they argue, you will perform your tasks more efficiently. What they are getting at is: Look after yourself before you look after everything else. I want to add something (I always do…): If you've got lots to do, *eat* before you begin. You will function better and happier as you efficiently cross off each "To Do" on your list. You function better when energy stores are full.

Besides, if you let yourself go too long without food, your body's heightened sense of hunger will propel you towards whichever food is hanging around as your resolve stands by the side. Breakfasting first ensures at least a fighting chance at denying yourself free reign into that marble chiffon cake you just *had* to make before 11am.

Having breakfast at the start of the day is like laying the foundations for a big building. Once the foundations are laid, the building is secure. Once you have breakfast, your resolve is more steadfast. The pressures and demands of the day may well attempt to hack away at your determination, but when you are well-fueled, you will be better equipped to resist whatever temptation comes your way.

A Little Goes a Long Way

If you still feel that you haven't got time for toast and tea (bentshing also takes time, you say) or Shredded Wheat (Al Hemichya[6] can "cost" an extra minute…), eating small amounts (of Borei Nefashos[7] after-brochah[8] foods) can often help to keep the tyrant of hunger at bay.

After eating light foods frequently, some people function even better than after partaking in heavy one-time sittings. Even if this does not tempt you, know that eating often can help to keep blood glucose levels high. This means you could be feeling energetic and fresh versus lethargic and low.

On the Go

If you are still shaking your head and wishing I'd "get real" in my expectations of you on erev Shabbos, know that even if you are a non-stop jitterbug, never-sit-for-a-minute kind of woman, it's still possible to eat properly on the run.

Fruit is a great winner if you find yourself in non-stop gear. Fruits are hand-held, which means they allow the other hand to continue with the current job. (Boy, do we live in a non-stop society or what?!) They only require a short after-brochah and are jam-packed with nutritional goodness.

If you find that, due to unforeseen circumstances, emergencies pressing, and life in general, you have (shock, horror) skipped breakfast…all is not lost. Apart from your one-hand-hold on a succulent pear, an alternative hand-free solution is sipping a mug of hot soup — either way, you'll still be on track. Besides, by 11:30am you might crave something more savory 'cause it's nearly lunchtime.

If you work outside the home, consider having a ready supply of "Cup of Soup"-type snacks from which to choose, stored in your filing cabinet under "E" for emergency in the event of finding yourself truly pressed. Some brands are free or low-pointed on certain diets. Warning: some are not.

Oasis Revisited (For those who have more time)

Seeing as our oasis was so pleasant to visit the first time (see above), let's go back for a second trip.

Remember, you'll need your all-encompassing tray complete with perfectly laid out lunch, cutlery, bentsher, and chilled diet soda ("on the rocks," i.e., with ice — we're going to an oasis and it can get hot).

If you integrate this little "treat" into your erev Shabbos scenario on a regular basis, you will also be increasing the association of erev Shabbos with something pleasurable. You will be less likely to dread erev Shabbos because it won't be associated with overwhelming busyness and a heavy workload. It will become something to look forward to and enjoy. This can be a delightful mental precursor to the event of Shabbos itself.

---

[6] Blessing said after eating wheat-based foods.
[7] Short blessing said after eating some types of other food stuffs.
[8] After-blessing.

Last time we covered the reasons why an oasis is a wonderful erev Shabbos stress-buster. Now we'll focus on why an oasis can also alleviate hunger and aid dieting.

☺ **Enjoy**

No one enjoys their food when they are only half aware of what they are eating, or are eating on the go. You will enjoy your food much more *and* be more aware of the fact that you are eating if you make a special point of getting away from it all.

☺ **Nutritious and Delicious**

If you are taking the time to rustle up a nutritious, cozy lunch for one, then you are going to ensure that your body gets the nourishment it needs and will therefore be better equipped to endure whatever demands/crises you place upon it.

☺ **Saying "No" to Nibbles**

When you have ensured that the chief chef, executive director-come-psychologist (you) has had a satisfying meal, you will find it so much easier to avoid those little nibbles on the go.

☺ **Gives You a Dieting "Booster"**

Each time you look after yourself by allowing yourself to have a proper, carefully balanced, attractive meal, you will find yourself less likely to stray from the dieting path. You are investing in yourself, so it seems such a waste to undo all that investment. And it is.

☺ **Center Yourself**

This oasis will create a haven of contemplation. If you have gone off the rails, it's not too late to get back on before Shabbos arrives. The peace and quiet will help you to center yourself.

OK, enough of the Bahamas, back to reality.

Tastes 'N' Testers

Everyone wants the food to taste delicious for Shabbos. It's such an integral part of creating its beauty. Besides, we want the peace of mind that comes when we can reassure ourselves that every dish is perfect. Now how on earth can we be expected to know if we put enough salt in the soup, if there's enough sugar in the cream, if the chocolate cake turned out *exactly* like mom's, if we don't taste it? Well, let's just say that there's tasting and there's…tasting.

The problem with those teeny-weeny tastes is that they are, by definition, usually eaten standing while hovering over the pot, baking tray, or foil container. They defy being placed on a plate, which would effectively give us the visual message that we are, in fact, eating. They insist on being performed in a pot-to-spoon-to-mouth style so we never get an accurate picture of what has just miraculously become invisible. If we can't see it, then it doesn't count. Right? Wrong. Here are some useful tips that can help you think twice before you dip in twice.

One-Time Tasting

Sure, go right ahead and taste the kugel. But if it does have enough salt, and it does taste like Bubbe's, then why are you having seconds and thirds? It's not quite a taste anymore, is it? Let's not make a taste into a mini meal. Once is usually enough.

Honestly…

If your tasting can potentially improve the quality of the dish you are preparing, then consider it well-justified. If there is nothing you can do to improve the lack of salt in the kugel, or the sogginess of the chocolate chip cookies, then, hmm…why exactly are you "tasting" it? Go on, be honest. Call it by its name. It's not a taste "l'kovod Shabbos Kodesh"[9] anymore, it's a real, true-to-life, sneaky little nibble — "honoring" yours truly.

Tasting When Hungry

What's going to happen to the apple pie if you are poised to taste it and you haven't eaten in over four hours? *Knowing* that yes, it really is delicious, isn't going to make it any easier to stop scooping your spoon ever nearer towards the pie's center.

Another reason to make sure you eat on erev Shabbos is that there's a lot of tasting to be done. Make sure your tasting and testing are done when you are not hungry.

Measured Pleasure

Measure the taste. If you know that you are unlikely to resist a full dessert-spoon taste of your favorite dish, use a teaspoon, or a measuring tablespoon. Let's know what we are doing. Tastes *do* count and are not invisible, even when they have been consumed. Note how visible they become when it's time to get on the scale again.

Find a Surrogate

Not a surrogate mother — a surrogate taster. I'm sure there'll be a line to try out that cake batter or to lick the spatula. If tasting your own good cooking is your particular downfall, leave it to someone else. They'll soon tell you if it's missing something and you'll be saving unnecessary calories. (Skinny husbands are good for this one.)

Discovering and Covering

To prevent a full blown shovel-full versus teaspoonful from disappearing down the hatch, try digging the teaspoon into the kugel, then covering the kugel with aluminium foil before you taste anything. This way you'll be less likely to dip in for seconds. As we are powerfully led astray by our eyes, if it's

---

[9] Literally translated: "In honor of the holy Shabbos."

all covered over, we will be less tempted. If it's still hot? Cover with a paper towel. It doesn't have to be airtight — just "eye-tight." It'll really have to need more salt/sugar/ketchup/whatever for you to have to "unveil" the temptation once again.

Budgeting Your Tastes

Every morsel that touches your lips has a price tag, especially those delicious for-Shabbos ones. Write down every taste test that you eat, lick, or bite. It's all calories and it all adds up. Knowing that you have to write it down can be enough of a deterrent to stop yourself from over-indulging. Try it out and see if you are surprised when you add them all up.

You might well feel that you have been especially "good" and that you have loads of points/treats/etc., to spend over Shabbos. One day's worth of tastes can easily equal all those extra points you were looking forward to spending. So, before you *do* go and spend them, make sure you still have some "money" in the bank.

Spit It Out

This one's for all those dieting die-hards who really mean business. Taking things quite literally, making a taste a taste, not a swallowed morsel, can knock hundreds of calories off an ever-increasing tally. And you won't even need to make a brochah.[10]

Lunchtime

If you've skipped the section where I harped on about the importance of having breakfast, it's not too late to hear me harp on about the importance of having lunch. If you are one of those whirlwind haven't-got-time-to-sit-for-a-minute types who frequently skips breakfast, then it becomes even more important to be fully prepared when it comes to lunchtime. That's because you'll be hungry by then and especially susceptible to lurking temptations.

The dangers of skipping lunch on a Friday are apparent in one client's Food Diary, which she shared with embarrassment. When she showed me (at the beginning of her "confession") that she had tucked into four big slices of challah as a kick-off into her Friday night meal, the first question I asked her, before she could get a word in edgeways, was, "What exactly did you have for lunch on Friday?" Sheepishly grinning, as if caught with her hand in the cookie jar, she admitted that she'd skipped lunch. When she had at last sat down to eat, her hunger had led the way. Her willpower didn't stand a chance.

Lunchtime is pivotal to maintaining a semblance of self-control. Because everyone is very involved with food at this point, it will be all over the place — counters, stove-top, table, etc. (under the table, in Shnocky's hair...). No matter where you turn it'll be there. If you are hungry and you didn't have time to prepare whole-wheat vegetable lasagna and salad, you'll be facing a lot of tempting nibbly-bits.

---

[10] Blessing (customarily recited before eating food), which is not needed when you don't swallow the food.

It's the time of day when everyone eats. And you should, too. It's a halfway-through-the-day pit stop. Just as breakfast is your kick-off into the morning, lunch is your kick-off into the afternoon. If you skip lunch, you are heading for a downward spiral in terms of energy, stamina, middos,[11] and dieting willpower. We need all of these so much more on erev Shabbos, so doesn't it make sense to make lunch a priority? It's all too easy to prepare food for the family, serve it, clear it, and forgo your own lunch amidst all the buzz. Don't. Either sit and eat *au famille* (they won't waste away if they have to wait for you to eat before they have seconds), or eat before you start serving.

Why don't I strongly promote the option of eating *after* the family? Because by then you are asking yourself to remain saint-like in resisting all those finger-licking french fries on an empty stomach. By the time you do serve yourself, it's quite likely that you'll actually have had generous pickings from their fare — a standard saboteur to the most nutritiously, low-caloried alternative lunch that you could ever prepare.

We're not focusing on the rest of the brood here. Although nutritionally they will benefit by having the same lunch as you, if necessary they'll survive quite nicely on pareve sausages and oven french fries. But Mom's another story…

What's for Lunch — for Mom?

It's no use to peer into the fridge at 1pm on a Friday to find only cream flans, pavlovas, and iced buns and then start thinking about what's for the dieter's lunch.

Below are some easy, healthy, low-calorie alternatives for a lunchtime menu. Don't feel restricted. If you've got more ideas than the ones I've listed, just add them to your selection.

Bread and Toast Fill You the Most

I'm so happy bread was invented. It can scratch the itch of so many different types of fancy. It can be sweet or savory; dense or light; white, whole-wheat, granary, raisin, spicy…you name it and someone will have made a loaf of it.

At approximately 80 calories per slice,[12] it can be a real dieter's delight. Obviously, you'll be increasing your fiber content if you choose the whole-wheat variety (as well as filling up for longer), but it is worth noting that a slice of white bread will cost you the same as whole-wheat bread in terms of calories.

Bread can be served straight from the plastic bag, or it can be toasted under the grill or popped into the toaster. It can also be made into those delicious edge-sealed triangle sandwich-machine toasties.

It's immediate (at worst it'll only take seconds either to defrost in the microwave or turn into toast); it's versatile (couldn't make supper?); it's wholesome (at least the whole-wheat versions are); and it's cheap.
Let's look at a few ways to capitalize on such a great find.

---

[11] Good character traits.
[12] 80 calories refers to boughtbread, not homemade, and weighs approximately 1oz.

On Top of the World

🍽 Don't know what to put on top of your bread? How about choosing from a selection of low-fat cheeses? Complete the open-faced sandwich with thinly sliced tomatoes, and you have an immediate meal prepared in seconds.

🍽 If you want a quick, nutritious for-the-family-too lunchtime meal, try rustling up an omelette or scrambled eggs. Use spray oil on the frying pan, add sliced onions, mushrooms, sliced tomatoes, and peppers (any or all) and, when they are golden brown, add your eggs. Adding veggies in this way helps to create a visually greater bulk of food for almost the same price in terms of calories. Cooking eggs this way will also warm you up if you are facing the winter chill.

🍽 Eggs can be cooked in many different ways. How about trying poached eggs on toast or soft boiled with "soldiers" (toast that's cut into finger-like strips); you dunk his head into the yolk and he's supposed to look like a soldier. OK, maybe he doesn't, but the kids'll love the dunking anyway.

🍽 How about borrowing one from the Brits, and spread marmite on your bread/toast? It's a tasty yeast extract, rich in B vitamins. Remember, it's a definite love-it or hate-it taste that English kids are raised on, so don't be surprised if you only score a fifty-percent success rate with the gang at lunchtime.

🍽 Craving something sweet? How about trying one of those reduced-sugar jam lookalikes? Reduced sugar means reduced calories, and you still get to stay friends with your sweet tooth.

🍽 Tip: Making an open sandwich (filling/spread on top of two flat slices of bread) can be more filling than a closed sandwich. Try spreading whatever you are having onto the bread, and layering cucumbers, lettuce, tomatoes, etc., on top. It'll look like you are having twice as much food as a closed sandwich. Maybe it'll feel like it too.

Warning: If you are using a high-calorie filler (smoked salmon/halibut spread/mayonnaise, etc.) you could end up using twice as much with an open sandwich (two slices spread with it, versus one). Therefore, you may want to choose a closed one, spreading only one side with the lick-a-licious luxury.

🍽 Not wanting to repeat myself too much, you can flip to "Sandwiches," page 226, for more exciting ideas on how to best utilize bread and the sandwich experience.

Inside Information

Got a sandwich toaster? Great for the winter. How about the following for fillers:

🍽 Spray oil the opened sandwich maker, pop in the bread, and scoop a few generous spoons of baked beans inside. If you want to make it really scrumptious, add reduced-fat cheddar cheese for the stringy, elastic-y extra special flavor.

🍽 If your frying pan is sitting on the counter all forlorn and unused, why not stir-fry, with spray oil, your onions, mushrooms, and garlic and scoop them into the sandwich? This way you only have to "pay" for the bread — the onions, etc., are free.

🍽 Old standard cheese and tomatoes (with or without tomato sauce/spices) is a real winner. Sandwich makers were created for these.

🍽 Apparently eggs are also yummy when cooked inside a sandwich maker. I've not (yet) tried them myself, so I take no responsibility for the results.

🍽 Although most people use their sandwich makers for dairy, you may be so enthusiastic about them that you want to get one for meat too. Spare chicken on erev Shabbos will come out great — you can even add some extra rice or ratatouille[13] with it for a completely satisfying whip-up. Works well for Shabbos leftovers too.

🍽 Basically you can put *anything* into a sandwich maker. Leftovers are given a new lease on life. Whereas the kids may have turned their noses up at a food presented earlier, they can easily tuck in when it is presented "incognito."

Cake of Rice Is Rather Nice

If you are still unpersuaded to dive into the bag of bread head first, maybe it's worth considering the versatile alternative of rice cakes.

Apart from offering many of the same lunchtime varieties (you can make them sweet or savory, add an egg, a salad, etc.) they can offer three advantages over bread:

✔ Because they are big, they give our brains the signal that we are eating a lot of food and we should therefore feel full afterwards (even though a lot of it is air — don't tell your brain this);

✔ If you don't have time to wash and bentsh, they offer a quick after-brochah alternative;

✔ If you are prone to eating on the go, dipping into a box of rice cakes can be a non-sticky, no heat required, immediate solution. (Just make sure you don't leave too many crumbs all over the car seat.)

---

[13] Eggplant, peppers, and onions vegetable mix.

Salads and Veggies, Salads and Veggies, and More Salads and Veggies

When you find yourself in the kitchen making salads and hot veggies for Shabbos, think ahead and make lots.

When it comes to those afternoon hunger pangs, you'll be able to dip into the bountiful supply that will be ready and prepared — just waiting for you. Not only can you eat them as a handy snack, but they can accompany you in your lunchtime oasis (see earlier).

Whether it's coleslaw (with light mayo), TCP[14] salad, string beans in tomato sauce, or garlic mushrooms, it pays to be generous in your quantities. Don't worry about making too much — Sundays were created for eating Shabbos leftovers.

While you've got the cutting board and knife out, why not make plenty of fresh fruit salad too? It's low-calorie and visually tempting. Besides, there's nothing like finding a huge bowl of juicy fruit chunks sitting in the fridge: Someone's already done all the hard work of peeling, de-pitting, and chopping for you. (Even if that someone *was* you.)

Here is a great timesaving tip for cutting up melon (it *is* erev Shabbos, after all): Cut a melon in half and scoop out the pits. Cut again into quarters. Holding one quarter in one hand and knife in the other, cut lines into the melon flesh — both horizontally and vertically — without cutting into the rind. Slice these "cubes" away by cutting flat-ways alongside the melon skin. Result: instant melon cubes.

Stand-by with a Soup Supply

Imagine it's chilly. You've got out all the sweaters, gloves, scarves, and hot water bottles, but you need to warm yourself up from the inside out as well as from the outside in. Hot soup is a great instant injection of wholesome warmth. Not to mention it's nutritious, (potentially) low-calorie, and assassinates hunger in its tracks.

During the week, when you turn your thoughts to making your favorite vegetable soup, make extra. Either liquidize and freeze a family-sized Tupperware container for Friday's lunch (you'll bring a smile to everyone's lips) or line your typical soup bowl with a plastic bag and fill it up till two thirds full. Knot the bag and freeze. This way, when you are in a hurry on Friday and haven't got time to make soup, you can just pull out your prepared plastic bag, pop it into a soup bowl, and microwave till piping hot. Three minutes and you're human again.

This tip is useful for whenever you find yourself making a soup, whether it's a split pea, lentil, mushroom and barley, or garden vegetable soup. You'll find you can select whichever kind you crave once you've built up a collection.

Even if you are not the organized type and can't seem to plan ahead so easily, all is not lost. There are quick 10-calorie soups available that will work as a dieter's aid just as effectively. Flick the electric kettle switch. Open the packet. Pour the contents into a cup and pour in the hot water. Stir with a

---

[14] Tomato, Cucumber, and Pepper.

spoon, or with the rear end of a pen if desperate. No stress, no time, and only one dirty cup (unless you use disposable and save yourself an extra ten seconds by the sink).

Alternatively, if you don't mind becoming fleishig and skipping the dairy coffees, you can dip into the chicken soup you made for Shabbos. Chicken soup is especially effective as a hunger reducer if you leave in some "free" veggies. See "More Please," page 163.

See also "Slurp Soup," page 93.

Lots of Pots

No, I'm not trying to create more pots and pans for you to scrub before Shabbos. I'm talking about potatoes. Baked potatoes — with soft, steaming flesh inside crispy, crunchy skins, to be specific.

By the time you've cleared up breakfast, made the beds, davened, had breakfast, and done two jobs on the "To Do" list, it's probably somewhere near 11am — the perfect time to pop a raw potato or ten into the oven. No peeling required. Just scrub, pierce with a sharp knife, place on a baking pan, and let the oven warm up the whole house — takes the chill off in winter and makes sure the air conditioner is working properly in summer.

This is such an easy Friday lunch it's worth considering it for a family lunch. Whatever you would normally put on bread can be easily transferred to baked potatoes. Think laterally and experiment — what's wrong with your five-year-old having peanut butter on a potato? There are restaurants that sell only baked potatoes with every filling imaginable. Try baked beans inside, or coleslaw, or the garlic mushrooms you just made for Shabbos. What about light mayonnaise, yogurt, or cottage cheese?

Apart from being a stress-free, zero preparation, easy, delicious meal, baked potatoes are high in fiber (that's good[15]) and are hot and filling. This means that in winter, you'll be getting warm at the same time.

Make a Meal of Cereal

Seeing as Friday lunchtime is not the time to start experimenting with the latest Cordon Bleu cookbook, if you find yourself at a loss as to what to eat, you can always reach for the cereal box. It's easy, convenient, cheap, and nutritious (we're talking Shredded Wheat, Fruit 'n Fiber, Bran Flakes, and Weetabix here, not certain nutritionally defunct rice and corn cereals which shall remain nameless).

Add some cut-up fruit for variety (bananas work well), or try pouring yogurt over the top instead of milk.

To really warm you up from the inside out (can you tell I live in England?), try making your cereal hot. Pouring warm milk or hot water onto porridge, oatmeal, or muesli can provide you with a welcome, filling, heat-permeating sensation.

Some people have fruit for breakfast and cereal for a meal later on in the day. Experiment, be creative, and see what works best for you.

---

[15] See "Appendix 5: Fiber".

Pasta's Faster

Considering that Fridays can become very busy, especially during the winter months (let's blame the clocks instead of our inefficiency), Thursday is none too early to start preparing and thinking ahead.

Making yourself an extra portion of pasta, low-fat tomato sauce, oregano (optional), and light cheese (also optional) for Thursday's lunch or supper may cut your workload in half when it's time for lunch on Friday.

Just open the fridge door on Friday at one.
There's a meal ready and waiting; all the hard work's been done.

Fishy Dishy

If you are already making fresh salmon, trout, or carp, etc., for an hors d'oeuvre for Shabbos, how about making an extra portion for Friday and serving it as a meal in itself, with some of those plentiful salads and veggies? You can always add a jacket potato to this (see above) to make your meal even more filling.

If you want to keep your fish "special for Shabbos," you can serve some of the fish "plain" on Friday, and make the rest extra special for Shabbos by whisking up a quick low-fat sauce.

When winter comes, it's more important than ever to capitalize on the healthy, invigorating fill-up called lunch on erev Shabbos. Because the afternoon is so much shorter, chances are you'll be running around doing last minute jobs right till candle-lighting time. Making sure you have "gas" in your "tank" will go a long way in helping you execute these jobs efficiently and, perhaps more importantly, happily as well.

There you have it: written permission encouraging you to eat. (Whoever said dieting was about *not* eating?!)

Erev Shabbos: Avoiding a Shabbos Dieting Disaster

So far we have looked at the first element of facing erev Shabbos, namely, how to prevent a dieting disaster on erev Shabbos itself. Now we are going to take a closer look at how erev Shabbos can be utilized to help us make Shabbos itself "diet-proof."

Be Prepared

Unfortunately, even those people who approach Shabbos with a high dose of resolve and resolution are not guaranteed to succeed. Why? Why is it not enough to be mentally "psyched" when facing the crunch?

Imagine Shnocky has a spelling test on Friday. Is it realistic to expect him to get high marks without studying for his test? Despite all the will in the world, his chances are low (unless, of course, he's naturally brilliant). He needs to prepare in order to actively boost his chances of success. So, too, in the world of dieting; preparation is crucial when facing a challenging situation. Unrealistic expectations ("Oh, I really hope I lose this week…") without the backup of being prepared leads to repeated failures and ultimate despondency. That's the bad news.

The good news is that there is something you can do to increase your chances of success. It helps to imagine that the amount of preparation (be it physical or mental) will directly correlate to your chances of Shabbos-mastery.

It doesn't always need to take hours of your time. It doesn't always need to cost the earth. It needs a mindset and a channelling of those vague desires into a plan of action.

So what can you do to prepare yourself practically? I'm glad you asked, because below are some tips that just might come in handy.

Alternative "Healthyotherapy"

We'll get down to the menus in a moment or ten. For now, we have to consider that while we are sometimes going to make the family all those favorite high-calorie dishes, we also have to make ourselves suitable alternatives. Although you don't have to be a gourmet cook to rustle up healthier alternatives that are tasty and low-fat, they may still need some time.

We're not talking about anything major here, just one or two dishes that you are making especially with yourself in mind because they are more healthful. (But you'd better make a decent-sized portion for the jealous munchkin who's bound to eye your plate at the table.)

Of course, you can always save yourself time and give the whole family a healthier menu. This way you get to reduce your workload *and* gloat about what a good mother/wife/hostess you are by looking after everyone's health (and waistline).

Thinking of You

Even if you haven't got the time or the inclination to get the food processor out especially for yourself, it's absolutely crucial to put a little time into thinking about what you are planning to eat at the Shabbos table.

Don't expect to resist all those yummy foods when there is nothing else on the table and you are at maximum hunger-level, having lit the candles hooooouuuuuuurs ago, as your stomach will loudly testify. The angels may well be accompanying your husband home to make Kiddush but they won't find any fellow angels sitting around the table past hamotzi.

So, think it through.

- Planning to make coleslaw?
  Have you got light mayonnaise in the house?
- Making apple compote for dessert to go with the ice cream? Have you got an artificial sweetener at hand for your own portion?
- Making kugel?
  How about reducing the amount of oil from your regular recipe and making your own alternative in a separate foil container?

It doesn't have to take extra time, only extra brain power (and you've got loads of that).

Automatic Pilot

Before Shabbos, write down what you are planning to eat *on* Shabbos to increase your chances of success. Why? Because making on-the-spot, under pressure, continuous decisions is much harder than cruising your way through the storm on automatic pilot. It just makes the journey a whole lot more enjoyable.

It doesn't take long to take out a pen and scribble your menu on Shnocky's Sedra quiz from last week just before the gang walks through the front door for lunch. It's a two-minute investment that reaps dividends many times over.

Although you can't read such a list on Shabbos,[16] you still stand to benefit from writing it. Writing the menu will put exactly what you are planning to have into your head, versus the vague sense of, "I hope I'll be careful."

It will also provide an excellent checklist for after Shabbos. Just tick off all those goodies you just knew you wouldn't be able to resist and had planned for accordingly, and then remember to add all those extras that snuck their way in, too. This way, you'll have a more accurate picture of how many treats/points/calories you either saved, canceled out, or overdid.

Save Up

In order to truly maximize your eventual enjoyment of Shabbos, not only is it important to know what you *are* having erev Shabbos, but it is just as important to know what you are *not* having.

We know for a fact that the Friday night seudah is coming up. We also know that our Shabbos meals have more courses, heavier courses, and more time in between courses than during the week. Because we want to enjoy our Shabbos, it's worth saving up calories on erev Shabbos and the week preceding Shabbos, so that you can spend them on Shabbos itself.

On Shabbos, we are more relaxed and able to fully enjoy all the dividends of our culinary labors. Why not take advantage of this potential enjoyment and save all those unnecessary erev Shabbos nibbles for a more fully savored experience at the Shabbos table?

Just as our Sages teach us to save that special Shehechiyanu[17]/fruit/dish/purchase for Shabbos to increase the honor of Shabbos, you can save up calories for Shabbos to increase your enjoyment of this unique day.

Saving up doesn't only have to be done on Friday. With Shabbos in mind (we know it's coming every week), you can minimize your intake throughout the week in order to take advantage of the increased sense of pleasure that culminates in your Shabbos experience.

---

[16] Although it is forbidden to read such a list on Shabbos, your local Orthodox rabbi may be able to help you write it in such a way that you will be permitted to read it on Shabbos.
[17] First fruits of the season require a special "Shehechiyanu" blessing to be said before enjoying them.

A word of warning is in order here: It is inadvisable to drastically reduce your overall daily calorie intake. You *need* food to keep your metabolic rate high. We're only talking about saving up 100–200 calories each day (that's about equivalent to one of those finger-sized mini chocolate bars). Besides, you could do with all those treats, rewards, and goodies to keep you going throughout the week (see earlier, "Rewards," page 51). So don't overdo the self-restraint (smile please, that was good news).

As a result of saving up, the food will taste better, you'll be more relaxed, and your enjoyment will be automatically enhanced. Plus, you will quite literally be enjoying the fruits of your labors (anything worked for brings an increased sense of fulfilment).

Beautiful Fruitiful

In the summer (or, if you live in a big, civilized city, all year round…), treating yourself to all those exotic and beautiful fruits for Shabbos will help to ensure a curbed appetite — and enhance your enjoyment of Shabbos.

When fruit is presented in an attractive display in a basket, glass bowl, or dish, you have created a forum for being stimulated visually, which will create a build-up in terms of desire. Our brain thinks, "It looks good, so it's bound to taste good too." You can't compare this type of pull to scrounging around in the fruit and vegetable box hidden somewhere in the pantry or fridge.

As we are all creatures prone to wanting an easy life (I was going to say lazy, but that's rude) we don't want to force ourselves to exert effort at every dieting turn. We want the food to be attractive, tempting, and immediately available. All this can so easily be accomplished with a little forethought. Just think how easy it is to nibble someone's leftovers because they are also tempting and immediately available (although probably not too attractive if they were left on the plate…). Let's counteract that tendency to nibble on all those undesirables by encouraging ourselves to nibble on what is good for us.

An additional advantage in preparing a beautiful, colorful fruit arrangement is that it will help to keep us focused during the meal. When we can see all those crunchy, gleaming, luscious fruits, we may be more likely to save room for them during the meal. In sight is in mind.

Last Minute Morsels

If you come into Shabbos already starving, we all know what's going to happen to that fluffy, warm challah thirty seconds after hamotzi. That's why it's so important to have a last minute snack and drink. A cup of tea with some jam-shmeared rice cakes or a bowl of cereal will do the trick just fine. The idea is not to fill up to the point of saturation, but rather to take the edge off your appetite. At least try to partake of a quick drink right before you light candles.

That takes us to the end of erev Shabbos. Next: Shabbos itself. (At least the white tablecloth doesn't have calories.)

Chapter 7

———— ◆ ◆ ◆ ————

Shabbos

Friday Night

The hustle and bustle of a typical erev Shabbos climaxes as we stand to light the candles. The atmosphere is magically transformed into peace and serenity as the last candle leaps to life. We can relax. There's no more work to be done. And boy, oh boy do we deserve a break. Shabbos. The day of rest and relaxation has begun. But this relaxation has been the undoing of many a determined dieter.

So let's go step by step through our Shabbos schedule and see what we can do to help ourselves stay on track even while relaxing.

The Twilight Zone

You've just lit the candles and the men scurry off to daven. The children are sprawled on the floor playing contentedly. You've done all you need to do. Ahhh. This peaceful time period is certainly what we need after all that running around, but it also has other advantages.

This "Twilight Zone," when we can't eat or drink before Kiddush, is the perfect time to prepare any food that naturally lends itself to being nibbled. The cream cake needs to be cut into squares and put into cupcake holders? The petit fours need arranging? The Twilight Zone is the time to do it. Not only will you be forced to resist all those tidbits, but you will also benefit later by being super-organized — you will be able to truly relax during the meal instead of taking time away from the table and missing all the fun.

If shabbos has been your dieting downfall, this chapter should be a real pick-me-up.

At the Ready

By the time you get to hamotzi, chances are that you will be hungry. Instead of downing three whopping slices of challah to curb your appetite, it is important to be able to jump straight into the first course. It should be this (low-fat) hors d'oeuvre that succeeds in filling you up, not the challah.

Make it easy for yourself. Prepare this first course before the meal, and have it already laid out on a tray right near you. The Twilight Zone is a great time to take those extra minutes necessary to become not just impressively efficient, but also full of vibrant resolve.

Mine, All Mine

If challah is your particular downfall, maybe it's worth considering making your own, pre-weighed-out challah rolls. Or buying your favorite ones and weighing them to see exactly how many ounces they really are. This way you'll have an accurate picture of the amount of challah you are having ("I had a 2oz roll, so now I've got x points/treats/sins to spend…") instead of guessing as you go on and on and on right to the bottom of the challah basket.

The challah roll provides an automatic portion sizing. It's round. It's self-contained. It's whole. And it's exactly x ounces. (You know, you weighed it yourself.) This is the amount you are allowed and have accommodated for accordingly. Extra will seem very much like extra.

Psychologically, knowing that this challah is "for me" means that it is easier to feel that "that one is not." Even if it is squishy, smells heavenly, and came out perfect.

At Arm's Length

OK, you've had your challah roll and you couldn't resist just a little piece of fluffy heaven. Let's get real. If that basket sits in front of you for a minute longer, guess whose arm is going to automatically reach for it? Best answer — push it away. Far away. Ditto for soup nuts, croutons, and mayonnaise.

It's one thing to munch through the challah basket's contents while you listen to your guest's life story; it's quite another to stop the flow of conversation by requesting that someone pass the challah. Take advantage of human nature and give the challah basket a shove in the right direction.

Rather Fishy (Gefilte Fish)

Although most white fish are an A1 low-fat source of protein, when you add oil, sugar, eggs and matzah meal, the calorie count can soar.

The solution? Be generous with the garnishing. Add extra carrot slices/cucumber/lettuce to fill out your plate and make sure to either serve yourself a kiddie-size portion or go "halves" with Shnocky.

If you're not so keen on gefilte fish anyway, serve yourself bowl number one of the chicken soup and have bowl number two with everyone else.

More Please

Not only does chicken soup purport medicinal properties, but it is also a dieter's life-saver. Still hungry after one bowl? Go on, treat yourself to another one. At minimal calories per bowl (not including all those extras like noodles, knaidlach…), you'll be filling up (and warming up, if you're feeling the chill) at the same time. Feeling full is one of the best deterrents to overeating.

Tip: Make the soup on Thursday, put it in the fridge overnight, and skim off all visible fat before reheating it for Shabbos. When the fat is cold, it changes consistency and turns from a liquid into a solid, which makes it easier to remove.

The Return of the Chicken Soup

Friday nights can be ultra-long in the winter, so you may get hungry again before bedtime. Instead of grazing at the open fridge, waiting for something just right to come out and grab you, why not dive into that pot of chicken soup again instead?

When you take the soup pot off the blech[1] to serve soup as part of the meal, hold onto the pot, pour most of its contents into a serving dish, and return the pot to the blech. This way you'll have something delicious waiting for you whenever you want it.

Remember, making it with extra vegetables means you're filling up on a really low-calorie treat.

Chock-A-Block At Chicken Time

I'll be the first one to admit that I love the main course. If you'd ask me if I'm hungry right then, I'd be forced to reply "no way." But chicken is the next item on the socially accepted agenda. And it's so delicious.

Below are a few tried and tested home-brewed tips to help you overcome an over-stuffed tum.

Small Plate

As we mentioned in "Small Is Beautiful," page 119, you can use a side plate instead of the regular sized main course plate to help you serve yourself smaller portions. There's a limit to the amount you can squeeze onto the plate, and, believe me, there's a limit to the amount you can squeeze into that skirt.

The Three-Quarters Rule

Make sure to fill your plate with seventy-five percent salad and veggies, and only twenty-five percent with chicken and rice or potatoes. Visually, you will still be looking at a lot of food; physically, you will reap the dividends.

---

[1] Metal sheet that separates the pots and the stove flame in order to refrain from the forbidden practice of cooking the food on Shabbos.

Cut It Out

Even if you are not on one of the Protein-Only or Carbohydrate-Only diets, sensible dieting advice, at least at this course, is to cut out one or the other. Having tried consuming food in all ways imaginable, I reckon this tip is worth trying at least once. Although it's a great tip in terms of dieting, I believe it's an even greater tip in terms of how you'll feel when it's time to clear the table. Having either the chicken/meat *or* the rice/potatoes prevents that heeeeeavy Friday night feeling of fullness so many people complain about. The waist-band isn't quite as tight, the force of gravity isn't quite as strong (to make you feel glued to the chair), and your body feels more comfortable to wear. Know what I mean?

Kugel Time

Since I worked out the calorie values for my favorite potato kugel recipe, every time I serve it I see "454 calories in one small piece." Even I got a shock at this huge number. Of course, anyone who's ever set foot in Diet Land knows kugel is a no-no. But now I had concrete proof of the damage incurred when the plate fills up. The black and white numbers make it more than a vague notion that we must steer clear — they're concrete facts. Don't make yourself round with one small square — substitute extra hot vegetables or salad or coleslaw or…ice cubes or carnations — *anything* except the kugel.

If you find your plate looks incomplete without the starch filling up its usual place to the left of the chicken and you just *have* to have a starch, how about choosing rice — at 248 calories per 3.6oz it's almost half what you would be consuming if you have kugel. Or how about new potatoes? Six small, boiled potatoes only cost you 175 calories.

Or you can try this low-fat, oil-free alternative to the real stuff. At 188 calories, it's still a winner of a substitute.

Suri's Healthy Potato Kugel

2 ½ lbs. potatoes
1 onion
4 eggs
1 cup soda water/seltzer
salt and pepper

Just prepare it as you would a regular kugel and dip in — guilt free.

Dessert Time

There are many different ways to do dessert. Sometimes all that's required is a little lateral thinking, and you get to satisfy both your sweet tooth and your conscience.

Enjoy

You can choose to enjoy that pecan pie with creamy vanilla ice cream on one of two pretexts:

- You saved up for it all week and now you can truly enjoy it, or,
- You're going to enjoy it now because your willpower has crumbled somewhere between the challah and the kugel, but you resolve to "pay back" the overdraft tomorrow by being extra careful.

No points for guessing which makes more sense.

Wait a Minute (or an hour or so)

As Friday night can be long (especially in the winter), there will be plenty of time to eat after the meal. I don't believe anyone will be staaaaarving after the main course, so why not capitalize on providing yourself with a well-savored dessert experience an hour or two (or three) after the meal (instead of during)? This way you'll know what you are peering into the fridge for, plus you have reduced the quantity of your overall intake. Not diving into the apple crumble both during *and* after the meal ensures that you'll only be having one dessert, not two.

Take "Mommy M'eiser"

Don't serve yourself a portion at dessert time, just take "m'eiser" from Shnocky — or Daddy, if Shnocky gets mean and vocal. You'll still get to finish off the meal with something sweet, but at a fraction of the calories.

Spoon Sense

Try eating your favorite dessert with a teaspoon instead of a regular sized spoon. Not only do you get more bites, but you also make it last longer.

Sweet Substitutions

Sometimes it's not the actual portion of chocolate cake that you fancy at the end of the meal — it's the sweetness that you are craving.

Try finishing off your meal with a black coffee and dark chocolate, or pinch a candy from the candy jar (you've been a good girl, after all). Sugar-free candies are even better. They're quantified, they're sweet, and they're not too filling.

Don't want to be singled out as being different from the crowd? Previously sliced fresh orange segments look attractive and can accompany richer dishes like chocolate mousse. The slices fill the plate without making your plate appear naked or sad. Most people enjoy a zap of juice at this point in the game — even if they are not on a diet.

After the Meal

I had a friend whom I would visit every Friday night. As I entered, she would aesthetically arrange the very finest fruits straight from fridge to fruit-bowl. They glistened and positively shone as they acclimatized themselves to the warmth of room temperature. We weren't always "on a diet" when we tucked in. But we always enjoyed the party, regardless of the fact that we'd opted for a low-calorie munch.

It seemed the perfect thing to eat after such a heavy meal. We'd digested enough food by then to make room for it. It wasn't too filling, it was full of natural juices, and we didn't go to bed with that overstuffed feeling.

In addition, if you are the one to host company on a Friday night, know that it's quick and easy to whisk up a delightful arrangement in seconds. You'll be staying on track and your visitor will bless you for helping her feel like a mentsh when she walks out your front door (instead of getting stuck in the doorway).

Sofa Settlers

Let's say no one is coming to visit you. The little kids are all in bed. Your husband and older boys are learning. The perfect opportunity has arisen for you to sneak to the couch, armed with the newspaper or the latest bestseller. And what exactly do you take along with you, strategically positioned at the perfect forty-five degree angle from your right elbow? — Pistachio nuts…chocolate candies…nuts and raisins…Bissli…potato chips. Who will be surprised when the bottom of the bowl is clearly visible and you're not even up to the last chapter?

I don't want to deprive you of your Friday night reward while you are tucked up all cozy and content. By all means, open up the stash of goodies. But measure out the quantity you are going to be happy with consuming *before* you get all ensconced and engrossed. Put the rest away. You can even tell yourself that if you get desperate you'll allow yourself some more. But, knowing human nature for what it is, you probably won't feel like getting off that couch for a while.

Even better, try this effective practical tip, a good, juicy, finger-dipping-into-the-bowl alternative to all those calories: Freeze grapes and place them by you as you read. I actually tried this one out when someone suggested it to our Group and I thought it was great. Refreshing, juicy, and sweet.

If you are reading this after adopting a decidedly horizontal position on the couch, know that now is as good a time as any to become fully conscious of what your nibble-hungry fingers are doing (apart from turning the pages). With this vision of you in mind, I can wish you a truly enjoyable Shabbos (and sweet dreams…). For those who like to finish something once they've started it, let's talk about Shabbos day.

Shabbos Day

It's Shabbos morning. The house rocks gently with the sounds of young children scampering. Shouting and hissing "don't-wake-Mommy" noises come from outside your door. The cholent's familiar aroma welcomes you as you plod slippered feet downstairs. No breakfast cereal boxes on the table today, only crummy remainders of a well-enjoyed Shabbos party. As you embark on the first session of clearing up for the day, your tummy begins to wake up too. Mmm, it's breakfast time. What should I have?

The answer to this question will largely depend on your particular stage in life. If all your children are old enough to go to davening, or have left home, or have not yet come into being, maybe you go to daven and come home at the same time as the menfolk. Maybe you're at the stay-at-home-and-wait-for-Daddy stage of life, or maybe you catch up on some lost sleep. Whichever way your Shabbos morning finds you, food will be high on the ensuing agenda.

Let's start with our first encounter with food on Shabbos morning. Kiddush.

To Kiddush Or Not To Kiddush — That is the Question

Let's look at our line-up of options for Kiddush time:

✔ When it's wintertime and Shabbos day is very short, maybe it's a good idea to skip the Kiddush-and-cake scenario and go straight to the Kiddush-before-the-meal scenario. There's so much food to get through within a very limited time span — one course less won't really be missed. Even if the men choose the Kiddush-and-cake alternative, maybe you can sit tight and make Kiddush on hamotzi a little later. It *will* only be a *little* later, because everyone has to have lunch sometime before Seudah Shilishis[2].

✔ Yet another alternative is for you to wash and have hamotzi while the others are having their kiddush cake. This way you don't have to wash again at lunchtime and can neatly sidestep the challah course. Don't worry, there's enough food to leave the table more than a little full even without the challah. Use a 2oz challah roll instead of starting (and seriously diminishing) a whole challah, and you'll really be ahead of the game.

✔ If you don't see yourself deviating from the norm at the cake 'n' Kiddush scene, let this time period find you well prepared. Have lower-fat options at hand — for example, Swiss roll or any sponge cake recipe. Whereas all cake fits nicely under the "extra calories" banner, some are worse than others, and sponge cake can be a low-fat, fluffy alternative to the real McCoy. (See also "Look After Yourself," page 201, for two lower-calorie cakes.)

---

[2] The third Shabbos meal.

✔ Less common again, although halachically[3] sound, is to make Kiddush and then drink another *reviis*[4] of grape juice to fulfill your obligation. Guzzling grape juice is not the same as downing gallons of diet drinks. In terms of calories, one big cup will provide you with approximately 100 calories. This option comes into its own when we consider that consuming cake can run into hundreds — plural.

✔ Another alternative is to make Kiddush and eat cereal (made of wheat, barley, spelt, rye, or oats). This may sit well with you if your tummy likes routine and has a tendency to object when deviating from its normal pattern.

✔ Even if you don't have the courage to be different and you didn't prepare any sponge cake or low-fat alternatives, remember that the halachah only demands that you eat one *kezayis*[5] of cake. Anything more is…how shall we say this nicely…unnecessary.

✔ If you are the sociable type and feel morally obliged to go to one of your friends' kiddushim every other week, know that the above tips may still be applicable before you step out through the door. Making Kiddush this way (before you go) will mean you are not asking a starving mortal to resist the most attractive, tempting, and delicious array of forbidden fruits (read: cakes) she has seen all week.

Looking At Lunch

Whichever way you make Kiddush, lunch is next on the horizon. It helps, especially in the winter months, to bear in mind that Seudah Shilishis is just around the corner, and we should therefore save a corner for it. There's nothing worse than being forced to consume food on a zero-appetite. Planning to avoid this discomfort starts with Kiddush, but seriously comes into play when we sit down to lunch.

Horsey Dorsey Coursey — Hors D'oeuvre

What a funny name. Why do we call it that? Wouldn't it make more sense to call it "The Appetite Awakener" or "The Precursor?" Anyway, the French won on this one and we'll just have to remember that this course is supposed to ignite hitherto dormant appetites. This means you're supposed to still be a drop hungry before the next course.

Bearing in mind the big food line up of the day, it's wise to choose something light for this course. Maybe skip the liver or eggs and instead choose melon or grapefruit segments, even if nobody else in your family will. If liver is your particular Shabbos delight, don't let me stop you — but serve yourself a child's portion and fill the plate with plenty of that pretty, color-contrasting garnish. Not only will you be reducing a potentially high-calorie intake by increasing the garnish greens, but your plate will look the same as everyone else's. It won't be sad and empty; rather it will be attractive and appetizing.

---

[3] By Jewish Law.
[4] Predetermined quota of fluid.
[5] Measurement about the size of a deck of cards or half a jumbo sized matchbox. It's best to ask your halachic authority to show you exactly how much this is.

Cholent[6] Quotient

There are as many different tasting cholents as there are balebustas[7] who make them. Never have two cholents tasted the same. Having said that, this all-time generation traveler has got *some* defining similarities.

Most people fry onions at kick-off, but try using spray oil or, gasp, no oil at all. See if anyone notices the difference. True, one tablespoon or two divided by the whole pot isn't going to do much damage, but when you're talking about a glug, glug free-handed bottle-pouring, well, that's another story.

Remember, cholent can be soupy or gunky. Maybe it's a good idea to develop a winter-time cholent that is a little less dense (stand-the-spoon-in-and-watch-it-stand-on-its-own) and a little more soup-like. This can lighten the heaviness of the meal quite effectively. If your in-house bochurim[8] sons complain, you can always separate the cholent into two pots and just put more water in yours. No extra work or separate recipes, just two pots and one big happy family.

If you are on a Food Combining diet, just choose whichever food group you are permitted that day (protein or carbohydrate) and leave the other food type for someone else.

Bear in mind that cholent need not be a course on its own, but can in fact be served with salads, which will also go a long way towards lightening the load. Treating it as a side dish in this way will automatically reduce its weightiness. (This one works especially well in the summer.)

Even if your particular weakness is cholent, think twice before cementing the stomach. Do you really need to have seconds?

Meeting the Meat

Some people skip the meat course completely in the winter because there's just so much food a person can stomach. If this is not applicable for your household (or it's summer), why not consider combining it with the cholent course? This way, you get to serve yourself a portion of cholent and a slice of meat, and fill up the rest of your plate with the crispness of the refreshing salads. Plus, you have one less course to serve and clear. This can also buy you more time to be at the table and conserve your energy.

---

[6] Shabbos stew.
[7] Housewives, homemakers.
[8] Male adolescents.

Desert Dessert

If your meal just isn't complete without this finishing touch, try substituting more filling desserts (plum crumble, etc.) for lighter, more easily digestible foods (low-fat sorbets, compotes, meringues, etc.).

However, if your end-of-meal stomach tells you it really doesn't want that apple pie and ice cream, do it a favor and listen to it. Partaking of dessert at the end of the meal is not one of the commandments. If you choose to skip dessert, or save it for later, you're bound to enjoy it so much more.

In the wintertime, some people choose to end their Shabbos lunch meal without dessert and serve dessert as the meal at Seudah Shilishis instead. Lateral thinking never hurt anyone.

Seudah Shilishis

If you find you've got an appetite for this meal (barely two to four hours after lunch in the winter), you're on the right track. If, however, you haven't yet mastered the art of eating small and often, it's mightily important to eat light to eat right at this meal.

This is for two reasons. One: that cholent is still very much in the pipes and two: Melaveh Malkah[9] is right around the corner. (On short Shabbos days, everything seems to be right around the corner.)

Fill your plate with all those light, crunchy, water-based salads like tossed lettuce salad or Chinese leaves. It looks like you are eating a lot. And you *are* actually eating a lot (instead of just sitting there) — but you're not packing in the calories. Cajole yourself into waiting till you've polished off that green lettuce mountain before allowing yourself something more substantial.

I have discovered something fascinating at this meal. In the winter, my whole family, right from tiny tots to strapping adolescents to my skinny husband, all want green salad for this meal — and lots of it. Even if they won't look at the stuff the rest of the week. And they're not even on a diet.

As I've mentioned before, in the winter some people have dessert as their main course at this meal. But even here the trick is to have fruit salad/melon wedges/pineapple slices/etc. rather than cake and cookies. Doesn't that sound nice — a big plate of tossed green salad with low-fat dressing followed by a tropical fruit selection.

Summertime Seudah Shilishis should see the table laid with mouth-watering, colorful, varied, plentiful salads. Try "doctoring" oily or high-fat dressings to lower-fat ones. Using half the amount of oil in a recipe can cut out hundreds of calories and doesn't have to compromise on taste or texture. For more ideas about salad dressing see "Dressing Down Salad," page 92. Try making a bean salad to ensure lots of fiber, or a three-colored (it's prettier) pasta salad with light mayonnaise to fill up. The summer months can be hot. Have pitchers of cold, refreshing drinks on the table — ready

---

[9] The customary meal enjoyed after Havdalah.

to offer everyone before kick-off. This will help to take the crabbiness off the kids (make that everyone), and will take the edge off your hunger (and headache from dehydration).

How Full is Full?

In the winter, you've just sat down after clearing up from lunch and suddenly it's time to set the table for Seudah Shilishis. You are not hungry, but it's a mitzvah to eat this meal. What should you do? Well, I'm no halachic authority, but the following is the priority list in terms of eats or don't eats as found in most halachah books.

- ✔ The best course of action is to wash for hamotzi and have a little more than a *k'beya*.[10]
- ✔ Next best, if one is not hungry and finds it difficult to eat bread at all, one should eat a food made from wheat, barley, rye, oats, or spelt. This would typically be your crackers or sponge cake (note: not rice cakes) or cereals (such as Bran Flakes, Weetabix, etc.).
- ✔ If that is also asking too much, one should try to eat either meat or fish.
- ✔ Failing that, one should try to eat some fruit or drink a *reviis* of wine or grape juice.
- ✔ Should one find it hard to eat or drink anything at all, one doesn't have to inflict pain on oneself to do so, since the purpose of the Shabbos meal is to give pleasure and not pain.

Melaveh Malkah

You've washed and dried the dishes, you've vacuumed the carpet and tidied up, and it's time for yet more food. Knowing what to have after all those delicious delectables have been devoured can be a real brainteaser. You want something different, something that you didn't have on Shabbos; something not too heavy, yet substantial. Perhaps something savory and healthy to return our systems back to their regular equilibriums…

If you've got time, motzei Shabbos is a great time to make a fresh vegetable/lentil soup. Make plenty, so you've got some for Sunday and through the week. That's one less job to do if your workweek quite literally has you working. We've all had nosh together with stodgy, heavy meals on Shabbos — soup can slip between the cracks, conforms to the opinion of having a newly-cooked food after Shabbos, and is kind not only to our tummies, but also to our battered resolve.

Sometimes winter can be a time for staying indoors and letting friendships slide by. Why not catch up with a few friends and invite them over? Maybe have each friend make a different diet-friendly dish. This might be a combined tummy- *and* heart-warming experience.

---

[10] Two kezaisim. See if that *kezayis*-defining halachic authority is still handy.

Whichever way you choose to bid farewell to Shabbos, take solace in the fact that it's only six more days till it comes around again. Shabbos doesn't have to be a dieter's disaster. Quite the contrary, it can provide a welcome change to a dry, routine, weekly menu. You can now look forward to a guilt-free Shabbos. You can experience the beauty and pleasure inherent in Shabbos without compromising on your policy of healthy eating, and you can use it as a spiritual and physical recharge to energize you for the week ahead.

Chapter 8

———— ◆ ◆ ◆ ————

Yom Tov – General

You might think that the foods we serve for Yom Tov are so similar to those we serve for Shabbos that there is no need for two whole chapters on Yom Tov. Argue though you may, this is only partly true. The problems and challenges we face when preparing ourselves (and our food) for a Yom Tov are different enough to justify two stand-alone Yom Tov chapters all of their own (this way Yom Tov doesn't get too jealous…).

Having said that, there *are* similarities. Therefore, in order to reduce the risk of appearing repetitive (perish the thought), I have listed those areas common to both scenarios with the relevant pages marked here for you to exercise your page-flipping abilities.

> *Here comes dieting advice that applies to all food-filled Jewish holidays.*

Before Yom Tov

Save Up

Yom Tov is coming whether you are prepared or not. Let's make sure we *are* prepared (in more ways than one). At least a few days before every Yom Tov, it shouldn't be too hard to remember to save up your treats/points/calories/etc. for whichever diet you are on. (It may be difficult to do, but it shouldn't be too difficult to remember.)

See "Save Up," page 159.

Be Prepared

Even if you are blessed with Herculean self-control, it's no good coming into a Yom Tov with the fridge stocked only with deluxe chocolate eclairs and hazelnut rings and the stovetop bubbling with fried schnitzel or roux sauces. Remember, you are human and will be hungry. If you don't prepare low-fat alternatives to all those goodies, no amount of resolve will be able to rescue you as you begin your munching.

See "Be Prepared," page 157.

Sensational Seasonal Fruits

When Yom Tov falls in the late spring/summer, that's the time to enjoy all those delicious spring fruits that are in their prime. Kiwis, strawberries, pineapples, passion fruit, melons…buy plenty — and treat yourself even if they seem a little pricey. Juicy, good quality fruits also count as Oneg Yom Tov, not just kid's nosh. So treat yourself and don't feel guilty. You are nurturing your body *and* your soul.

See "Beautiful Fruitiful," page 160.

Think-Drink

Especially in the late spring/summer, it's a good idea to have plenty of low-calorie drinks in the house. Remember the best, lowest calorie drink is always accessible and free — water from the tap. Refrigerated, cool water with ice and lemon is thirst-quenching and immediately refreshing. Hot, cranky kids are also easily calmed with cold drink, so stock up.

Freezer Teasers

While we are still talking about the heat…why not freeze reduced-calorie juice into popsicle molds or plastic disposable cups with plastic spoons dug in? You can also try freezing low-fat yogurt into lollies (especially useful for Shavuos if your custom is to eat milchigs[1]), or try freezing bananas for a cooling, fiber-rich treat. Stock up on low-fat ice cream alternatives: Tofutti ice creams/sorbets/etc. This way, when your neighbor comes to you shvitzing[2] and complaining that she put the heat on for Yom Tov, you can open the freezer door, graciously offer her something from your selection, and sit down and share it with her.

Cool Food

Being prepared when it comes to mealtimes can mean winning half the battle. Try making hot, low-calorie soup for hors d'oeuvre (or in the summer, cold fruit soup, cold gazpacho soup, fruit kebabs, or attractively arranged summer fruits). This way you have filled up on something low-calorie right at the start of the meal and your resolve will not crumble from starvation. (See "Hors D'oeuvre," page 168.)

---

[1] Foods made of milk or milk products.
[2] Perspiring.

Remember to make plenty of salads. This is very helpful in the summer when the afternoons are long. It's a good move to have some real food at your fingertips when your tummy reminds you that suppertime is usually scheduled for 6pm, not 10pm or later.

Plan of Action

Writing menu lists before Yom Tov is a great tried and tested way to reap concrete dividends from all your overflowing willpower. Write down exactly what you plan to eat (and any alternatives).[3] (See also "Automatic Pilot," page 159.)

A typical menu list would be something like the following:

Food	Points/Calories	Notes
Points/Calories accumulated:		
Challah		
Mayonnaise		
Fish		
More Mayonnaise		
Soup		
Matzah Ball		
Roast Beef		
Boiled Baby Potatoes		
Mushrooms		
Coleslaw		
Fruit Salad		
Ice Cream Scoop		
Drinks		
TOTAL POINTS		
POINTS/CALS REMAINING		

The notes section should be written to remind you, for example, to defrost a dish, or to open your low-fat mayonnaise before Yom Tov.

---

[3] Note that these lists cannot be read as a list on Yom Tov for halachic reasons, so ask your local qualified halachic authority how to solve that problem.

The top of the chart shows the total number of points/calories accumulated so far. Writing this down (before you spend the points) will help in your conscious distribution of them. Note that if you don't use up all your allowed points, they are tallied at the end and can be spent at the next installment.

Erev Yom Tov

Eat!

In all the buzz and bustle of erev Yom Tov, don't forget to eat. If you have something to eat before Yom Tov you won't be so hungry when you come to the Yom Tov seudah itself. Otherwise, you might end up watching your resolve for self-control, together with the challah crumbs (or matzah specks, depending on the season), crumble onto that newly vacuumed carpet. We feed the baby, we feed the plants, let's not forget to feed ourselves as well.

See "Hunger," page 146, and "Lunchtime," page 151.

Sleep

Try to sleep on erev Yom Tov. This one can be tough, I know, but it's worth its (and your) weight in gold. Not only will it enhance your Yom Tov experience, but you will also be able to control yourself better if you are not too exhausted. (At least we can dream on…) (See "Shuteye," page 142).

Mindset

One Course Less

If a one-day Yom Tov is a challenge and a two-day Yom Tov is a hurdle, then what's a three-day Yom Tov? One thing is for sure: It involves a lot of heavy meals that we wouldn't normally be consuming. Just compare a microwaved baked potato with cottage cheese and side salad to your Yom Tov menu list. To waylay the risk of eating more than your body requires (on any Yom Tov — even a one-day kind), why not choose to skip a course altogether? We are creatures of habit. If we are used to eating whatever is put in front of us, we continue to do so without thinking about whether we really want/need to eat. Make a conscious decision about what you do or don't want to consume. We shouldn't just do things because that's how we have done them for years. (After all, that's probably why we need to diet in the first place.) So, let everyone else pick up their forks and knives and plow their way through that course while you sit tight and act right.

Treat Yourself Versus Blowing it

Don't try to be "better than good," thinking you are superhuman and will speed your weight loss by abstaining. After you've seen all those delicious Yom Tov delicacies one too many times, you'll blow the whole thing with an "in for a penny, in for a pound" party.

Rather, save up points and spend them wisely over Yom Tov — but *do* enjoy your Yom Tov and *do* spend the points.

If you forbid yourself indulgences, you suffer the risk of blowing the whole concept of controlled eating when you finally *do* succumb to temptation. And we all know that if you do go and have a deliciously fattening time, it makes it so much harder to revert back to dieting. You will feel that going back to a diet is a negative step ("Oh no, now I will have to stick to my whole-wheat roll/2oz bread instead of chomping away on moist, squishy challah…"). **If you never completely "come off" the diet, then you never consciously have to summon up energy to go back onto it either.**

Listen To Your Body

If I would be asked for my one, most important piece of advice in terms of healthy eating it would be this: Listen to your body. So simple, and yet so ignored.

If you are hungry, then by all means, go and eat. Yes, be careful in choosing what to eat, but if you let yourself get hungry you suffer the real risk of getting grouchy and aggravated, not enjoying the Yom Tov, and then going wild when you finally do get the chance to eat. Your self-control is lessened because the impulse is stronger. The decision over what you are eating becomes harder to control and willpower goes out the window.

In practical terms, this means if you are hungry on Yom Tov afternoon and the seudah is not until 10pm, you should have a light snack, or even the seudah's hors d'oeuvre. When you get to the seudah, you should skip that course. You will be able to, because you won't be starving.

But remember, when your tummy tells you it is full, you have already eaten too much. The ideal is to feel pleasantly un-hungry, not full. That feeling of needing to unbutton the skirt is a sign that the stomach has exceeded its natural capacity. We all know how uncomfortable that feeling makes us. Let's avoid it. When you are satisfied, you should stop.

It's even a wise move to stop just short of feeling satisfied. This is because the food takes a few minutes to reach the stomach and your brain needs this time to register its fullness.[4] So you won't really feel full until several minutes after you have finished eating.

---

[4] See "How to Eat, Eat Slowly," page 120.

We are creatures of habit. I bet the idea of stopping halfway through a seudah never even occurred to you. People just don't do it. But people who want to lose excess pounds would be wise to learn this skill. Sounds obvious, but so few people exercise this as a real option. Better yet: Eat less at every course and enjoy the whole seudah.

See also "Practice Feeling Full," page 122.

Stay in Control

There's nothing worse than being organized and prepared and following all these recommendations to the tee — and then watching your resolve disintegrate over the Yom Tov itself because now is your chance to capitalize on all those saved-up treats. As your hand dives into the jumbo package of potato chips, know that one handful is not the same as five, and that one piece of cake is not the same as finishing off all the kids' leftovers as you clear the table. Control means awareness — of what you are doing and what you are eating.

During the week, it might be easier not to go astray because you can write down all your indulgences to help keep you on track. On Yom Tov, try counting your treats by putting toy counters — or marbles, or candies — into a cup (careful with that one — the candies go into the cup, not the mouth).

Enjoy

Eating is a wonderful sensation. Our senses are tickled and excited, we smell the aromas, we see the beautiful colors, our tastebuds savor the lingering flavors. But we live in such rushed times that we tend not to savor the moment. To truly enjoy what you eat, you have to slooooooow down and smell, taste, and chew your food properly.[5] All year around this might be a tall order, but Yom Tov is an ideal time to practice. Besides, the food is so much yummier then. You have worked so hard to shop, cook, and prepare it — why not take the time to enjoy it too? Besides the enjoyment, your digestive system will bless you for chewing your food properly, plus, you'll end up eating less and enjoying it more.[6]

Whichever diet you are on, or even if you aren't on any formal plan but are interested in healthy living, the most important thing is to be healthy and happy and to enjoy yourself while you achieve this goal.

---

[5] See "Concentr-eat When You Eat," page 121.
[6] See "Eat Slowly," page 120.

On Yom Tov Itself

Move

Yom Tov meals do not lend themselves to hyperactivity — at least not for anyone over age three. We sit to eat, we sit to listen to the beautiful Divrei Torah,[7] we sit to bench…. So grab the opportunity to go for a Yom Tov walk. You'll feel "aired-out," you'll burn a few calories, you'll raise your metabolic rate, and you may even get to have a good shmooze with someone.

After the Schloff[8]

You wake up. Your mouth is dry. You're in need of something revitalizing and juicy. Don't blow the opportunity of giving your body what it really needs by stuffing it with cake and chocolate.

Keep crisp apples in the fridge so they can help to wake you up and make you feel refreshed. Try cutting a Granny Smith or Washington Red into slivers attractively laid out on a plate, sitting down like a lady, and reeeeally enjoying them (instead of the hand-to-mouth, casual, on-the-run style of eating).

If you're looking for a light snack, how about trying diet drinks, frozen ices (in the summer), frozen bananas, frozen yogurt (if you're milchig or over Shavuos), compote, frozen grapes, chilled melon cubes, slices of fresh pineapple, salads…The list is endless. Only your imagination is limited.

Chocolate

Sometimes when we have just woken up from our Yom Tov schloff, we will find ourselves raiding the cupboards for "something good." Ahhhh…chocolate. With a cup of hot coffee. It warms us up and provides that deliciously intense sweetness we seem to crave during a long afternoon.

Chocolate does not need to be your downfall over Yom Tov. (See "Don't Choke on Chocolate," page 99 for four helpful tips.)

You can enjoy your chocolate, or, better yet, have healthy alternatives ready (see below).

Nibbly Bits

Who doesn't find themselves grazing at the fridge on those long Yom Tov afternoons? We smack our lips and strain our eyes over every shelf, looking for just the right thing to scratch our tastebuds' itch. Having the right types of food at hand can make all the difference.

---

[7] Insights from the Torah.
[8] Nap.

Here are some suggestions for those lip-smacking times when you don't know quite what to have:

- ¡●¡ Rice cakes with low fat mayonnaise and sliced tomatoes;
- ¡●¡ Sticks of vegetables (with dips of cottage cheese/yogurt/chopped herring or on their own);
- ¡●¡ Extra portions of chicken or fish (cooked without skin and no oil);
- ¡●¡ Cereal;
- ¡●¡ Pasta salad (cooked pasta with light mayonnaise and tomatoes, pickled cucumbers, corn, and whatever else you're in the mood to eat).

Be creative, think laterally, and plan ahead (heard this before somewhere?).

Trick Your Tummy

When deciding on what to have during those long "in-between" times of day, trick your tummy into feeling full without high calories by filling up on fiber-rich foods. Remember berries, whole-wheat crackers, and fruits and veggies (including salad) can all be wonderful fillers.

Drinking also tricks the stomach and takes the edge off the appetite. It will rehydrate your body, which may have consumed an above average amount of sodium in the salty foods served over Yom Tov.

Seudah Shilishis

When Yom Tov falls on Shabbos, even if you choose to serve dessert as the seudah, make sure you have plenty of light, fresh, crispy, water-packed foods from which to choose (e.g., lettuce, bean sprouts, apples, melon, etc.). Chances are everyone will be feeling a little full and will appreciate the chance to have something refreshing and light instead of dense and heavy. Maybe wash and serve a fruit salad, or apple/pear compote.

See "Seudah Shilishis," page 170.

The Second-Night Seudah

If you've been right on track throughout the rest of the day and have paced yourself accordingly, you might even find that you are actually rather hungry. That would be great 'cause then you could sit down and enjoy yourself. Food tastes so much better when you have an appetite for it (note: not uncontrollable starvation). However, if you find yourself facing mountains of food without an appetite, do yourself a favor — think minimal and eat even less. Skip it or small-scale it. There may be a commandment to partake of this beautiful Yom Tov meal, but there's no commandment to feel like an overstuffed potato knish.

Menus Under Scrutiny

Now that we have suggested some tips to make Yom Tov easier and more enjoyable, let's take out the microscope and scrutinize a typical Yom Tov meal in order to get a realistic picture of where the calories are actually coming from. When your chin sags into your chest after reading this menu, we'll try to look at some ways that we can hack away at such a horrific number until it becomes less menacing (and more palatable).

This is Mrs. Average's menu plan...before she reads this book. Here goes.

FOOD	CALORIES
Kiddush	
Slurp of Grape Juice (¼ cup)	25
Challah (2 big slices)[9]	470
Honey (2 Tbsp.)[10]	86
Mayonnaise — homemade/full fat (2 Tbsp.)	200
Meal	
Fresh Salmon (palm-sized piece)	197
More Mayonnaise (1 Tbsp. with salmon)	100
Challah (1 medium slice for a hefsek)[11]	150
Unskimmed Soup (2 ladles)	100
Soup nuts/croutons (1 handful) with soup	150
Soup nuts/croutons (1 handful) with Divrei Torah	150
Matzah Balls (2)	90
Roast Beef (2 thick slices)	284
Tzimmes (fried onions, carrots, sugar, honey)	150
Potato Kugel (3" × 3" piece, i.e., a ninth of a deep square pan)	445[12]
Coleslaw (with homemade mayonnaise)	100
Apple Pie (1 slice)	290
Vanilla Ice Cream (1 scoop)	97
Chocolate Syrup (2 Tbsp.)	110
Drinks throughout the meal[13] (Coca Cola/pure fruit juices/etc.) (4 cups)	300
TOTAL	One fat lady (3,544)

---

[9] This number is based on a thick, squishy, generous slice of about 3oz.
[10] This one applies from Rosh Hashanah till after Succos.
[11] It is customary to have a different food to make a separation between fish and meat.
[12] That's about 74 calories per tablespoonful!
[13] Coca Cola, pure orange juice, and pure apple juice are all 75 calories per 7 fluid ounces/200ml.

Even I had to swoon at that total. Unbelievable. One meal and you're nearly 1,500 calories over your whole day's allowance (that's almost an extra day's calories snuck in there). And we wonder why we feel fat over Yom Tov.

Now let's go through the menu again, trying to shave some of those awfully big numbers so that we can enjoy Yom Tov without having to add inches at the same time.

Kiddush

We'll stay with the grape juice — after all, we're Jewish aren't we?

Challah

Now we're getting down to nitty gritties. Store-bought challah is usually fluffier and lighter (high-powered bakery machinery kneads the dough more efficiently). That means that one big-looking piece of bought challah contains fewer calories than your homemade same-size equivalent. No, I'm not telling you to stop baking your own yummy family favorite. I'm just awakening a new challah consciousness.

Although you may well be truly hungry when you face your Yom Tov meal, there's no better time to exercise self-restraint than right from the starting line. You can certainly go ahead and have your big slice of challah — but note the singular tense. And make sure that whatever you are serving for hors d'oeuvre is right next to the table, ready and waiting to be served (see "At the Ready," page 162). This way you can enjoy your challah but continue to curb your appetite with the next course. When you are not so hungry you will invariably find it easier (I didn't say easy) to make more healthful choices throughout the meal.

Have you ever seen a 1oz slice of challah? I once presented our Diet Group with different sized slices of challah and asked them to guess their weight. The overall majority underestimated entirely. Try it out yourself — a 1oz thin slice of homemade challah is smaller than the size of the average palm. Although you're not allowed to whisk out the scale at the Yom Tov meal, a mental picture of exactly what a slice of challah looks like can be a powerful tool in making you aware of what you are consuming.

In the sample menu above, two big slices will give you 470 calories. I estimated that a big slice was about three ounces (3oz = 235 calories). 470 calories is cliff-edge close to providing a quarter of your calories for the day. And that's *before* the real food. If you would substitute your two slices for just one, you'd be saving 235 calories. Better yet, how about going for a medium slice (2oz) and saving 313 calories?

Honey

Although from Rosh Hashanah onwards the honey jar and challah are inseparable, a little bit of honey is not the same as bumblebee belly-flopping headfirst into the jar. Enjoy the taste of a smear on your challah and refrain from extra spoonfuls. Besides, it's bound to get *something* sticky (your fingers, outfit, left ear…). Let's have one tablespoon versus two, and save 43 calories.

Mayonnaise

Some people enjoy their challah with mayonnaise almost as a course in itself. Either you do, or you don't. Must be genetic…or minhag or something. If you are from the school of thought that challah was created to be eaten with mayonnaise, try a simple substitute: Use light mayonnaise over regular or homemade and shave off 50 calories per tablespoon.

An additional tip: Try spreading it onto the challah without taking a mini Mount Sinai onto your plate. Tastes the same, with fewer calories.

Hors D'oeuvres

Fresh salmon is a great fish — high in Omega-3 fatty acids (the good guys), low-fat, filling, and tasty to boot. But whereas he might be a firm favorite for a main dish, he adds extra calories to an already jam- (honey?) packed line-up.

Let's look at a couple of alternatives. One big slice of honeydew melon will give you 63 calories. An hors d'oeuvre of half a cantaloupe melon (in "plaice" of the salmon) will give you 57 calories, saving you 140 calories. And don't forget, if you are a mayonnaise woman, you can eliminate the extra 100 white 'n' creamy calories from the total, too. Melon and mayonnaise just doesn't have the same ring.

Also, if you go for the melon you won't need another slice of challah for a hefsek. (Sorry, you can't justify that one on religious grounds.)

Soup

Remember, skimmed soup is free (or near enough); the extras are not. This includes any potatoes, parsnip, or kreplach[14] that might have found their sneaky way into the pot.

Soup Nuts/Croutons

Whatever you call them, I'm talking about those yummy, can't-stop-once-you-start, tiny, bright yellow, crispy (mouth watering yet?) squares. You know, the ones the kids love to party on and then scatter all over the kitchen table and floor till you hear the crunch underfoot. Anyway, those little critters weigh in at 150 calories per ounce/handful (I weighed them) and just seem to seep into the cracks of the best dieter's armor. In terms of real food, it's like having eaten three apples or two thin slices of bread. You'd notice eating those — but do you notice you're finishing off the bowl of soup nuts?

Tip: Let's aim to be conscious that we are nibbling on them. In practical terms, the best way to do this is to pour one spoon into your bowl and tuck in to the soup while it's still hot and the croutons are still crunchy. Let them get soggy and you may be tempted to go for another spoonful to increase the crunch. When you have taken your turn, pass the croutons around the table — hopefully they'll end up out of arm's reach.

---

[14] Dough-based delicacy.

Matzah Balls

If matzah balls are your Yom Tov enjoyment, don't let me stop you. After all, 90 calories for two isn't going to break the bank. But if you don't really care for them and you're only eating them because the ladle scooped them in anyway — why "waist" the calories? Save them for something you really will enjoy later.

Roast Beef

There's a big difference calorically between meat that was first fried (seared) in oil, and meat that is roasted in the oven or cooked on the stovetop. The above number is for meat that is roasted — if you fry it first, you can add a whole bunch of extra calories to that number.

Don't worry, I'm not going to advocate depriving yourself of this special Yom Tov food. But two thin slices can easily be substituted for two thick slices without really seeing the difference on the plate. So instead of 284 calories, you could easily reduce this number by a third and cut out 95 calories. There, that wasn't too painful, was it?

Tzimmes

I reckon I could be sued for apikorsus[15] if I advocated skipping this one, so I won't (I like peace). Instead, how about frying the onions in calorie-free spray oil instead of the real stuff — you can still use the sugar and honey but you will have reduced the calories significantly. We're talking about cutting out an extra 135 calories per tablespoon of oil, so if you're the type of cook who free-pours the bottle without a care in the world…think again.

Potato Kugel

See "Kugel Time," page 164, for a calorie-saving (188 calories per portion) kugel alternative.

Coleslaw

Once again, a simple substitute of using low-fat mayonnaise instead of home-made/high-fat mayonnaise cuts the calories in half. Think low-fat mayo is too tart? Try adding a no-calorie artificial sweetener. Taking this easy-peasy alternative route to the tastiest coleslaw in town will shave off 50 calories per tablespoon of mayonnaise (per estimated portion) and no one (except your bathroom scale) will notice the difference.

---

[15] Apostacy.

Apple Pie

It'll come as no surprise that apple pie is full of not just apples, but calories too. If your sweet tooth will give you no respite until he gets his "just desserts," try substituting this high-calorie delectable with the following.

	Calories
Fresh fruit salad, in pure juice (3.5oz)	48
Canned fruit in juice (3.5oz)	50
Sponge cake, fat-free, filled with jam (1 slice)	181

Alternatively, you could get creative and substitute the pie dough for a sponge cake base. Add the apples on top and presto, you have a low-fat apple cake.

Ice Cream

I know someone who religiously savors her Friday night ice cream treat each week. She works hard for it and only after a "good" controlled week will she allow herself this scoop of heaven. Indeed, if this is your particular soft-scoop-spot, go right ahead and enjoy. The problems come when it's not just the ice cream that's your particular delight, but it's the challah, the mayonnaise, the soup croutons, the apple pie…. In short, if you've spent your allowance wisely all day then I'll be right behind you as you pat yourself on the back with a well-deserved reward. Remember, it works both ways. If you've let loose and made willpower part of history, then sorry, I won't be joining in with a pat (and nor should you).

Sometimes it pays to compare the calorie values for different types of ice cream. They can vary quite considerably. While you've got your head in the freezer, take a look at sorbets too. They have fewer calories, as the fat content is usually lower (or non-existent) compared to ice cream.

If it's something cold and sweet that you crave, how about trying one of the kids' popsicles? At about 30 calories per stick, they can make an excellent substitute and scratch the itch.

Chocolate Syrup

I know it looks really deliciously gooey to see all that dark brown liquid dripping over your dessert, but there goes an extra 110 calories that could've been saved for another day. How about using multicolored sprinkles for an alternatively aesthetic zap?

And if you avoid the ice cream altogether, you'll also probably avoid the chocolate syrup — two for one.

Drinks

Although I'll be the first to advocate drink, drink, and drink some more, there's a huge difference between drinking the real, high-calorie fizzy sodas or going for the low-calorie equivalent. Seems a shame to spend extra calories on a millisecond gulp as opposed to spending the same number of calories on a food that you can smell, taste, savor, chew, and enjoy for longer.

If you can't stand Diet Coke, try experimenting with other low-calorie flavors. They're bringing new ones out all the time. It's worth the investment, considering you can save an approximate 300 calories *per meal*. If you have three meals in one day, that's 3 × 300 = 900 calories — nearly half your daily allowance. So, think low-cal when you think drink.

Now, let's see all that translated into an at-a-glance menu plan.

FOOD	CALORIES
Kiddush	
Slurp of Grape Juice (¼ cup)	25
Challah (1 big slice)	235
Honey (1 Tbsp.)	43
Mayonnaise — Light (2 Tbsp.)	100
Meal	
Half a Cantaloupe Melon	57
Soup (with extra veggies, e.g., large carrot)	35
Roast Beef (2 thin slices)	189
Tzimmes (fried onions,[16] carrots, sugar, honey)	50
Kugel (no oil variety)	188
Coleslaw (with Light mayonnaise)	50
Fresh Fruit Salad in pure juice (3.5 oz.)	48
Diet Drinks	0
TOTAL	**1,070**

Conclusion

Making conscious decisions along the way to substitute, skip, or enjoy your food goes a long way in streamlining not only a potentially disastrous 3,000-plus calorie menu, but will also help to streamline you as well.

---

[16] Fried with spray oil.

Considering that Mrs. Average is only supposed to consume 2,000 calories to break even (she's not even on a diet!), when she sits down to only one Yom Tov meal without care, she can easily consume 3,500 calories. It's not as if she'll cancel food for the rest of the day. She'll still be wading through calories at the other meals, which may potentially lead to a dieting disaster. The bottom line? You need to think ahead to think thin.

Get Back on Track

If you find that your diet is the first thing to go when faced with all the extra preparations, Yom Tov goodies, and treats, know that there is a big difference between blowing it for a few days or blowing it for a few weeks. A short "stop" in the overall journey is not as bad as getting off the train altogether. As soon as you feel more in control, get straight back into it. The difference in weight could be the difference between a couple of pounds or at least three to four times that amount.

Whichever Yom Tov you are anticipating, you want to be able to enjoy yourself, your environment, and your food without having to pay the heavy price of being heavier. You want to schep nachas from your children, your husband, your family members — and yourself. Let's not disappoint ourselves with unfulfilled dreams. Rather, let's make our Yom Tov experience part of the journey in actualizing those dreams to become better, happier, and healthier people.

Wishing you a healthy, happy Yom Tov.

After Yom Tov Pick-Me-Up

Yom Tov is now behind you. You have guzzled grape juice and munched on matzah/challah till you can't zip your skirt anymore… Now you are left in its aftermath, feeling fat, despondent, and fed up — both literally and figuratively. Maybe you've put on the amount you lost before Pesach/Succos/etc. and are feeling that you are back to square one. Maybe you are still moaning about starting that diet that you meant to start weeks, months, or even years ago.

Well, negative thoughts run counterproductive to positive solutions, so now is a great time to throw that negativity into the garbage can. Don't be so hard on yourself. Yes, you had a lovely Yom Tov, and yes, you put on weight — tell me who didn't put on weight (and how did they do it?!) — maybe a pound or two, or more realistically, three or four (or more…). But our old excuses about being "too busy," "too far gone," etc., are just that — excuses. We need to recognize them for what they are and zap them accordingly with a brand new resolve.

We must be especially alert after a Yom Tov not to fall prey to the comfort of wallowing in self-pity and apathy in relation to weight loss. It is hardly constructive to be depressed about the damage done. It's over, it's past, gone, history. That is not the issue. So what exactly *is* the issue? Quite simply: what are you going to do about it *now*?

You've got a choice. You can either dwell on your fatness and be depressed about it and continue to eat to "feel better," or you can pick yourself up and go forward.

Any Olympic gold medalist, any billionaire, any accomplished inventor, or, for that matter, any successful person, will tell you that his way to success was not one smooth, straight path. Not even a tzaddik[17] is born to greatness, strolling along a red carpet to heaven. No, it's really hard work with plenty of stumbling and even failures. Any accomplishment is an accumulation of accomplishments. There are highs. There are lows. It's what you do after a low that determines your ultimate success.

We have to learn how to lose a battle and win the war. We have to stop dwelling on our failure and use it as an opportunity for growth — in effect, change it into a learning experience that will catapult us forward. When you *have* put on weight, when you are feeling low and despondent, *that* is the time to pick yourself right up and move forward, because that is exactly how you will succeed in the end.

I am sure you have read or heard success stories of how a lady lost 100+ pounds and look at her now — all skin and bones — yes, you too can look like this, you can make your dream come true…it's sooooo easy. What they don't always dwell on, but what is *always* the case, is that she also had her peaks and valleys, her highs and lows, her successes and failures. ***Everyone who has ever successfully lost weight and kept it off, has had failures.*** But what did this lady and all like her do about it — there's only one choice — she kept moving forward, she kept picking herself up after each lapse, after every failure, until she turned her failures into a success story.

I once read a story about a professor of medical students who was giving the students their mock final examination. They had all worked really hard because they all knew the paper was going to be extremely difficult. They took the exam and the professor took them away to mark. When he came back the following week, he was carrying a glass milk bottle full of milk. He said to them, "Today I am going to teach you a lesson that you will remember for the rest of your lives." He went over to the lab sink and smashed the bottle into tiny pieces, with milk splashing all around. He continued, "Five words I have to say to you all — DON'T CRY OVER SPILT MILK! — You have all failed. But it was the mock, and we still have time to learn from our mistakes. Now, let's go over the paper together."

So, too, with us: We are not going to dwell on how much weight we have put on, we are not going to raid the pantry for all the goodies to drown our sorrows. We are going to go forward and do something positive about our weight, and in this way, and ***only*** in this way, will we achieve success.

Tell me, what better time is there to strengthen a resolve or embark on a new project than right now? So let's just go through a few reasons why now is the perfect time to motivate yourself to trim down and shape up.

---

[17] Perfect, righteous person.

No Big-Time Yom Tov Approaching

Whereas Pesach, Shavuos, or Succos may well have taken days or weeks of preparation and foresight, possibly distracting us from looking after ourselves, we now face a relatively calm period in the calendar. We can use this quiet time to re-channel our energies.

Yummy Fruits 'N' Veggies

It's true we live in spoiled times in terms of gashmius[18] and can get strawberries in winter and carrots in the summer, but boy oh boy, don't the strawberries taste better in their right season? The summer is the time to enjoy all those nice juicy mangoes, nectarines, berries, etc. — a dieter's paradise.

Light Makes Light

When it's hot outside, we don't crave heavy-duty hot meals. We naturally gravitate towards lighter food. How does a light, crunchy lettuce salad with a low-fat dressing sound versus your standard wintertime fare of heavy meat and potatoes? Or what about snacking on crisp, fresh, chilled, Washington Reds versus good ole veggie soups while you picnic in the shade in the garden. (Ahh…)

Long Days-y, No Lazy

Not only does summer bring heat, but it also brings light, long days. That means we are more active and busier for longer. When we move we burn off more calories, providing a further incentive for us to kick-start our weight loss campaign.

And when it's bright outside, we are more inclined to get out and about. We'll take the kids to the park, we'll go for a walk, and we'll leave the car behind. All this exercise counts.

Less time indoors also means less time to face the temptations lurking inside the kitchen. So get out, enjoy the sunshine, and leave the car behind.

A "Spring" in the Step

It never ceases to amaze me that as soon as it's sunny outside, out come the smiles, the "Hi there! How are you?"s. People seem happier, more upbeat, and even more energetic. The impetus for starting a new project is in the air together with nature's renewal and vibrancy. Let's tap into it and focus that energy towards building a new you.

---

[18] Materialism.

Looking Good, Feeling Good

Who wants to run around with her skirt's top button undone or held shut with a two-inch diaper pin? Wouldn't it be lovely to wear that blouse tucked in instead of sloppy-style out? Who wants to wear a full-length coat in tropical heat with sweat pouring down her face because she is too embarrassed to take off her coat? Don't forget, you can't wear your coat in the swimming pool!

Last year's summer clothes really might have shrunk in winter storage. But it's not comfy to wear warm winter clothes that *do* still fit when it's ninety degrees in the shade. We want to fit into (and look good in) our summer clothes. So let's do something about it and not be embarrassed once again this summer.

Take Up a New Activity

Don't make the mistake of thinking winter is a good excuse to give up on yourself. There is a massive long stretch from after Succos till Chanukah. It's a great time to join an exercise class. (I notice my classes are fullest at this time.) Getting out during the winter may take an extra effort, but the physical and social dividends are worth it. Who wants to be stuck inside, glued to the radiator, when you can be out there having fun and seeing old friends at the same time?

In a nutshell, let's sum it all up:

- ✔ We are not going to get down about our weight or cry over spilt milk;
- ✔ We are going to do something about it. We are going to use the past as an impetus for the future;
- ✔ We are going to do it *now* — right after Yom Tov, so that by the time we thaw out of the Ice Age and enter a bright, light, glorious summer, we will also feel bright, light, and glorious;
- ✔ We are going to take full advantage of the upcoming weeks of routine (after Succos) to concentrate on our new project of focusing on ourselves and trimming up.

Chapter 9

— ◆ ◆ ◆ —

Yom Tov – Specific Yomim Tovim

Y ou might have noticed that some issues, such as fasting (Yom Kippur) or partying (Purim) have not been neatly cubbyholed in the previous general section on Yom Tov. Therefore, this chapter aims to provide a comfortable new cubbyhole for them, so let's address some of the specific scenarios that arise with particular Yomim Tovim.

After Rosh Hashanah

Fasting After Feasting: Concentrating on the Misconception

I can just hear that little voice in your head saying, "It's OK to eat whatever I want on Rosh Hashanah because the day after Rosh Hashanah is a fast day." But let's look at the logistics of losing weight after overeating for two days by abstaining for one:

Mrs. Average (average weight, height, shoe size, hair, etc.) only needs about 2,000 calories per day to maintain her weight. We all need to burn off, lose, eradicate, or zap 3,500 calories to lose one measly pound. This means that it would take *two* **fast days**, not just one, to burn off one pound. (2,000 × 2 = 4,000). Most of us will eat well over 2,000 calories on each day of Rosh Hashanah, so we would probably need a week's worth of fasting. You'll be relieved to know that I don't suggest you try this. I'm just trying to put things into perspective.

> *This chapter should help make each Jewish Festival the elevating inspiration intended — not the dieting disasters they so often are.*

Erev Yom Kippur

When I was a naïve newlywed, a friend who was well-versed in such matters commented that erev Yom Kippur is one of the busiest days of the year. I had no idea what she meant. We went out for the seudos, came home to an immaculate apartment, and perused the ArtScroll handbook about Yom Kippur. Many years later, I can nod in assent at the truth of her statement.

Preparing, serving, and clearing two meals; cooking something else for the children to eat on Yom Kippur itself; making 101 phone calls to 101 busy phones (they're all doing the same thing) to convey your "fast well" and "please forgive me" wishes; making the house look Yom Tov-dik; shlugging kapporas[1]; davening; and trying to keep the decibel levels below ear-splitting is quite a tall order. Some might even call it stressful. And whenever faced with stress, we have an increased tendency to forego our good intentions. (Yes, it's a shame that happens on the day before Yom Kippur.)

On top of being busy and sending our resolve on a mini-vacation, on erev Yom Kippur we are assured that it is a mitzvah to eat. Talk about enticing. Not just to eat one meal, mind you, but the mitzvah lasts *ALL* day. So whatever morsel, mountain, or munchie you crave, you have the assurance that you are creating angels with each bite. (They don't tell you about the extra pounds you are also creating.) What better excuse do we need in our holy pursuit of such easy mitzvos?

Although it would be wonderful to eat our way into Paradise, we don't want to eat our way into the next world prematurely, G-d forbid. Therefore, some degree of control is in order. We don't want to undo all our good work so far. And, in our heart of hearts, we know that the mitzvah is not a blanket statement enforcing an ultra fress-out.[2] So, how *are* we going to face the temptation of overindulging? Let's start by addressing the temptation of *under*indulging…(I always did like being contrary).

Look After Yourself (and Don't Feel Guilty About It)

With that busy schedule taking place all around you, some might even protest that they are too busy to eat (it takes all sorts…). Although we may laugh at this supposition, it can happen that with all the hullabaloo of jumping up to answer the phone and "Who wants more chicken?" and "Stop that right now or you don't get dessert!" etc., you might risk facing the fast either not as satisfied as you would have liked, or, worse still, thirsty from the minute you light candles.

Although I know it sounds like a tough policy, it's worth prioritizing your own needs before your children's. Remember: *You* are fasting — your kids are not. To win over the softies amongst us, think of it as a long-term investment for your childrens' sake — no one wants a grumpy, grouchy mother because she's overly hungry and thirsty before she even begins the twenty-five-hour countdown.

---

[1] An ancient custom involving chickens or money, customarily performed the day before Yom Kippur.
[2] Binge.

So, let Shnocky cry a minute while you finish your plate; take a minute longer to drink an extra glass of water *before* you feel thirsty; and let someone else answer the phone (or, dare I suggest, just let it ring?) so that you have time to chew your food properly instead of knocking it down the hatch so you can talk to Auntie Miriam.

Listen To Your Body

Yes, it's a mitzvah to eat on erev Yom Kippur; yes, you are going to need to eat in order to manage the fast well, BUT that does NOT mean that you should overload your stomach.

Feeling uncomfortably full (when you can feel the skirt digging into your waist; when you are fully conscious, almost painfully so, of your stomach and its contents), is not only a big, bad policy for dieters (see the finger-wag?), but it is also unhealthy.

It is unhealthy because overloading any organ in the body puts excessive strain on it. Just like a weak knee joint will complain to you by making you feel pain when you walk or jog (in order to make you stop), so, too, an overfull tummy will ache when you have put too much food in it. We all know that glumpy feeling after the second bowl of cholent. This is the body's way of warning you to stop abusing it. (And you just thought you were full.)

If you eat an excessive amount before the fast (i.e., more than your normal daily fare), then you may feel even hungrier than usual after you have digested the food. (Although there are several reasons for this, we shall avoid digression and remain stoically relevant.) Suffice it to say that the more you have expanded your stomach with food, the more you may feel hunger as it empties.

Therefore, *do* make sure to eat, just keep an eye on the internal barometer and don't overload the ole tum. (See also "Listen to Your Body," page 177.)

What To Eat (and What To Avoid) Before the Fast

Everyone will tell you something different when it comes to what will ensure a smooth-sailing, easy fast. If you've been doing the same thing for years and fasting merrily along, stay with good old tried and tested. Don't spoil the good for the perfect. But if you're the type who hasn't yet tuned in to the way your body likes to stoke its fuel, then try one or two of these tips.

The foods listed below have specific reasons why they can help reduce hunger, tiredness, and irritability.[3]

---

[3] As Yom Kippur is a long fast day, a certain level of hunger, fatigue, etc., can be expected. Even the most nutritious of food eaten before the fast is going to be digested, leaving your stomach empty. Our aim is to try to be realistic in our expectations, and therefore try to diminish, not eliminate, the negative effects of fasting.

Grapes

Grapes have a high level of natural sugars called fructose. These sugars are readily absorbed by the blood and have a beneficial effect on the body, particularly before a fast day.

Grapes are also a relatively water-packed fruit. So, not only are you getting a whack of natural energy-boosting sugar, you're also getting extra liquid.

Carbohydrates

Carbohydrates (rice, pasta, whole-wheat bread, etc.), which are foods high in complex sugars, provide the body with long-lasting energy. They also provide the body with glucose, which is turned into energy. This glucose *slowly* dissipates into the blood stream and helps to keep your energy levels raised, or at least on an even keel.

Note that when carbohydrates are eaten exclusively on their own, they are not particularly satisfying by themselves, nor do they satisfy for long. Therefore, eating too many calories from carbohydrates is easy. By adding protein and a bit of fat to every meal (e.g., tuna fish with low-fat mayonnaise on toast), including snacks, you will feel satisfied for longer.

Some people maintain that it is especially conducive to a good fast to eat plenty of carbohydrates on the days preceding the fast in order to bring the glycogen (energy) levels up to the maximum. Similarly, they promote the idea of drinking grape juice just before the fast, to help start the fast off with a high blood sugar level. Just take care not to overdose on the stuff — at 92 calories per cup, it can be "expensive" water in dieting terms.

Proteins

A word about those fashionable protein-exclusive diets…

If you eat only protein just before the fast, bear in mind that to process the protein, your body needs lots of water. As a result, you will be drawing water away from your body cells, drying them out instead of packing them with water. While you *will* lose weight, most of the weight you lose will be liquids your body needs for those essential functions like breathing and digesting and…well, all those other healthy activities.

Therefore, to avoid the ill effects of fasting, you should try to avoid eating an excessive amount of protein in the twenty-four hours directly preceding the fast.

The bottom line? Skip the exclusively carbohydrate or exclusively protein menus in the lead up to Yom Kippur and go for a satisfying mixture of both, with a dash of fat for good measure. (I can see you smiling already.)

Avoid Chocolate, Sweets, High-Sugar Desserts

Getting déjà vu? Yep, you've seen this one before — it's written in all that boring literature you pick up at the doctor's office (and we also mentioned it earlier in "Sweet Treats," page 98). Here, however, the reasons for avoiding these temptations are slightly different.

Besides providing calories without much nutritional value, this type of sugar also provides artificial highs. These highs inevitably lead quickly to energy lows, which are devastating for a fast. This is also detrimental to a diet, because when you are on that low-swing you feel that the only way to get up high again is to have more sugar which, of course, means more calories. This is a vicious circle. You want more chocolate and then more and more.

Although sugar is rapidly converted into glycogen and carried to the muscles, you don't want "straight" sugar (sweets, honey, chocolate bars) because it's *hydrophilic* (hydro=water; philic=loving), which means that it pulls water from body tissues into your intestinal tract. That can increase dehydration and make you nauseous.

In other words, avoid what's no good for you, especially before a fast.

Fats

Fats have double the amount of calories (energy) per gram than either proteins or carbohydrates. That's why it's usually a good idea to avoid too many of them when dieting. But before a fast they can come in really handy, because fats also take longer to digest than proteins and carbs. Longer to digest means feeling fuller for longer. And that's a good feeling for a fast day.

Hold it right there…just in case your hand went zooming towards those french fries and pizza…we're talking moderation (as always) when it comes to fat. A dollop's OK, especially before a fast, but fried fish and chips, well, that's kinda cruel to your digestive system.

Drink

You know this one already,[4] but because it's sooooo important and relevant to fasting, I'm going to take the liberty of expanding on it just a "drop."

Boring but important fact: It's very important to drink enough before the fast.

This is because your body needs water to stay hydrated (i.e., the body cells need to be buoyant and full of water) to function at optimal levels. As we can't drink **on** Yom Kippur, it is even more important to try and drink **before** Yom Kippur.

Yes, it is true that some of the liquid you ingest will automatically be lost during normal bodily functions (like going to the bathroom), but the body will retain some of it. It will therefore take longer to feel dehydrated and suffer from its nasty little followers called fatigue, I-just-can't-get-off-the-sofa, and not-now-I've-got-a-headache.

---

[4] See "Think-Drink," page 174.

An added bonus of drinking a lot is that you will feel full on calorie-free liquid. This will help to diminish the need to eat every single amazingly delicious dish that you have prepared.

To help the body combat thirst, you should drink plenty of non-sweetened liquids before the fast, but also spend the fast in a cool place to cut down on perspiration, and refrain from activities that raise the body temperature (you get the day off from aerobics).

Bites, Licks, and Tastes

No prizes for guessing where to find Mommy on erev Yom Kippur. Just open the kitchen door. You may well find yourself puttering about your kitchen for the day's duration. This means that you will automatically be surrounded by food: its preparation, its serving, and its clearing up. This is asking for trouble when it comes to B, L and T. (See "BLT," page 105).

Here are three new tips for the price of one (always one to give you value for money…): **Know *what* you are eating. Know *when* you are eating. Know *that* you are eating.** Pin it on your fridge. It's a good one.

Even if it is a mitzvah, it's still calories. (Like any mitzvah, you need the right intention).

Fasting and Weight Loss (What Fasting Does To Your Body and Why it's Not a Good Long-Term Idea)

Fasting results in low energy, weakness, and light-headedness, not real weight loss. Any loss is water and muscle, not fat, and you will regain the weight when you start eating again (I know, it's sad). Contrary to some popular trends of thought, fasting does not clear toxins from the body either — just the opposite: Ketones can build up when carbohydrates are not available for energy, and that amassing of ketones stresses the kidneys and can ultimately be harmful to your health (see "The Complete Scarsdale Medical Diet," page 23).

In short, don't be deceived by your bathroom scale, even if you see your weight reading plummet. After the fast, you can expect to regain that weight when you start eating normally again. Sorry about that.

All Change

In order to reduce your suffering from withdrawal symptoms that can make it even harder to get through the fast, from Rosh Hashanah onwards make a conscious effort to reduce your intake of coffee, tea, cigarettes, chocolate, or anything else you consume habitually or compulsively.

Some people recommend varying meal schedules in the days preceding the fast. The hunger most of us experience may not really be caused by a lack of nutrients, but rather by having been conditioned to receive food at expected times.

After Yom Kippur

It is not unusual to find that you are not even hungry anymore at the end of a fast. No, sorry to disappoint you, you haven't turned into a living angel. Your body has merely adjusted to the state of starvation and has made the necessary modifications. However, you do have to eat (music to your ears). But before we unleash our desires upon the entire remaining contents of the fridge, we should note the following:

Eat Slowly

Be gentle to your digestive system: it's been through a lot (haven't we all). First you stuff it as though you were going on a ten-month world tour without so much as a soup crouton; then you abruptly tell it to go into complete hibernation for twenty-five hours; then you resume eating again, in the middle of the night, with rich Yom Tov foods. So, be gentle and kind to your stomach and it will be kind to you. Eat slowly.

Chew

Sounds obvious, but how many of us take the time to chew our food properly? Chewing is especially important when breaking a fast, as we want to gently rev up our digestive system to cope with food again.

There are important enzymes in the saliva that act on the food and start off the whole digestive process.[5] If you skip this stage, you are asking your other organs (including the stomach) to compensate for this and they may well complain (sometimes quite embarrassingly — be warned) about being overworked.

Pause

Let your body readjust to the demands you are now going to place on it.

Give your stomach a chance to tell your brain that you are full. If you eat too quickly, you will end up eating more than you really need. Who wants unnecessary calories?

Pause in between courses, and pause after a drink. Take it easy.

Besides for the physiological benefits (of you feeling comfortable and in tune with your body's needs), pausing also aids dieting.

Stop When You Are Full

We have a section "Listen to Your Body" in our Yom Tov chapter. We have a section "Tune in to How Your Body Feels" in our Practical Tips chapter. So here, we'll call this section "Stop When You Are Full." Variety's the spice of life.

You are not morally obligated to eat everything that you could have had on Yom Kippur and didn't. Just because you have made a banquet suitable for your whole tribe of in-laws doesn't mean that you **have** to have every course.

---

[5] See "Digestion," page 396.

I know it's a lovely feeling to have all those points/treats in the bank just waiting to be spent, but try to remain in control — remember, Succos is just around the corner.

Again, listen to your body; if it is telling you that it is full (even if your brain can't believe you are really full after a cup of tea and a cracker), it's telling you for a reason — so stop.

Wishing you all an easy lead-up to the fast (without stress or indigestion), an easy fast on Yom Kippur itself (every minute is a mitzvah), and an easy fast-break (although not quite breakfast). G'mar Chasimah Tovah and a Gut Gebentshte Yahr.

Nine Tips for Chanukah: One for Each Candle

(Plus one for the Shammash)

It's dark and cold outside (unless you are on the sunny side of the world, down-under or in South Africa). It's warm and light inside. The menorah is lighting up the darkness and the aroma of freshly fried doughnuts and latkes wafts through the house. It's early evening. You're decidedly hungry. You're probably going to sit around the table for at least a half-hour's break. You crave a nice cup of tea or coffee. It'll warm you up. How can you have a cup of tea on its own? It's somehow too wet without something to go with it...and those mouth-watering doughnuts are just being brought to the table...

Let's add some serious rethinking to those aromas if these doughnuts are going to form the basis of an extra special early supper.

How can you resist temptation? How can you maintain any semblance of restraint when all those oily goodies are going to stare you right in the face for an entire week?

Here's a list of tips to keep next to the menorah, somewhere between the matches, candles, oil, and Maoz Tzur[6] cards. Holding on to it may be just the thing you need to keep your hands off all those fluffy latkes.

Time-Bound Sit-Around

We are not talking about a major Yom Tov, where we have two heavy meals each day and nosh in between. We are talking about a cup of coffee, a treat, and a little sit down for half an hour. This means that in the worst-case scenario, you will only have to exercise supreme self-control for thirty minutes (OK, forty, if you include cleaning up).

For those of you who are reading this and thinking, "Not in my house! We have at least an hour-long suppertime followed by games, sketches, and family entertainment...all while 'polishing off' the dining room table." Although your exposure to forbidden fruits may be slightly longer, it still doesn't compare to the repeated, lengthy sittings of a major Yom Tov. (Besides, you can clear the table before you bring out the dreidel/newest board game...)

---

[6] Probably the most famous Chanukah song.

Putting this into perspective can help us summon up the necessary reserves of willpower. Most people, when pressed, can concentrate on their teenager's mental arithmetic, run in place, or enthusiastically clean their stove for a half-hour period. It's not so long. Therefore, it's also not so hard.

If, however, you do happen to have long, drawn-out sittings at this time, you can try clearing away any high-calorie foods before sitting down to a game or shmooze. Leaving healthy snacks and fruit bowls on the table will still give a festive atmosphere.

Got boys coming home at different times? Leaving food around for hours at a time is asking for trouble. Why not prepare a dinner plate for each of them and then execute your clear-up?

Rewording Rewarding

We know menorah-lighting is coming up later on in the day. If you are the sort who zealously guards your chocolate bar (hidden and locked away in the fridge) for an end-of-day, well-deserved treat each night, think again.

Although rewarding yourself on a regular basis is an excellent means of utilizing a sense of positive reinforcement (see "Rewards," page 51), rethinking exactly when that reward is a reward and when it is an outright excess is a timely pursuit at this particular mini Yom Tov. Having chocolate at menorah-lighting time as a reward *in addition* to other Chanukah treats falls into this latter category.

As we know full well that our resistance will be low when we serve all those for-Chanukah treats, maybe it's appropriate to utilize the "reward concept" at this time. This means skipping the midnight chocolate and substituting it for a lighting-time yum-yum instead. You'll be rewarding yourself for "good behavior" dependent on the previous twenty-four-hour period from candle-lighting to candle-lighting, instead of celebrating it at the stroke of midnight.

A word of caution. A reward is a reward when the goal has been accomplished. If you managed to forego all other temptations since the last candle-lighting ritual, then you deserve the reward. If not…guess who ends up with a carrot stick with her cup of tea.

Be strict to be successful.

Daylight Saving

Making Chanukah the official time when you are going to reward yourself means that it's worth saving up calories/treats during those other times, so that you can truly enjoy yourself while you bask in the warm glow of family and friends.

Knowing, right from breakfast time, that you are planning to spend your daily treats at candle-lighting time means you have an incentive to exert self-control for the entire time leading up to the big event.

Due to the oily nature of the goodies involved, it's particularly worthwhile to save up calories with this in mind. As a general rule, frying will double the calorie content of a food. For example, three slices of toast contain 235 calories, but three slices of fried bread contain more than 500. One gram of oil/fat contains twice the number of calories as one gram of carbohydrates. In fried doughnut language that could mean 250 calories, versus nearly half that amount for an equivalently sized baked bun.

That's the cost for *one* doughnut. Not the extra one that somehow landed up on your plate because the first was so good, nor the other half of Shnocky's because he couldn't manage to finish his. Subsequent mental arithmetic required.

Caution: Portion

One of the most effective ways to counteract such tendencies is to control your portion size.

Yes, you can afford to have a treat for Chanukah without it impeding your weight loss. Yes, you are serving doughnuts. And when you serve yourself, it's OK to make sure it's the most mouth-watering one. But maybe cut it up (when you see two halves, it can seem like more food quantitively). And definitely adopt the mindset that "what you see is what you get," i.e., that chosen doughnut is for you, but the rest are totally off limits. Likewise when serving french fries: Know that the controlled quantity you serve yourself is totally in order and may very well not impede your weight loss. Not so for all those extra unaccounted-for french fries that wiggle their magical way down the hatch.

Imagine you are shopping. The controlled portion you put into your cart is paid for. Everything else in the shop is not. If you take anything extra, you're stealing. So, too, with your plate: When you have specified your permitted portion, you can relax and enjoy it. It's been accounted for, saved for, and "paid for." When you start dipping into everyone else's portions (including the free-for-all mass of plates in the middle of the table), you are, in fact, *stealing* yourself out of a weight loss.

When it comes to serving everyone else, if you've got the courage, try persuading a big daughter/seminary girl/husband to serve in your place. (That way you might feel too embarrassed to ask for seconds.)

Fill Up During the Day

Another effective suggestion to help counteract the tendency to overindulge at menorah-lighting time is to be wise during the day.

Remember that foods high in fiber are low in calories and will satiate your appetite for longer. Choose whole-wheat bread, whole-wheat pasta, jacket potatoes with baked beans, spinach, broccoli, or leeks for lunch, and a banana for dessert.

Try not to let yourself get hungry. It's so much harder to maintain your resolve with a growling tummy (besides, you'll end up growling as well).

Drink Something First

Take the edge off that desire for latkes and make sure to drink two glasses of water before you tuck in.

Have a Mini Snack Before the Goodies

You know you are going to have your treat in a minute, but you really are quite hungry. Sirens should be going off at full blast. Be warned. We can rarely make logical decisions when we are hungry. So try having a healthy snack first (rice cakes with topping/jacket potato/fruit/low-fat yogurt) or a mug of vegetable or mushroom soup, and then you can allow yourself a guilt-free dessert. This way, you can savor the treat instead of utilizing it to satisfy your hunger.

Look After Yourself

In keeping with the good old tradition, most yummy delectables that are served over Chanukah are fried. Need I say more? Basically, when we are talking about cake or cookies being high in calories, we are talking about cosmic-heights when it comes to frying.

It's all too easy to adopt an "all or nothing" frame of mind when it comes to anything remotely resembling cake. You might want to plonk all forbidden fruits in the same basket. When you feel that you have dipped into this bounty, you might think, "What's the difference, it's all calories?" True, even low-fat cakes will cost you calories, but we're talking serious overdraft when we talk about frying.

Whereas it is possible not to feel deprived and to still "have your cake and eat it too," you might want to take the time to make an alternative to the standard greasy fare. This way you will be able to enjoy yourself without the excessive extra calories. One never knows, maybe your family will also like the alternative. (Make sure to save some for yourself if they do.)

Here are two lower-calorie alternatives to start with:

Swiss Roll

  2 large eggs
  ⅓ cup superfine sugar
  ⅓ cup self-rising flour

Directions:

> ✔ Break eggs into bowl, whisk lightly, add sugar, and whisk thoroughly until thick, creamy, and almost white in color.
>
> ✔ Lightly fold flour into mixture.
>
> ✔ Place in a Swiss Roll cake tin lined with parchment paper.

✔ Bake at 425 degrees Fahrenheit for about 7–8 minutes (do not overbake or it will crack when rolled).

✔ Turn onto sugared parchment paper. Remove lining paper, and trim edges.

✔ Spread warm jam onto the surface area quickly.

✔ Working from the narrow end, make the first roll with your fingers, then continue by drawing paper away from you over the Swiss Roll.

✔ Leave to cool, resting on the seam. Dredge with sugar.

1 Medium Slice[7] = 135 Calories[8]

Rugelach

2 cups water
¼ cup fresh yeast
8 tablespoons sugar
½ cup oil
2 eggs
2 lbs. bread flour
spray oil
cocoa/cinnamon sugar

Directions:

✔ Pour two cups of hand-hot water into a bowl, add yeast and sugar, and leave for a few minutes to ferment.

✔ Put oil and eggs into the mixer, add the yeast and water mixture, and then add the flour. Knead well.

✔ Leave mixture to rise for 1 hour.

✔ Roll out dough, spray oil the surface, and cover with cocoa or cinnamon sugar.

✔ Roll into a log.

✔ Bake at 350 degrees Fahrenheit for about 20 minutes or until golden.

1 Small Bun (and I mean small)[9] = 142 Calories

As additional measures for siphoning off all that extra oil, try the following alternatives:

◆ Fry your latkes using spray oil or, better yet, bake them;

◆ Try making potatoes into french fry-shapes and spraying them with oil and then baking;

◆ Make up some microwave "light" popcorn for a handy nosh.

---

[7] Thickness equivalent to a squashed-down thumb.
[8] This is a general guide only, as these figures will vary depending on the recipe used.
[9] Pinch index finger to meet thumb and you have the "OK" size of small.

Watch out for marzipan,
Cakes, nuts, and cream flan,
Although they don't qualify as oily as some,
They pack in the calories quite royally on mom.

Leave the Leftovers

You've controlled yourself all the way from Maoz Tzur to Al Hanissim. But now comes a real killer: What will happen to all those remaining french fries and squishy bits of cake and tiny, hardly-there leftovers?

Psychologically, it's hard to see our own hard work go into the garbage. At least someone should get pleasure from our efforts. After all, it's such a waste, such *baal tashchis*[10]…But it's worse *baal tashchis* for **you** to be the garbage can, so scrape them all away.

Better yet, if your lovely kind daughter is still around, ask her to clear those remains with which you will have problems.

All those leftovers seem much more inconsequential when we are embarking on the journey from table (clearing it) to kitchen. Answer me honestly, how many french fries have you eaten on such a journey when no one was looking? I rest my case. (See also "BLT," page 105.)

The joy of Chanukah is not just inherent in the doughnuts and latkes. There's a lot to be grateful for…the miracles that occurred at this time, our health, our community, our families. We have each other. You'll remember the smile you received when you hugged Shnocky as the candles cast a warm glow across his face for much longer than you'll remember the taste of those oily treats. Let's create memories we can cherish — not nightmares of lost opportunities. Let's take ourselves in hand so that we can truly have a *LIGHT* Chanukah. Gut Chanukah.

Purim

Purim is the day that defies the force of sanity.

Let's picture the scene. From the minute the semi be-costumed children pound at your bedroom door at the first signs of dawn, the spirit of the day is intensely joyful, mixed together with liberal doses of exuberance and excitement. Shpielers[11] who have had a drink or ten leave their reticence somewhere next to their shtenders.[12] Children are in permanent hyper-mode. Serious people smile, dance, and sing. It's party time-come-carnival in one.

This whirlwind of buzzing activity and surprises around every corner can undo the resolve and self-control of even the most stalwart, carrot-loving dieter.

---

[10] Wastefulness.
[11] House-hopping merry-makers.
[12] Lecterns.

Then there is the nosh. Boy, is there nosh. Every counter, table, chair, and carpet is covered with the most beautifully presented, attractive, and enticing pleasure-parcels. Each one contains more calories than the last. There's not even the option to hesitate to open up a closed package, because the kids have gotten there first. Chips spill out, chocolates sit within inches of reach, cream cakes wait in bite-size pincer-grip cupcake holders, just begging to be picked. The aroma of Bissli and Pringles hangs in the air, further awakening an already alert desire.

Oh dear.

Not much comes through the door in the way of tasty, low-calorie, tempting, diet-proof goodies (unless it's from someone trying to give you a hint).

What are we going to do? Should we give up before we start (and undo all our hard work till now)? Or should we see what we can do to help brace ourselves for the avalanche of temptation that's right around the corner?

Let's not give up — at least not without a fight. Let's take a closer look at the practical side of preparing ourselves so that we can still enjoy the day for the fun-day that it is, without having to contend with any extra unwanted pounds in leftovers (besides, there'll be enough leftovers to last till next Purim).

Our greatest battle-planning strategy advantage is that we know that Purim is coming. (Yes, I always say this. That's because I always have to.) It's not as if the owner of your favorite delicatessen has shown up on your doorstep for a surprise visit, laden with free samples. You know the time and place of Purim (even if that's about all you know to expect). Therefore, you can plan ahead. It doesn't have to catch you off-guard, arms up in surprise, exclaiming, "Well, what could I do?" You can do plenty. At the very least, your efforts might curtail your overindulgences; at the very best, your efforts may be well rewarded.

Our plan of attack starts as early as…

The Day Before Tanis Esther

OK, let's resign ourselves to the fact that this is our last day of "normal" for forty-eight hours. The kids are still in school, we can still hear ourselves think, and our resolve is not yet shaky. We are still feeling fit and well (we're not fasting yet) and we've taken the phone off the hook for a break. Let's chap-a-rein.[13]

 Lists

If you are the list-type (if you're not, it's a good time to start), you'll find your lists invaluable. Not only are you less likely to forget something important (like Shnocky's green face paint), but you'll also feel more in control (of a control-defying environment).

In addition to the obvious lists of "Things to Do," "Mishloach Manos Recipients,"[14] "People to Call," etc., let's add another list (list-people are already getting excited — they just love making new lists): "My Eating Plan."

---

[13] Let's take advantage.
[14] Food package recipients.

This will definitely require a little of that lovely peace and quiet that still finds you in a tidy, calm kitchen so that you can think it through. When you're done, post the list on the fridge so that you'll pass it throughout the day on Purim.

While you are making this list, you might find that you will need to buy something that you are planning to eat. For example, checked chopped lettuce, fresh pineapple, your favorite spring water with a hint of lemon, etc. You've still got plenty of time to shop so that you don't end up without any healthy alternatives to all that junk food. True, you'll still have to decide whether or not to eat the right food. But if it's not even accessible by being in the house, you won't even have a decision to make.

You can try breaking down this list into something resembling the following table, bearing in mind the upcoming changes to routine:

Before Tanis Esther		Check
Breakfast		
Lunch		
Supper		
Snacks/Extras		
After the Tanis		
Supper		
Snacks/Extras		
Purim Day		
Breakfast		
Lunch		
Supper		
Snacks/Extras		

I know what you're going to say — "Since when do we have breakfast, lunch, and supper on Purim…?" We'll get there in a minute (or as fast as you can read…); for now, let's just fill in the gaps in terms of what would be ideal.

Once you have filled in all the healthy alternatives you plan on having, you can quickly check-box your way through your day. It's easier to check exactly what you are eating, as you go along, than it is to write it down; remember, it's going to be a wild day. If you know what extras you have had (or have resisted), you'll know what leeway you have left to spend. This type of consciousness will preempt the "Oh I've blown it now so I might as well continue splurging" mentality.

Shopping

When you are making your lists of things to buy, consider adding light, water-packed foods, such as celery sticks, or fiber-rich snacks, such as whole-wheat crackers, to your list. Low-fat yogurts are another good in-between food. Why not make these foods a family affair? After all, the in-house fasters may also appreciate having light snacks available a couple of hours after they have officially finished breaking their fast with the meal. If they're out on the table for everyone, you'll be more inclined to go for them yourself.

Remember, there's lots of in-between snack times over Purim. There's Purim night, after you've heard the Megillah and find yourself hungry again; there's all those awkward non-breakfast/lunch/suppertimes on Purim day; when your tummy reminds you at 3pm that you haven't eaten any real food since you woke up; and there's motzei Purim, when the house looks like it's been hit by a tornado (it has) and it takes you till 2am to tidy up. (Guess who's going to be hungry at 2am when the last time you ate was 5pm?)

 Make Soups for the Troops

Seeing as we are at war with nosh (also, with Haman, *et al.*), we need to keep everyone well fed, warm, and happy. Making double portions of soup before or even during the fast can cut your work in half. This way you can serve half to break the fast, and the other half in the Purim seudah itself. Try to save a little soup for yourself and you will have an easy, instant, ready-for-repentance recipe for Shushan Purim.

 Stress-Busters

Bearing in mind that one of the most compelling reasons why we turn to food is stress,[15] it makes sense to focus on stress-busting a potentially stress-bursting time.

Mishloach Manos:

Although you're busy, it's a good idea to try to make headway by preparing the essential Mishloach Manos (i.e., the ones that will get you the mitzvah) in advance. Once you have taken care of these, you will be free to concentrate on helping the rest of the family with theirs. Doing this while your tolerance-tank is still full (as opposed to when you're not feeling 100% over the fast) means that you will be working more efficiently (and more happily) than leaving the bulk of the work for Tanis Esther.

I know some really (sickeningly) efficient people who make up their Mishloach Manos weeks in advance. (You know, the type who've been collecting all those used vanilla essence bottles since last Purim). Listen, if you can start Pesach cleaning in Shevat, you can start Mishloach Manos making by Rosh Chodesh Adar.

---

[15] See "Stress," page 64.

Forget-Me-Nots:

With all the buzz and clutter it's easy to forget some of the most important mitzvos of the day. Therefore, remember to put wine on your shopping list and visit the bank for small cash denominations for the shpielers. Better yet, make a "his" and "her" list (like those cute matching towels), and stick this one on his. Allocate an envelope for Matanos L'Evyonim[16] (and put it somewhere safe and accessible). Believe me, you don't want to have to go to the bank on Tanis Esther, when there's another 101 things that demand your immediate attention and you're facing an ever-nearing deadline (even more so on Purim).

Take it easy, don't deny yourself a break from the mounting demands, and be as kind to yourself as you are to others. Oh, and if you're making everyone a cup of coffee, don't forget to make one for yourself as well. You deserve it.

Tanis Esther

Uncle Moishy's Purim tunes are blasting at top volume. The kids, like wound-up springs, are getting more and more psyched with each passing day. Mommy's busy stocking up the freezer with all the Purim goodies while wiping chocolatey hands on her apron to appropriately "oooh" and "aaaah" at Shnocky's made-in-school Purim costume.

D-Day (or should I say "P-Day?") is getting nearer. The excitement is as tangible as the newly blossomed springtime buds. But before the party begins, we need to brace ourselves for a fast day. A day of introspection and abstinence automatically calms the frenzied build up and helps us focus. Let's see what we can do to help ourselves on Tanis Esther.

For what to eat before a fast and other useful tips, see earlier in this chapter, "Erev Yom Kippur," page 193.

 Consider the Children

Remember that the children may be at home part of the day and will need their energies channeled, even if your energies have gone to bed without you.

Some people save the children's Mishloach Manos for Tanis Esther. This keeps them occupied and involved in the anticipation of the day (as if they need any more anticipation…). If your children are all young, it's a great time to invite an older girl over to help supervise that all those winkies and chips find their way into the bags and not the tummies (at least not yet). She might welcome the break from school, or an opportunity to take her mind off the fast. Either way, she gets a mitzvah and you get an extra pair of hands.

If just the thought of all that last-minute packaging sends your blood pressure up (G-d forbid), and you prefer to do it all well in advance, maybe you could get the children to design their own "To/From" cards. The only mess this entails is scissors, crayons or felt tip markers, and clear tape. Easy entertainment. Easily cleared.

---

[16] Gifts to the poor.

Another idea: Involve them in your baking. Kids love rolling dough and making their own cookies or Hamantashen.[17] If you're baking anyway (for all those shpielers), now is a great time. Besides, by baking on a fast day, your decision to taste and test has already been conveniently made for you. (Remember, it's easier to clean up a mess than it is to deal with cranky, hyper-excited, high-strung, bored kids — and it's also quieter.)

Tiny Tots Tea-Time

I found this one scribbled down on a scrap paper last year, to remind myself to do it this year. It's a noise-reducing investment to give supper early to anyone not fasting. Yes, I know it can mean two messes, but let's loosen up on the mess-stress and resign ourselves to a messy house for the next two days. Expecting it helps with accepting it.

If the younger ones are fed in the first shift, it'll be easier for you to sit down and break your own fast with peace of mind in the second shift. If you have an externally calm environment, you are more likely to stick with your self-control in terms of food choices. Besides, you might need the time to make sure you actually do break your fast, and are not just serving food to everyone else. The older children are more likely to understand that Mom also has to sit down and eat something — now. These mature, sophisticated, caring individuals may even be able to help you with serving and clearing up (especially if you show them this part with all those compliments).

If you want your little ones up for the nighttime excitement, that's fine. But if you'd rather they weren't kvetch-pots[18] the next day, on Purim day itself, it'll be easier to get them settled into bed if you start bedtime before all the action begins.

Breaking the Fast

The fast day itself has pretty much been taken care of for us, in terms of food choices — zero. With that easy decision behind us, let's concentrate on exactly how we plan to break our fast.

See earlier in this chapter, "After Yom Kippur," page 197, for some useful tips, but while we're here, let's add a few more…

For those of you who only hear Megillah after the men come home, it's really important to make sure that you do eat *something* before you leave the house. The more you patchke[19] in the kitchen to prepare the meal for the returning men, the less time you have to refresh yourself with some timely nutrition.

Although it's lovely to be the gracious hostess and serve the men when they come home, etc., it's still important to look after yourself. In the worst case, they can continue without you if you need to go to the Megillah reading. So don't worry if everyone hasn't finished the whole meal (or even started it) by the time you have to leave — just make sure you've had something yourself.

---

[17] Triangular dough-based pastries.
[18] Crabby, cantankerous…
[19] Fuss.

If you're going to break your fast when you and the men return from Megillah, take the first twenty seconds to drink a full 8oz cup of liquid. Then you can start to serve everyone else *and* have a smile on your face at the same time.

And when you do sit down to eat, break the fast slowly, listen to your body (and waistband), and try to overcome the impulse to eat just because:

☹ Everyone else is eating;

☹ There's food right in front of you and it's the first time you've sat down all day (plonk);

☹ You feel pressured to get to the Megillah on time;

☹ You've still got so much left to do;

☹ You're stressed;

☹ You're really thirsty as opposed to hungry, but you haven't got time to distinguish between the two.

Maybe you're not hungry anymore (it can happen, especially after a fast). But it's never a good idea to let yourself go without water beyond the timespan of a fast.

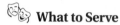 **What to Serve**

Considering our water deprivation, in addition to actually drinking, we need to focus on consuming foods that have high water content. How about having various platters of fresh vegetables cut into strips surrounding dips? Different colored peppers look so pretty, as do thin carrot sticks and cucumber sticks. They're light on the digestion, appealing to the eye, and kind to the tummy. Craving light carbohydrates with the dip? Why not display some low-calorie (high in munching value) breadsticks? At 10 calories per stick, they're light, savory, and festive looking.

How about trying the following dip, which is low in fat and calories but is tasty, savory, and healthy. When I made it for my Diet Group, they went wild over it:

Eggplant Dip

1 medium eggplant (it's the big, black vegetable somewhere between the carrots and the celery in the supermarket)
¼ raw onion
2 Tbsp. light mayonnaise
salt, pepper, and garlic powder to taste.

✔ Slice eggplant lengthways and place on baking tray (can spray-oil the top for a really roasted effect).

✔ Bake for about 45 minutes at 350 degrees Fahrenheit.

✔ In a food processor, chop the onion using the blade attachment, and add the baked eggplant when it's slightly cooled.

✔ When cool, add light mayonnaise and seasoning.

✔ Place in airtight container and refrigerate.

These dips 'n' sticks are a great food to have on the table for the ensuing hunger-attacks that come later on as well.

Labor Effective Mechanisms

That's just a fancy way of saying let's save ourselves some time and double up on our production. If you've decided to make a fancy Waldorf Salad for the Purim seudah, why not make double and serve some after the fast as well? A side dish in time, saves nine.

Set on Satisfaction

Although it's never a good idea to overfill ourselves, it's also not a good idea to be overly hungry, especially after the fast. Let's bear in mind that we'll be putting out all those frozen cakes and goodies for the shpielers and family — calories that will be sitting out looking ever-so-innocent and beautiful. If you are hungry when you're hanging around them, they're bound to disappear really quickly.

Constant Control

Although you might reason that since you've fasted you must be entitled to free reign once the party starts,[20] this mentality can easily carry over into Purim day (and beyond). There is no substitute for control. A useful aid to maintain this ever-elusive control is to keep checking off your menu plan. Keep a pen handy so it's easy to track.

Since the day lacks order, routine, or stability, it's doubly important not to let your wild external environment effect your controlled internal environment. (Basically, that means you're still in Diet Land even if your surroundings tell you otherwise.)

If you've gotten this far and can still hold your head up high, let's stay with the flow and look at how we are going to manage Purim Day.

Purim Day

First, take a deep breath and hold onto your hat. This can be a hair-raising day.

Essentially Essential

If there seem to be too many things to remember, too many things to do, and too many things to sort out, just remember the one following piece of advice: If I could fill the whole page with this tip in big, bold, 100 pitch letters, I would. It's absolutely vital to the flow of the whole day. It's this: **EAT BREAKFAST**.

Sounds simple? That's only because last Purim was a year ago and you've forgotten what it's like.

---

[20] See earlier in this chapter, "After Rosh Hashanah," page 191, where we got rid of that mistaken theory.

It's such a busy day. We're so rushed. Food is flying everywhere, and it's all the "good" stuff too. Temptation knows no bounds. Don't get me wrong: I am not saying that it's all off limits (I *am* human), but it's one thing to indulge and enjoy the taste, and it's quite another to *fill up* on chips, nuts, cake, and chocolate in place of a good square meal (on a round plate?). Besides, if you are hungry before you start indulging, chances are that you will only start tasting the yumminess after the third cake — the first three were consumed to assuage your hunger. No one wants to have to embark on a two-week program of repentance because of a one-day lapse. It's just not worth it.

Having breakfast will ensure that you have the reserves to handle all those unexpected happenings with equanimity, grace, and even a smile.

This tip goes for the whole family, by the way. No one needs additive-injected kids overdosed on sugar from the minute they wake up till bedtime. Providing them with something nutritious and proper will stand them in good stead. (Besides, then you don't have to feel guilty that they've eaten garbage for the rest of the day.)

What's easy? Mezonos rolls[21] with spreads; cereals; yogurt on its own or poured over fruit salad; crackers and herring; a selection of crackers you don't normally buy; cottage cheese inside half a melon…the options are endless. Just plan it ahead of time.

 ### No-Lunch Lunchtime

Don't know about you, but when it's one o' clock, I don't even have to look at the clock: My tummy tells me it's lunchtime. Just because it's Purim doesn't seem to make a difference, either.

Let's skip the kids this time and focus on you.

If your Purim meal is not going to start before 4pm, at lunchtime it makes sense to serve yourself (and anyone still sensible) the first course or two of what you have prepared for the seudah. The truth is, any nutritious and filling food is OK, but it might be easier to access what's already been prepared and is waiting in the fridge. If you got lucky and received some good old fashioned whole-wheat rolls and assorted dips, dive in, and make sure to invite the children to join you. They might be sick of all that junk food by then and be delighted to tuck into some real food.

Becoming overly hungry doesn't just mean low resistance to high calories. It also means headaches, fatigue, and low functionality.

 ### The Meal

If you've managed to stay on course so far, more courses are on the way.

You've cleared up a bit (oh, *there's* Shnocky, underneath the debris of chip bags…I wondered where he was), you've banned any more nosh (till tomorrow), you've set the table, and you finally get to sit down. It's this act of sitting down that I'd like to

---

[21] Haven't got time to spread hundreds of rolls for the gang? Try spreading big, fresh, long rolls and then sandwiching them together before cutting them up into bite-size pieces. It's quick and easy and just as delicious.

focus on. Or, more precisely, what exactly is next to you as you are sitting down. When you finally get to drop onto that chair, make sure all those beautiful dips and vegetable sticks are right next to you for company. Push the mayonnaise, extra challah, and soup croutons away — well out of arm's reach. Bring all those diet drinks near and take a moment or two to savor a refreshing liquid injection. Although we've said this before, it's even more appropriate at this particular time, because our feet will be begging us to stay put for a while.

Even if you chose to dip into the soup pot earlier on in the day (i.e., at normal lunchtime), there's nothing to stop you from enjoying it again. This way you will fill up on a low-calorie food with the seudah company. The fuller your tummy feels, the less the inclination to go headfirst into the chocolate mousse and apple pie (that's the theory, anyway).

The Clear-Up

The guests have gone home, the children are (at last) tucked in bed, the streets have quieted down, and you're left with the mess. It's rather like that motzei Shabbos letdown, when you feel the blues over the fact that the party's really over. It's at low times such as these that the urge to pick up and pop in all those leftovers might be too much for you to resist.

What can you do to avoid this last-of-the-day's dieting trials?

Music

I know, there's been so much noise, it might be quite nice to sit back and listen to the sound of your own breathing, but no one's going to do much sitting down now. Not in the face of cellophane, soggy cake, and trampled chips. Put the music on and lift your spirits with a tape or CD that you like. Choose something really upbeat so that you'll be inspired to wipe down the counters in time with the fast beat, or vacuum the floor to its rhythm. Make it loud so that it can permeate your soul and give you the lift you need. Don't worry about waking up the kids; at this stage, they'll sleep through anything.

Speed

Don't like cleaning up all the mess? So do it anyway — just do it quickly. Try to motivate yourself with a deadline — "Let's see if I can be finished with the kitchen in under an hour…" Or how about racing a friend — first one to finish calls the other. (The winner gets to gloat — *and* come help the other person finish up.)

Reward

No one's immune to the power of a reward. Tempt yourself with a hot bubble bath, or a cozy cup of tea with your husband, when you've finished.

Talk

Some people like to work and shmooze at the same time. Why not pick up the phone for a good ole gabfest with someone whom you haven't spoken to for a while — or choose your best friend to grumble with. By the time you've both had a laugh, the work'll be all done. (It's also rude to eat and talk at the same time, so your mouth will be busy talking instead of munching those leftovers.)

Delegate

Anyone big enough to still be awake is plenty big enough to help clear up. Unpacking the Mishloach Manos can be fun. Make piles: one for keeping (put into cupboard); one for giving away (see below); one for the kids to devour sometime before Pesach…

Distribute

If you find yourself drowning in every conceivable nosh known to mankind and realize that you are not going to be able to resist this treasure stash past tomorrow's breakfast time, give it away. There are plenty of bochurim who will gladly help you dispose of it all. If there are no bochurim near you, maybe you can take it all to a nearby hospital so that the patients (and staff) can have a party. You can create a lot of good will if you choose to give your leftover stash to your cleaning lady. (After all, it's worth buttering her up with only four weeks left till Pesach.)

Let's not get bogged down by all the things we have to do. Let's not look at the negatives of all the nosh we're denying ourselves. Let's change our mindset from the outset. It's going to be a glorious day. Our children are going to have fun. Our husbands, friends, and family are going to have fun. We're going to have fun. Purim is not about nosh. It's about the joy of the day. And there are no calories in that. Here's to a happy, jolly, freiliche, healthy, stress-free Purim. Gut Purim!

Pesach

Making Pesach is a wonderfully rewarding, fulfilling experience. The house feels clean, the children are buzzing with excitement, the fridge and freezer are stocked with mouthwatering Pesach food, and you have the deep-seated satisfaction of knowing that you were the primary catalyst in making it all happen.

But as my grandmother always used to say, "You don't get aught for naught." You don't get something for nothing. Pesach also brings with it deadlines to meet, upheaval, lack of sleep, and a seemingly insurmountable workload piled onto an already existing tight schedule. Any ensuing stress will usually result in mommy prioritizing everything and everyone else other than herself. And as dieting requires focusing on oneself, guess what's first to go? The kitchen resembles a war-zone; no one can find the bag of sugar; the milk next to the front door (the fridge is now

Pesachdik) has gone sour; and everyone wants lunch. Enter tired, hassled, hungry housewife, exit plateful of oven fries and pareve sausages — from table to tum.

Ever the advocate of forewarned is forearmed, let's break down the potential areas of trouble and try to find some soothing solutions.

Let's kick-off with a very timely strategy to handle the befores, durings, and afters of Pesach.

Before Pesach

For all the weeks of physical labor and head-work that go into making Pesach, we still have one advantage (while we flick, panic-stricken, through the weeks turned days on the calendar): We sure know it's coming. (I know, we've said this before, but the truth is that it's worth saying each time.) We can utilize this awareness to provide some very positive dividends.

The tips below don't take up much time, energy, or mental space (there are too many lists in there anyway). They just require an attitude. Let's not throw caution to the winds over these final days of crème de la crème busyness. Let's hang on (for dear life) and adopt a positive mental response to our present situation.

Cook Before You Leap

If your first steps to Pesach usually find you with scrubber in one hand and Mr. Clean in the other, stop in your disinfecting tracks. Try cooking for the "week before" Pesach as the first step towards making Pesach. No, I don't mean walking into the Pesach kitchen. I mean making extra quantities of nutritious, healthy meals in the days when opening the kitchen cupboards still finds flour and pasta.

This way, you will be able to fill up on something low-calorie while enjoying the ease of not having to make the meal from scratch amidst all the pre-Pesach hullaballoo. You can either double the family-size spaghetti with meat sauce (serve half, freeze half), or portion out individual meals, all wrapped and ready to go into the oven or microwave — especially for you. (Remember to label them well, especially if they contain chometz.[22]) If the family is going to dine on fried fish and oven latkes, you can sit all smug (and slim) and dip into your airplane-style low-fat alternative. Even if you're not on a plane, you're still getting somewhere.

Here are some good, one pot, low-fat, easily frozen meal ideas for the balebusta who means business when it comes to dieting before Pesach.

---

[22] A general term for all food and drink made from wheat, barley, rye, oats, spelt or their derivatives. Chometz is forbidden on Pesach because it is leavened.

Spaghetti Bolognaise (Serves six)

spray oil
4–5 medium onions
2 lbs. chopped meat, extra-lean
2 cups water
4½ lbs. frozen carrots
2 cloves garlic
2 cans chopped tomatoes
salt & pepper
1 lb. spaghetti

Directions:

✔ Spray oil over bottom of a big (pressure cooker-size) pot.

✔ Chop onions and fry until golden brown.

✔ Add meat and continue to fry.

✔ When the meat is brown, add the water and remaining ingredients except the spaghetti.

✔ Bring to a boil and then simmer for about 2 hours.

✔ Turn off heat and set aside.

✔ About 20 minutes before you want to serve, reboil and add spaghetti.

Rice Stew (Serves six)

spray oil
4–5 onions
2 lbs. cubed stew meat
6 cups water
4½ lbs. frozen carrots
1 lb. mushrooms (optional)
spices, salt & pepper
3 cups rice

Directions:

✔ Spray oil over bottom of big (pressure cooker-size) pot.

✔ Chop onions and fry until golden brown.

✔ Add meat and continue to fry.

✔ When the meat is brown, add 2 cups of water and remaining ingredients except the rice.

✔ Bring to a boil and then simmer for about 2 hours.

✔ Remove from heat.

✔ About 30 minutes before you want to serve, add the remaining 4 cups of water and bring to a boil.

✔ Add rice. Bring back to a boil and simmer for 15 minutes.

✔ Turn off the heat and let stand for ten minutes before serving.

Soup-Er Suggestion

You can even freeze family or individual portions of vegetable soups in advance. (After all, who's got the time to make a delicious veggie soup erev Pesach?) Try portioning it out into soup bowl sized portions so that you know the frozen soup will fit your bowl. (Tip: See "Stand By with a Soup Supply," page 155, about lining a soup bowl. Alternatively, freeze the soup in individual plastic cup portions.) Make sure to put them into the freezer in such a way that you have easy access to them (and that they don't fall over before they've frozen — ugh). There's nothing more off-putting to good intentions than having an argument with the freezer shelves full of UFOs (Unidentified Frozen Objects).

Breakfirst

Just like a car needs gas to function at optimal performance, so, too, do busy Pesach-making people. Don't kid yourself that it's worth saving the calories by skipping breakfast, or justify its omission by claims of being too busy. It's an investment. If you can start the day with a full "tank," you will have more energy, be less irritable, and have greater willpower when it comes to sorting out those leftover Mishloach Manos.

Eat At Mealtimes

Even if it's crazy busy and the drawer contents of the entire kitchen are screaming for your attention, make sure to eat throughout the day. One of the best ways to do this is to sit down with the family at mealtimes. The food is hot and at its best and you can optimize the time to take a well-deserved break. It's too easy to skip the meal (thinking you'll heat yours up later), become ravenous as you sort, sift, and scrub, and then pounce on the goodies at the back of the cupboard. Besides, everyone will be happy to have mom sit down with them.

Treat Yourself

While overcoming temptation during the day, don't forget to reward yourself for all your hard work. Put a treat aside for the end of the day, when you can finally sit down with that hot coffee and enjoy it. And make sure you are sitting and actively enjoying it — not sorting, cooking, making lists, etc.

What To Eat

When wondering what to eat during the days preceding the Sedarim, try filling up on fresh fruit by leaving a fruit bowl on the table (it's easier for everyone to access, plus it provides an easy appetite-reducer-come-stress-reliever if the meal isn't quite ready on time because you've been scrubbing inside the oven). Snack freely on vegetables (zucchini in tomato sauce, TCP salad, etc.) or soup. If you've got a pot of soup on the stove and don't know what to have, try adding those cute tiny pasta shapes that only take four minutes to cook and hey presto, you've got a meal in minutes (that can last for hours).

If you can face the bombsite of a kitchen on a full tummy so that you are physically satisfied, **and** if you can hold your head high with the knowledge that you are still on track with your diet, it will generate a lot more positive energy all around.

Drink

Exercise works up a sweat. Scrubbing and scouring can sometimes classify as exercise — at least they sometimes make us perspire. It's getting warmer now that spring is upon us. And all that kashering (of sinks, etc.) is pretty steamy business. All these factors mean that your body may be in even greater need of a drink or two as you go along.

Therefore, make an especially concerted effort to drink during these busy days. This will take the edge off your appetite while rehydrating your body and reducing the chances of those nagging where's-the-Tylenol-and-are-they-Kosher-l'Pesach headaches. Water is best, but decaffeinated coffee and tea still serve the same purpose. (Tip: Try leaving a pitcher of water on the counter to remind you.)

Seder Nights

Bearing in mind that we don't usually sit down to a four-course meal around midnight after a veeeeery busy, long day (which has already included a day's worth of calories), it is especially important to make a concerted effort when choosing which foods to eat during the day of erev Pesach.

There are potentially enough calories during Shulchan Orech[23] alone to last a whole day. That's not including all the matzah and wine or grape juice. Basically, that amounts to eating two days worth of food in one day. And we wonder why we feel bloated after the Sedarim…

---

[23] The Seder Night festive meal.

The Meal

By the time you get to Shulchan Orech, chances are that you probably won't be so hungry any more. Remember, you can always fill up on morror (joke, but lettuce *is* a source of fiber). Choosing low-calorie hors d'oeuvres like fruit instead of fish will also alleviate hunger without sabotaging weight loss. By the time you get to the main course, it won't be hunger that propels you towards the kugel and roast potatoes — so try substituting these with a salad or hot veggies. Or even serve yourself a half-portion sized helping. There is no mitzvah to leave the table feeling like an overstuffed tomato with popping buttons before finishing Hallel.

Drink

Remember to drink during Shulchan Orech. It's been a while since you last drank (we're talking about water, not grape juice). If you have been busy serving the meal or dealing with the little ones, you may forget to drink — especially if you have to race against the clock to finish by midnight.

Dessert

Dessert — well, some have the custom to skip dessert, and it's never too early to adopt a custom or two, especially if it's ice cream at the table and not pineapple. Alternatively, make lighter desserts: fruit salad, low-fat mousse, or dietetic ice cream (whisk strawberries with sugar and freeze). You could even skip the dessert-on-the-plate scenario and opt for a black coffee with a small piece of chocolate. The sweetness might take the edge off your craving and you get to reduce the overload to your stomach (which is probably feeling mightily overloaded — and that's *before* the afikomen[24]).

Fiber

If you have been eating a healthy, nutritious, low-fat, low-calorie diet prior to Pesach, you've probably also been having a diet high in fiber. Some of the main sources of fiber are whole-wheat bread, whole-wheat pasta, cereals, and brown rice. Without these (on Pesach) we must make a conscious effort to try to increase our fiber content in other ways. Alternative sources of fiber are: baked potatoes, carrots, parsnips, beets, broccoli, leeks, bananas, prunes, rhubarb, and most fruits[25].

Spreads

For those who don't eat gebrochs,[26] you've got it easy. For those who do, place a slice of bread next to a square matzah (no, not at the Seder table…) and the difference in surface area becomes immediately apparent. If you still have an appetite for matzah after the Sedarim, watch out for the extremely high-calorie value of shmearing mayonnaise all over the matzah's extensive area. The same caution should be taken on Chol HaMoed when spreading butter,

---

[24] The obligatory final matzah eating.
[25] See "Appendix 5: Fiber, chart," page 402.
[26] Matzah eaten together with other foods.

margarine, or jam. Try letting the butter get soft and scraping it on very thinly so you can hear that dry, crispy, scraping sound. Alternatively, try spreading only half the matzah and use the other half to cover it — sandwich style. Or try the matzah with only jam and no butter (or the other way around). This way you dramatically decrease unnecessary calories while still savoring something sweet and crunchy.

Let's get real. Since when did matzah (with whatever spread you use) ever fill you up? Certainly not before the fourth piece. Go easy on it — all those extra calories in the shape of innocent spreads can soon add up. It's one of those mindless, munch-'n'-crunch-more-'n'-more foods (like peanuts and Pringles…). Addictive without being satisfying.

Motzei Pesach

When the Pesach dishes are all clean and locked away, when the aluminum foil, garbage bags, and surface linings have all been ripped off, and when the chometzdik cakes and cookies make their return from the bakery, looking all too fresh and yummy…take extra care not to undo all that hard work of self-control you just exerted over Pesach. Order the whole-wheat rolls and crackers instead. Remember that chometz, although tantalizing after a week of abstinence, is going to be around for the next 51 weeks — so relax and enjoy yourself till then!

Chag kosher v'someach!

Shavuos

We have eagerly counted the days turned weeks right up to Shavuos. We remembered to count the Omer[27] each day and in good Yiddishe tradition we feel we have duly earned our cheesecake. I can just hear you say, "Now she's going to tell me not to have my cheesecake!" Oh, no, I'm not. What I will say is that one slice of cheesecake is not the same as finishing off the whole thing when the kids aren't looking, and controlled indulgences over Yom Tov are not the same as wild extravagances. It also helps to keep in mind that Weight Watchers attributes the same points for full-fat cream cheese as they do for margarine. So biting into that cheesecake is calorically almost like biting into margarine. Yum.

Cheesecake

Incidentally, I once worked out *my* favorite cheesecake recipe (it uses Tofutti versus real cream cheese) and one slice (⅙ of a pie) worked out to be over half of my daily calorie allowance. Knowing what we are having is definitely worth *knowing* (and not just guessing), or else we face the shock-horror-gasp scenario at the scale the following week.

---

[27] The customary counting of the days between Pesach and Shavuos.

While I don't want to be the party-pooper and deprive you of your well-deserved treat, it's worth noting that there are fewer calories and less saturated fat in different kinds of cake than in cheesecake — sponge cakes lead as a real low-fat winner, and rugelach aren't too bad either. So try tasting the cheesecake and fulfilling your mezonos/cake obligation with sponge cake — see, you *can* still have your cake and eat it!

As an addition, below is a delicious, tried, and tested low-fat alternative to the real stuff.

Very Low-Fat Cheesecake

> 1 lb. very low-fat cottage cheese
> 1 lb. very low-fat fromage frais
> 6 Tbsp. powdered artificial sweetener
> 2 large eggs
> 1 tsp. vanilla extract
> squeeze of lemon juice to taste

Directions:

> ✔ Blend cottage cheese (in a dairy blender) till smooth and thin.
> ✔ Add all other ingredients together.
> ✔ Blend for a few seconds.
> ✔ Pour into baking pan (can line with baking paper).
> ✔ Bake for 25–30 minutes on 350 degrees Fahrenheit until just set.

Delicious covered with sliced strawberries and kiwis.

All these tips specific to each Yom Tov might well take us on a world tour round-the-year. But our sightseeing tour through the seasons takes other detours along the way and we need to handle them as well. Summer vacation may be your oasis of relaxation within the buzz of routine, but you don't want to come back home with only the memories of a weight loss mirage. Let's look at how we are going to pack our resolve, as well as our suitcases, to go on vacation.

Chapter 10

———— ◆ ◆ ◆ ————

Summer Vacations

Introduction

In between dusting off the sunglasses and shaking out the maps and backpacks is the budding, antsy anticipation of the upcoming summer vacation experience. As we prepare for this international exodus from routine, maybe we can take this opportunity to similarly prepare ourselves for some of the common dieting pitfalls that we may encounter along the way.

The Theory Side

From a weight-conscious perspective, there are three types of people who go on vacation. Hands up if you see yourself fitting into one of these categories:

- You expect to lose while you are away.
- You will aim to stay the same or only gain a small amount. You will definitely "let go" and give yourself leeway, but will remain in control.
- You are going to blow the diet and enjoy yourself.

You can put your hands down now.

> This chapter should help you enjoy your vacation and your diet at the same time.

Everyone has to know herself. Being realistic in terms of which category fits your style will reduce your frustration and will contribute to your sense of control.

Let's address these categories one by one.

■ Expecting To Lose

Expecting to lose weight when placed in a challenging situation indicates high levels of that magical, ever-evasive willpower. That's great. What's not so great is that this expectation may well be unrealistic, and you may be setting yourself up for failure.

That's not to say that weight loss is impossible — staying at home and doing day-trips allows you the comfort of a very familiar kitchen and lifestyle. If your diet is up and running, you can capitalize on the direction it is taking you and continue upwards and onwards. In addition, you will probably be exercising during your day trips, and may automatically be avoiding nosh on your outings. Maybe these factors will contribute to a few pounds off after all. Of course, the downside is that when you return from your exhausting outing to all those home comforts (ice cream cone, any-one?), it's all too easy to raid the cupboards and blow the whole thing.

If you're touring around or traveling long distances by car or minivan, you will have to face the demands of trying to keep everyone calm, content, and quiet. Nosh comes in handy to keep little mouths busy, but must Mommy fit into that category too? Driving necessitates less exercise, so there isn't much chance of burning off all that ingested Bissli and corn chips.

Going away, however, is a different kettle of fish. It might be realistic for someone to expect to see herself pounds lighter in September if she is the type to choose to leave the nosh behind (or count out exact portions for children only) when visiting outer Mongolia. The limited access to anything remotely kosher (or caloric) may work in her favor. But this may not be a realistic scenario for Mrs. Yiddishe Mamma; she packs the entire contents of her nearest delicatessen weeks in advance, as if preparing for world war or famine. Inaccessibility of nosh is similarly inapplicable for those going to bungalow colonies or kosher hotels, or who find themselves near kosher grocery stores just bursting with the stuff. For them, nosh is as prevalent as the mosquitoes.

Another point to consider when away from home: Many people are thrown off balance with the changes in routine, location, and lifestyle. Putting your hands on fresh salad or vegetable soup doesn't seem so simple anymore in a vacation cottage. ("Where's the knife? Is this side dairy?") Taking time out to rustle up something nutritious seems impossible when you find yourself hungry three-and-a-half miles away from civilization with only a backpack of pretzels and cake (and a dozen or so children) for company.

Whether staying put or facing adventure, the fact that your phone and doorbell won't ring (as much) automatically lends to a relaxed atmosphere, which may also be more conducive to letting down the dieting guard. Since you are not working, and therefore have no pressures, deadlines, or working buzz but are "off duty," you might well fall into the lure of being "off duty" when it comes to being food conscious as well. Forewarned is forearmed.

The key to all of this, of course, is to be realistic and fully aware of the temptations and scenarios that will face you.

▪ Aiming To Stay the Same/Small Gain

Let's paint a realistic picture of what summer vacation means for moms. The kids finish school just about when you need to sit down for two days straight to write all those packing lists that keep you from sleeping at night. They are oh-so-excited and therefore oh-so-noisy, wild, or hyper (take your pick or choose all three). Plus, they're going to need occupying for the next eight hot weeks.

With the extra demands of having the kids around, increased temperatures, and a noticeable lack of routine, from a dieting perspective it would seem that you might not have so much time (make that remaining strength) to take those few extra minutes to look after yourself the way you routinely do throughout the year.

That's not to say that exerting some level of control is impossible. It *is* possible, it's all a question of juggling while remaining joyful versus seething while getting stressed. And don't think the answer to all your problems lies in going to a hotel — see "Fully Catered, Fully Caloried" later in this chapter.

Why am I talking about stress when I should be talking about sunbathing? Because vacations are for fun. Vacations are for family. They are for enjoying, relaxing, re-energizing, and letting off steam, so that when we come back to our routine, day-to-day living, we feel refreshed and happy. (Getting itchy feet, huh?) If you are going to prioritize your diet *at the expense* of your vacation, then think again.

For most people this two to eight week time capsule is a once-a-year opportunity to unwind. Don't blow it. If you have to put your diet on hold (note: not down the drain), so be it. Allow yourself the flexibility to maintain control without the stress. But remember, there's a big difference (psychologically and on the scale) between breaking a diet and bending it. So you won't lose your four pounds, and you might even put on a couple — but the chances are that you will be able to take this new, energized feeling with you when you begin your program again in earnest. Capitalize on the long-term investment and put your dieting in perspective.

▪ Blowing the Diet

In stark contrast to the previous option, this mindset has serious negative repercussions. Many long-term dieters adopt an "in for a penny, in for a pound" mentality when faced with challenging situations that find them not quite meeting the challenge. ("I've had the mayonnaise with the challah already, so I might as well have the fried schnitzel, roast potatoes, non-dairy ice cream sundae…") The downward spiral is a frighteningly fast route to undoing all the hard work that has taken so long to achieve. With this mentality, the dieter releases herself from any semblance of self-control. Because she has broken the diet, she can now officially indulge to her heart's content. It's this feeling of a release from the "shackles and chains" of dieting that catapults her into her no-holds-barred banquet and shoots her up into the next weight-bracket.

This all-or-nothing mentality is also in evidence when a person faces a situation like vacation times and makes a *conscious* decision beforehand to blow it. She may well overindulge only because she is now not on any formal diet, and is, in a way, rebelling against the rigidity of her program. She knows deep down that she will probably end up going on the diet again and is fearful of the potential restrictions; she therefore justifies that she had "better enjoy life now." Even though a couple of chocolates would have satisfied her sweet tooth, she now finishes off the entire box.

As if all this wasn't bad enough, when you go for the "blow it all" option, it is *so* much harder to resume control and start again. Somehow, the energy required to start a program *yet again* evades us, and we just continue to overeat recklessly because that has become the status quo.

This is such a shame. We all know the results of such an attitude; we all know who is going to pay the price for such recklessness. All I ask you is: Is it really worth it? If you have been losing weight successfully till this point, just remember how you feel now. Maybe your skirts are looser, maybe you can move more easily — maybe you are enjoying the feeling of being in control of what you eat and also of your life. Do you want to lose all that and start from scratch?

When we go away, we take photographs to remind us of what a wonderful time we had. How about taking a photograph of yourself before you go — without the camera. A mental photograph or freeze-frame of how you feel now might be enough. This is the mental picture that you should take with you to carry you over the hurdle.

If you have managed to lose a significant amount of weight prior to your vacation, try taking a real photo (the flattering one, where you look a size smaller) with you on vacation. Pin it up somewhere prominent as a constant reminder of what you want to achieve.

To Conclude

✔ We must be realistic in our expectations of what we can achieve comfortably during this period (to reduce our frustration);

✔ We must take responsibility for our actions;

✔ If we "blow it all" it will be harder to succeed in the long run;

✔ If we maintain control but remain flexible, we will stand the best chance of succeeding — both in enjoying ourselves and in our long-term goal of losing weight.

The Practical Side

Having covered the theory side, we now know how to pack our minds with the correct attitude. Now let's focus on how we're going to pack our bags…

Advice for All Vacation Scenarios

You are packing your bags, so pack a tailor-made diet bag as well, just for you. What are you going to include?

A handy-sized water bottle

Refillable, easy to access, and a good idea when you are climbing all those mountains, traveling on long trips, or even just going for a long walk/jog. Try keeping a supply of treat-yourself expensive low-calorie drinks on hand. You know, the sort they serve at Sheva Brochos. You can refill your personal handy-sized bottle with these delicious drinks or with cool water.

The Diet Book

If you are on a formal diet plan, take the plan's book with you. Maybe it's been a while since you read it — the refresher can motivate and remind you of potential stumbling blocks or forgotten rules. Taking it with you physically can mean taking it with you psychologically.

Sneakers

Having a good pair of supportive sneakers can help you overcome the inertia to exercise. There's nothing more off-putting than going for a long walk in high heels or uncomfortable shoes. Treat yourself to a decent pair. The investment will mean that you'll feel obligated to get your value-for-money out of them, and your feet will bless you after each outing (see "Choosing the Right Sports Shoe," page 322).

Swimsuit

Take your bathing suit even if you don't think you'll need it. If you get to where you are going and find out that, yes, there is separate swimming, you'll kick yourself if you haven't got a swimsuit with you. (It's not an easy item to substitute…)

Another water bottle

What? Another one? Yes. This one is for filling up with low-cal juice and freezing the night before, so that you have a cool, refreshing slurp-alicious drink when you come back exhausted after a long outing, or even when you are on the road. This may also help you keep your cool in the front seat as the kids keep losing theirs in the back.

Sandwiches

It's the spread, not the bread, that piles on the pounds. If you are a peanut butter lover, know that a scraping versus a generous smearing can significantly reduce the calories. Try smooth peanut butter instead of crunchy for just as much taste, with better ability to spread and less nut (read fat).

Here are a few suggestions for Mommy's special sandwiches (or try them out on the whole family and see if you find a new favorite):

- Hard-boiled eggs, processed with raw onion. The juice from the onion binds the egg into a good spreading consistency. If you want a deliciously savory tang, try adding pickles.
- Hard-boiled eggs processed with tomatoes (light mayonnaise optional);
- Tuna (in brine or water, skip the oil) with light mayonnaise and spring onions;
- Chopped herring with sliced tomatoes. This is a tasty, low-fat spread that makes a change from the usual.
- Jam without the margarine or butter;
- Reduced-fat triangle cheese/Cheddar cheese/cottage cheese/low-fat soft cream cheese;
- Light mayonnaise scraped with thinly sliced tomatoes on top (spices optional);
- Banana (not just for mush-faced babies — my mom has had this on her bread every lunch for years!);
- Cocoa mixed with water to a paste consistency. It's low-fat, sweet, and cheaper than the regular chocolate spreads (you might just find that you don't want that chocolate bar after all...), and has fewer calories;
- Ketchup with oregano sprinkled on top;
- Low-fat yogurt spread over the bread with sliced strawberries on top;
- A salad sandwich;
- Toasted or barbecued bread with barbecued chicken/tomatoes/sausages.
- Egg and cress;
- Lean beef and horseradish ;
- Low-fat cheese and chutney;
- Cottage cheese and pineapple;
- Chicken and pickles;
- Salmon and cucumber;
- Turkey and cranberry sauce.

Old habits (the good ones)

If summer vacation threatens to jolt you out of the good practices you have learned in Diet Land, don't let it. Yes, it may seem a contradiction to be sitting down to pizza, fries, and a *Diet* Coke, but stick with the Diet Coke anyway. Ditto for all those junky sugary cereals with low-fat milk. Don't trade in your skim milk for whole fat just because you are bending the rules.

Hang on to the good habits as well as you can — it'll make it that much easier when you decide enough is enough and take up the reigns of true self-control again.

Sense of humor

A sense of humor is probably the most vital piece of equipment when facing any vacation period. It can turn the most trying of situations into a warm, life-long memory. If all else fails, laugh.

Conclusion

Our vacation period doesn't need to set our dieting goals back to square one. We can still have a refreshing, rejuvenating, relaxing respite, complete with happy, wholesome vacation highlights — and still maintain our chosen diet. All it requires is a little forethought, a little preparation, a little substitution — and a lot of positive attitude.

Advice for Different Summer Vacation Scenarios

Although we all go on vacation for more or less the same reasons (to relax, refresh, bond with the kids, get a suntan, etc...), there are different ways and means to achieve these goals.

Let's take a look at three different vacation scenarios and focus on the trials, tribulations, and advice specific to each of them.

- Vacation Number 1: Civilized Base With Day Trips
  - Staying at home;
  - Going to a family camp;
  - Going somewhere semi-civilized away from home;
  - Going to a bungalow colony;

  (And, in all four cases, using them as a base for day trips).
- Vacation Number 2: Fully Catered, Fully Caloried
  - Going to a fully catered hotel (and wishing you could stay there forever).
- Vacation Number 3: Beyond Civilization
  - Going to the back of beyond and hanging out with the trees;
  - On-the-go: traveling long distances by car/minivan/camper.

■ *Vacation Number 1: Civilized Base With Day Trips*

Trials and Tribulations

- Easy access to cupboards/shops for kosher food;
- Easy to use convenience foods because of kosher kitchen;
- Pressure from people to indulge;
- Informal meals;
- Informal dress disguises our weight gain;
- More shmooze-time means more cake recipes;
- Not as much exercise incurred.

Advice

Stopping Shopping (Access to cupboards/shops for kosher food)

Give yourself a break from daily shopping; try to be organized and only go grocery shopping once a week. It's always harder to resist the chocolates at eye level and it's certainly more frustrating when you've only gone in for a package of rice cakes. Getting shopping out of the way frees up more of that precious vacation-stuff called relaxation time. And remember, the purpose of the day is to relax.

An even better alternative to standing in all those lines with hot, cranky, hungry kids? Call or fax your order in to the store. This not only saves time and avoids spontaneous buying (and desire awakening), but is also better on the pocketbook as well. Alternatively, if you've got a sensible-aged kid just hanging around shooting the breeze, send him on a shopping trip so that he can be doing something useful at the same time.

Box Under Locks

If your downfall is grazing at the cupboard shelves, how about making a specially designated "nosh box" and put it up high (ask your husband to do the honors if he's tall, or ask any unassuming passing giant) so that you will need a chair to get it down. You could, quite literally, put it under lock and key, so that you have to find the key and unlock it each time. This "bother" might help to curb the frequency of each trip. Hopefully this will be a little more off-putting than finding a "healthy" supply of chocolate bars at eye-level.

Hot Pot-ato (Convenience foods)

If your stay-at-home vacation is synonymous with oven fries and pareve schnitzel, try putting your own potato into the oven at the same time. A baked potato takes less time to prepare than oven fries (you don't have to open the bag); will automatically reduce calories; will fill you up for longer; and can bake at the same time as the fries. (You can slice it and spray it with spray oil if it's a large potato, so that it's ready at the same time as the family's meal.) See "Lots of Pots," page 156.

Fast Food

Alternatively, in the days leading up to vacation time, take advantage of the peace and quiet of having the children still in school and cook batch quantities. This involves making whatever healthy, dietetic food you normally make, only making more of it. Portion it out into individual microwavable/ovenproof aluminum foil containers, and hey presto, you have your own low-fat version of fast food.

Bar-B-Que

Another great, low-fat, high-entertainment cooking method is barbecuing. You can get disposable barbecues from most supermarkets and can cook up all sorts of delicious, nutritious, fun foods. How about trying corn on the cob, fish, pre-cooked potatoes (it's quicker), chicken schnitzel, onions, tomatoes, and peppers. There's supper taken care of — and you won't have any pots to clean!

Peer Pressure Preview (Pressure from people to indulge)

If you experience pressure from your fellow neighboring campers to "just have one" when you are sitting outside together watching the children, don't buckle just because of peer pressure.

Practice your refusal lines in advance: "Sorry, they don't agree with me," "No, thank you, I'm full," or "Thanks, but I'm on a diet — please don't tempt me again, because I might not be able to resist the second time around!" They'll admire your guts for trying to stick with it in unfavorable circumstances and will ask you for your recipe for willpower. See also "No-No's," page 80.

Alternatively, you can always bring along your own low-fat/calorie snack or a cup of tea or coffee (with artificial sweetener) to enjoy, while you enjoy the company.

Easy-Peasy-Meals (Informal meals)

In the case of the bungalow colony, there's no hubby around to formalize mealtimes (appetizer, set table, napkins...), or force us to make nutritious choices in our menu planning. We want everyone to be happy and everyone loves pizza, hot dogs, hamburgers, and fries. Who in their right mind can summon up the extra energy to swim against the tide and provide vegetable lasagna when hot dogs keep the gang fed and happy?

Just because formal mealtimes are relegated to the memories of yesterday doesn't mean it's impossible to modify your chosen changeover to slap-dash menus.

✔ You can try to choose whole-wheat varieties of any bread product — it's still a hamburger even if it's brown. The theory behind this easy substitution is that the fiber will help to fill you up so that you'll eat less of the high-calorie foods.

✔ You can pile up your plates with plenty of salad. It's fresh, crispy, refreshing, fills up an empty plate, and still tastes great with a low-calorie dressing.

✔ Substituting high-calorie products with the comparable low-calorie version is an easy-to-implement measure. Plonking light cheese in the shopping cart instead of the real thing can knock off calories and no one (except the scale) will notice — especially if they've just come in from a baseball game.

✔ Even if you are not making the pizza, macaroni, or lasagna yourself but are buying every convenience food imaginable, check out the nutrition label for exactly how "bad" the food is per serving (see "Food Labels," page 112). Maybe the pizza package sitting next to it isn't as bad and still provides an oven-to-table style meal. If it is truly "evil," try filling the plate up with a lower-calorie food to supplement it. For example, one slice of high-calorie pizza can be accompanied by a baked potato and side salad instead of indulging in two or four slices of pizza alone.

✔ If all this informality of chimpanzee-style-mealtimes sends you into a tizzy and you find that you simply can't think straight and certainly can't think "diet" at such a time, try having your own meal at a quieter time. Maybe you can start eating after all the little ones are in bed and the bigger ones give you fifteen minutes of quiet for you to have your own meal in peace. You can arrange all the food that everyone else is having at the time they are having it — so that you don't have to spend extra time preparing the food. This tip is especially useful for those who find they are picking at everything and losing track of exactly *what* they ate because of the general hullaballoo.

✔ Don't forget cereal. If the slap-dash meal you just prepared is not only high in calories but you actually don't even like it, don't be tempted to dig in for an easy life. You can have just as easy a life by opting for a crunchy, filling, nutritious cereal.

Pinch an Inch (Informal dress disguises our weight gain)

If the bungalow colony lifestyle has you shlepping around in a housecoat all day and you've forgotten what getting dressed feels like, beware. Loose, baggy, and comfortable housecoats are still (generally) loose, baggy, and comfortable even when you have put on weight. Not so with tailored, fitted business suits without elastic waistbands.

Not only will you not feel the "pinch" in such informal, relaxed attire, but your psyche also feels more relaxed, loose, and unconstrained. Although I'm not going to suggest you wear your best suit in the sun, perhaps the following will help to keep you more conscious of how your body is going to feel once you're back to normal routine.

✔ Take along one skirt that fits perfectly. Look at yourself in the mirror at the start of your vacation. Notice how the waistband fits without having to undo the top button (no elastic waists, please), how the material falls smoothly over the hips, and also notice where exactly the skirt hem reaches. Now sit down in front of the mirror and pay attention to the same areas.

While you're away, try this skirt on every two weeks and compare your findings. As some people will notice weight gain in different parts of their body, it is important to pay attention to the tummy area, waist, *and* hips. If the skirt has become tighter at the hips, it may well mean that the material puckers at waist-hip height and will appear shorter (that's why you're looking at the hem length). While a skirt might appear to still fit OK when standing, the proof of the pudding is when you sit (note: It's not a good idea to sit in it if it already proved to be too tight when standing…).

(I once went away for two weeks and in the second week I put on a skirt that had fit perfectly before the vacation…it ended up going back into the suitcase and I ended up skipping dessert. Although appalled, I was happy to have experienced such a good and effective stop-gap).

✔ If an extra skirt just will not squeeze into the already-bursting suitcase, an effective gauge (although not quite as accurate) is to use a belt, and note which hole feels snug without being tight. Another option is to take a piece of string or wool, tie it around your tummy, and (shocking!) leave it there. Loose clothing may be more comfortable, but something snug around your middle can serve as a reminder to stop eating when it feels tight. (It'll soon tell you when you've had enough fries.)

In terms of this loose, casual, let-it-all-go mentality, there's no surer combatant than the good ole faithful Food Diary (see "Dear Diary," page 108). Keeping careful tabs on what you are eating by writing it all down (yes, *every* french fry, potato chip, and ice popsicle…) is a sure-fire winner in ensuring self-control. Beneath that carefree 'n' comfortable exterior could be lurking a cool, calculated control.

Brooding Over Food (More shmooze-time means more cake recipes)

I've never been amongst a group of women who had nothing to talk about. (Guess that's just not one of the problems of being female.) Although there are the usual favorites of kids, general gripes, and clothes, no one will argue that food can be listed as one of the top ten favorites.

I know one lady who was swimming away quite happily on her bungalow colony vacation, when someone by the poolside started talking about this *fabulous* chocolate cake recipe. So emphatic was she in her conviction that this was simply *the* best chocolate cake ever, that our swimmer dragged herself out of the pool, sped along to her house for a pen and paper, and recorded it for posterity. (We should all be blessed with such drive and energy.)

Instead of exchanging recipes for cookies and cakes, why not start up a dieter's recipe session? Hold competitions — the best salad/low-fat dessert/fruit creation wins. At least this way you'll end up with a bunch of diet-proof recipes for when you get back home to all that serious repentance. In addition, you could hold weekly Club Meetings — each person brings a course or part of a low-fat supper. You only have to make one dish, and yet you get to enjoy the variety (and recipes) of everyone else's.

Initiating such a venture will automatically help to steer the conversations towards more healthy food choices ("What did you say you added to that salad last week?"), plus, you stand to benefit from the potential group support system to help you keep on track.

Loving Moving (Not as much exercise incurred)

Inquire whether the camp or town you find yourself in has swimming facilities (and remember to swim — don't just shmooze). If you are near a gym, ask about dance/aerobic classes. How about setting up a daily walk with the big daughter whom you never see, or finding a "walking buddy" from the camp? Chances are they might also need the exercise and will bless you for dragging them along. Good fun vacation alternatives are badminton, volleyball, softball, and basketball — who says you're too old to play ball?

■ Vacation Number 2: Fully Catered, Fully Caloried

☹ Trials and Tribulations

- Yummy food and big portions;
- High availability of food;
- Strong social pressure to eat;
- More time, more relaxed, and therefore "more eat;"
- Want to get value for money;
- Not much exercise.

Advice

Catering to Catering (Yummy food and big portions)

You sit like a lady, the food is served, you don't see a pot, pan, or sponge, and you are presented with an enticing selection of all your favorites. Sounds like a restaurant? That's because basically it is. So see "Chapter 11: Eating Right When Eating Out," where you'll find lots of relevant tips to counteract the tendency to over-feast.

Taking Care When Food's Right There (High availability of food)

While facing the delights of a sumptuous, freshly baked continental breakfast, it can be difficult to bear in mind that sumptuous, freshly baked lunch, high tea, dinner, and after-dinner coffee and cakes are all to follow. The sheer availability of beautifully arranged, aroma-wafting delicacies can require Herculean self-control to resist. Here are a few tips to help keep you in control of food and not the other way around.

✔ If you manage nothing else this vacation, promise yourself that you will rate your level of hunger on a 1–10 scale (1=not hungry, 10=starving) before sitting down to any meal or snack. This simple stop-check should provide you with an effective measure of how much food you should be consuming how often. I'm not saying that you should never have a nibble unless your tummy's growling (would I?). I am saying if you rate yourself as being number 2 at about 4pm, you will face your own honest assessment and may choose to have only one cookie instead of the automatic three or four.

✔ As the potential calories around you on any given day may exceed two or three days' quotas, try asking the waiter to serve you half-size portions. (You won't go hungry after a three or four course meal.) And now that you have read ahead to the restaurant chapter, you'll have plenty of good ideas for this trial as well.

✔ Remember, the key is to take control of your environment and consciously *choose* what you really want to eat and how much of it you want to eat.

Social Graces (Strong social pressure to eat)

When faced with the tea/coffee-time social pressure to eat because everyone else is eating (and persuading you to do so), apart from the advice above (listed under "Vacation Number 1: Civilized Base with Day Trips"), try the following:

✔ Move the plate of cookies away from where you choose to sit (before you sit down). This should act as a deterrent because it will mean that you will have to ask someone to pass them to you. Not only will you have to interrupt the conversation to do so, but it's kind of embarrassing to draw attention to our desires (unless we are sitting with only best friends, when anything goes).

✔ Let your neighbors know that you are trying to stick to a diet. (They'll help you and you'll be too embarrassed to fress-out in their company.).

✔ If the plate looks more or less demolished before you arrive, secretly find a waiter and ask him to please clear the table — out of sight, out of mouth.

✔ Keep drinking. Not only will you rehydrate your body from all that stair-hopping exercise and be taking the edge off your appetite, but you will also be keeping your hands busy as well.

✔ Speaking of busy hands, why not pull out that half-finished sweater and your knitting needles, or start crocheting? Busy hands are too busy to go prowling for food.

Prime Time (More time, more relaxed, and therefore "more eat")

Having more time to relax may mean extra time for extra indulgences. When occasional treats become everyday staples, not only do we gain weight, but the heightened enjoyment of the food is reduced. (A Shabbos treat eaten every day is no longer a Shabbos treat.)

People always ask me whether I still enjoy my food (as if fat people have a monopoly on food enjoyment…), and I reply that I enjoy my mini-chocolate bar now more than when I used to finish off a whole regular-sized bar. Does anyone experience the same enjoyment during chocolate number six as she did during chocolate number one?

While on vacation, make a conscious effort to fill the time with other relaxing pursuits. Take up a new hobby. Finish the knitting you started the last time you went away. Read. Socialize (without food). Listen to music. Have a facial, manicure, or massage. Vacationing isn't just about food. We can treat ourselves in other ways as well – credit cards, watch out.

Value for Yummy (Value for money)

Most fully catered vacations cost a pretty penny or thousand. Feeling like you want to get your value-for-money can easily turn into getting fat-for-each-yummy. Just like the leftovers at home are better off in the garbage can rather than in your tummy, so, too, it is preferable to refuse food rather than to over-stuff yourself. We are not human garbage cans. When considering the concept of getting value-for-money, think of it in terms of quality, not quantity. Imagine that you are paying for each taste, not each full plate. Remember that you've paid for it once, and you don't want to pay for it again — on the scale.

Galvanize and Mobilize (Not much exercise)

Although you may well be making the trip from bedroom to dining room many times throughout your day, unfortunately, this does not qualify under the banner of healthy "exercise." You don't even get to burn off one or two calories by jumping up and down to serve each course. As you are pretty much glued to your chair, it's going to take a concerted effort to mobilize those limbs.

If you have access to a pool, take the opportunity to swim daily. Remember that the real benefits of exercise are only accrued when you swim, not while you shmooze in the shallow end. Some hotels have gym facilities on site. Don't be embarrassed to try one out even if it's your first time. Everyone has to have a first time at some stage. You can always watch for a while before launching yourself onto the bike, or better yet, ask someone in Reception to show you the ropes.

Remember that every little bit counts. Try using the stairs instead of the elevator. You can't use the "I'm too busy, I haven't got time" excuse 'cause you are on vacation and you've got plenty of time (after all, that's the whole point of the vacation). If you start off the vacation by avoiding the elevator, you'll soon find yourself automatically choosing the stairs. Compete with yourself.

Time how long it takes to get up or down the stairs and try to beat your own record. Wherever you are, I'm sure another family member will be only too glad to accompany you for some one-on-one attention on a daily brisk walk. Setting a fixed time (between Minchah and Maariv?) will help you overcome the tendency to wait for the elusive urge to get moving.

■ Vacation Number 3: Beyond Civilization

☹ Trials and Tribulations

- Being so hungry you eat the next morsel that comes your way;
- It's easier to have what everyone else is having;
- Being too frazzled for self-control.

☼ Advice

Bag of Tricks (Being so hungry)

All that countryside and earthiness seems to awaken an even heartier appetite than usual, and hunger can thwart the strongest of intentions. The answer: Don't let yourself get too hungry. Be prepared for any eventuality. Have your own special bag of nutritious snacks easily accessible in your backpack. Your bag should contain goodies such as:

✔ Crackers (whole-wheat/fat-free matzah crackers);

✔ Low-fat pretzels;

✔ Rice cakes;

✔ Low-fat potato chips;

✔ Fresh fruit;

✔ Peeled carrots;

✔ Bottle of water/low-calorie drink;

✔ Sugar-free candies/sugarless gum.

Got A Hot-Pot? (Having what everyone is having)

When it comes to mealtimes, you may not feel that you have what it takes to make separate food for yourself (like an extra pot, the energy to wash it, the inclination to make two separate menus, i.e., one regular, one dietetic…), so don't. Try serving one-pot meals (chopped meat, carrots, and spaghetti) and helping yourself to extras of the veggies and less of the meat. Maybe it's a good idea to take along that Slow Cooker that's waiting for winter at the back of the cupboard. This way supper can cook all day and be ready, piping hot, and filling for when you return tired, hungry, dirty, and wet (OK, let's hope, not so wet). Stews are nutritious, filling, and economical. Try adding barley or soup mix packs to thicken the stew, and beans and lentils to make the food stretch. This way you can enjoy it, guilt-free just like everyone else — and you've only got one pot to wash in the treife[1] sink.

---

[1] Not kosher.

Shortcut Musts (Too frazzled)

If you are too frazzled for self-control, then rethink your vacation. You may well be busy with the family, but it's a shame for the vacation to turn into a stress-attack. Try taking shortcuts. For example:

✔ Keep meals simple (see above);

✔ Serve meals outside whenever possible. This way you don't have to sweep the floor or wipe the table;

✔ Keep laundry to a minimum (the cows won't mind if Shnocky's got a mark on his sweater, or his shirt isn't ironed);

✔ Turn a blind eye (or close the door) to the mess (unless your husband objects). No one's going to pop in unexpectedly, so you don't have to worry about impressing anyone. It's all going to be tidied up for Shabbos anyway, so relaaaax and fix your eyeballs on a good book instead;

✔ Don't bother making the beds — they're only going to get into them and crumple them again at night.

Conclusion

Summer vacation is a well-deserved oasis of rejuvenation. We need to utilize it as such. When we come back to our homes and routines, we should be feeling well-refreshed, not well-fressed. Let's take the relief and space from which we have benefited so tangibly, together with our new sense of calm vitality, right into the rest of our year.

Boost for After the Summer Vacation

So you've come back from your vacation, you've washed all the muddy sneakers and cleaned out the pretzel crumbs from the backpacks. Wouldn't it be nice, you muse, to be able to unzip those extra pounds just like we so easily unzip our windbreakers? 'Cause chances are that with all that relaxation, we relaxed in terms of food as well. That's the bad news. The good news is that there *is* something you can do about it.

If you take only one piece of advice for the after-vacation-let's-get-back-into-routine scenario, take this: BEGIN AGAIN. At the risk of stating the downright obvious, this means getting right back on the bandwagon. Don't we always tell Shnocky to get back on his bike when he falls off so that he doesn't get scared off for life? The longer he leaves it, the harder it is to get back onto the seat. Same with a car crash. Same with those who bend their diet till it breaks. Somehow it's easier to give Shnocky this advice than take it ourselves. But hey, that's the scoop with all advice. **In a nutshell — the longer you leave it, the harder it is to begin again.**

Just so that you know it's a human and not an angel who wrote this book…I also put on weight with all that fresh air, hearty appetite, and tempting coffee and cake by the hearth. My skirts feel just that bit too snug, the zippers don't slide up so easily, and I feel really yuck.

Although it's refreshing to taste "forbidden fruits" to excess once in a while, I can honestly say that by the end of the vacation I look forward to some healthy eating and to feeling light again. It would be only too easy to continue the pattern of what has become the status quo: *not* counting the calories/points/sins/etc. But I try to take myself in hand and decide that I had better take my own advice and get right back into the swing of things.

The result? I try to leave the table after a piping hot, filled jacket potato without feeling like platefuls of soggy fries are sitting for hours in the confines of an overfull stomach. I try to tuck into a crunchy, fresh side salad without feeling grease coming through the pores of my skin after an oil-drenched lookalike. I might not immediately lose what I had put on over vacation, but I sure feel better immediately — knowing that I am in control again and feeling a new spring in my step.

I want you to feel good about yourselves too. The answer lies (as Granny always used to say) in not putting off till tomorrow what can be done today. Put your few pounds behind you and start now, before they turn into a dozen or more. Go for it!

Chapter 11

— ◆ ◆ ◆ —

Eating Right When Eating Out

For eating out at a wedding, Sheva Brochos, or any social event or celebration, see earlier, "Socializing and Celebrating," page 81. In this chapter, we are focusing on restaurants.

Why Go Out?

Unless your husband's the mashgiach[1] or you're the chef, most people tend to visit restaurants for special celebrations or occasions.

After you make reservations, you spend the rest of the day in simmering anticipation of the candlelit dinner for two (or ten, if it's a family affair). Even a last minute "Oh I didn't make supper, let's go out for it" dash is a pleasant respite from the disaster site dinner table and dirty dishes stacked in the sink.

Going out for a meal renders some serious advantages. Not only is it a mess-free option, it's also stress-free (apart from finding a baby-sitter. We can usually cope with the stress of what to choose from the menu). It's also an ideal way to extricate ourselves from our humdrum routine. It shakes us up — out of that bad mood, or away from that nagging problem. We can change the pace of our day (ahhh, that's better…) and come back to our lives with renewed vigor, vitality, and a fresh perspective.

> *Do you leave your diet at the door when you go out to eat? After this chapter, you won't have to anymore.*

---

[1] On-site Kashrus supervisor.

At a restaurant, you can catch up on a relationship that you've let slide. No interruptions mean quality time conversation. (Remember to leave the cell phone at home.) Or you can go alone and enjoy the harmony of your own company.

Psyching Up To Go Out

Whenever we are faced with a celebration/special occasion scenario, we seem to have a built-in automatic reaction to overindulge. We'll anticipate rich creamy pasta sauces or gooey chocolate desserts. We tend to equate restaurant hopping with forbidden luxuries. "No one's watching…I can let go, it's a one time deal…How can I waste the opportunity to have such wonderful food…" etc.

Let's just stop a moment and think. Cast your mind back to the last time you ate out. Which comes to mind most vividly — the food you ate or the experience you enjoyed? Is it the roast duck with fried rice that springs to mind, or do you remember whom you were with, the laughter you shared, the atmosphere of togetherness, the relaxing ambience?

Yes, we want to have a good time. Yes, we want to create memories together with our loved ones. But we don't want to be reminded of our extravagances by a pinching waistband for weeks to come.

We want to remember the occasion, not the consequences. And the best occasions are about people, not about food.

One of my clients was planning to go away with her husband for a few days of quality time together. Throughout the entire trip she maintained control and resisted all unaccounted treats and delectables that came her way. She told me the thought that kept going through her mind was "the food was not the focus — they were." She reminded herself that she wasn't going to remember what she'd eaten three weeks from now, but that she would remember the special time of togetherness that they had shared.

I asked her if she regretted not having indulged, or if her policy of control had hindered her enjoyment of the trip. She said, "No way. This way I got to stay on track while having a wonderful time. I've got no regrets."

Planning Ahead

While we do want to exert care in our eating (read: be in control), we don't want to feel so restricted that we won't enjoy ourselves. We need to look at the meal in the context of the entire day or week's way of eating. Balancing an anticipated eating-out celebration with super-low-calorie eating at home a few days before the big event will go a long way towards helping to counteract those little extras and overindulgences. It will also give you the freedom to enjoy the meal itself without paying a heavy penalty for it.

A word of caution is in order here. Some might be tempted to go for another option: not to be careful *beforehand*, but just be super fantastic afterwards for a few days/weeks. Although on paper this may sound like an option, in practice it gets the thumbs down. Why? Number one: To be so restrictive for so long is incompatible with self-control. Number two: Even if you can manage this enforced starvation mode, it makes dieting such a restrictive burden that it might cause a ripple effect later on that will lead to giving up the whole diet, 'cause who can live like an angel, anyway? And number three: Many diets exclude unlimited "paying back," i.e., your points/calories/etc. can only be stretched out over a certain *limited* time period.

These days the world is becoming so much more health-conscious. It's a big bucks industry. People are wanting and demanding healthier food options, and restaurants are responding. Nowadays you'll see "Healthy Salad," "Dieter's Special," "Low-Fat Choice" as standard options on many menus. There's no excuse anymore to blow your diet for lack of choice. Even if your favorite restaurant does not offer healthier alternatives (yet), there's still plenty you can do to enjoy yourself without paying any penalties.

Adapting the Menu To Your Diet

If you are following a Food Combination diet (each meal consisting of either protein-based foods or carbohydrate-based foods) or an exclusively protein diet, then you can quite happily diminish hum-and-haw-what-to-choose-time by a good half hour. You'll either be saying yes to the fish, chicken, or meat dishes and no to the rice, potatoes, starchy veggies, and pasta dishes, or vice versa.

Note: If you are following a low-calorie, low-fat, high-fiber, high-carbohydrate diet, you'll need to leave the house half an hour earlier to study the menu more closely.

Potential Problem Areas

Let's look at the most common pitfalls when dining out and see what we can do to prevent falling into them.

There are five main stumbling blocks.

- Confusion
- Being too hungry
- Portion sizes
- Hidden extras
- Too many courses

■ Confusion, Confusion (Confusion)

The first time I went into a Chinese restaurant, I thought I'd gotten the wrong menu. The words were in English, but that's where the similarity to my mother tongue ended. They were transliterated from Chinese, so it had things like "Moo Goo Gai Pan" and "Tim Suyn Gai Kow." I nearly asked for the English menu, but my embarrassed husband stopped me in the nick of time.

Not knowing what is available, or how it is prepared, served, or cooked, can result not just in frustration ("Eek. This is yuck and it costs $30!"), but also in zillions of extra hidden (or so you think) calories.

 Tips

Be Assertive (And I Mean *ASSERTIVE!*)

Being typically English (read: not usually assertive), I had to learn this one from my American husband. (Americans are usually good at this.)

Listen, it's your menu choice, it's your meal, and it's your money. You have a right to ask for whatever you want. Sure, we all have to remember what our mothers taught us and ask nicely, politely, with a smile, etc., but it doesn't cost extra to ask a few questions — either for clarity or as a means of request.

So if the menu seems to be written in double dutch, Chinese, or Swahili to your untrained eye, take the time and trouble to ask for a running commentary from your knowledgeable waitress. Make it part of your restaurant experience. You might have a friendly laugh or two over what the dish is versus what you thought it was.

Apart from the obvious question of "What exactly is this?" other questions you might want to ask are:

✔ How is the dish cooked?

✔ Does the chef use any oil in the preparation/cooking process?

✔ Are the portions large? (Ask to see the size of the plate it is served on.)

✔ Is the accompanying vegetable assortment a generous portion, or should I order an extra portion of vegetables?

✔ Are the vegetables marinated or served in any oil-based dressing?

✔ What low-fat alternatives do you have on the menu?[2]

✔ Will the chef steam some vegetables especially for me?

✔ Can the chef cook this dish without any oil?

Rather the devil you know than the devil you don't.

Being pleasantly assertive and requesting what you truly want is a habit worth cultivating throughout your meal (let's make that throughout your life…) (as we'll see later on in this chapter).

---

[2] Even if the restaurant does not provide any low-fat alternatives, your question is still worth asking. When the restaurant managers realize that people are requesting healthier options, they may respond to demand and introduce new dishes. This is always worth mentioning to the manager when you thank him on your way out.

■ I'm Staaaarving! (Being Too Hungry)

You've starved yourself since lunchtime in anticipation of tonight's occasion. You are ready to devour any morsel that comes within hand-reaching radius. Remember our lesson in self-assertion? Now's the time for another opportunity to get what you truly want.

 Tips

Clink a Drink

No, sorry, not of the alcoholic variety. Let's bear in mind that alcohol before a meal will weaken an otherwise steadfast resolve and add about 100 calories per glass — and that's before you've even started lifting the knife and fork.

Right as the waitress brings you the menu, ask her if she would be so kind as to bring you a carafe (fancy word for pitcher) of iced water. Whatever you decide to order, it's going to be a waiting game before the food makes its way to your fork (or chopsticks…). Take this opportunity to clear the palate in anticipation of all those wonderful nuances of tastes and textures. You'll be taking the edge off your appetite as well as rehydrating your body with some refreshing liquid.

Start Smart

It's important to set the meal's nutritional tone right at the start. We all know what happens after choosing fried garlic mushrooms with cream sauce as an appetizer — the spiral is positively downward right through to dessert.

Know that you can have all three courses — but only if you kick off at the starting line with the right type of appetizer. What's that? Clear soup (or vegetable based), grilled vegetables, or salads with reduced/low-fat dressing (see upcoming section "Sauces to the Sideline").

Starting in this way enables your resolve to remain steadfast throughout the entire meal. If you can manage to start off on the right foot, when you are at your hungriest, then the rest of the meal should be a breeze.

Pass The 'Pas' (Bread)

Presumably you are going to a restaurant because you are hungry and want to eat. You want to be fully conscious of all that you are about to choose. In order to do this, while you are playing the waiting-for-food-game, it's important not to fall into the trap of consuming unconscious nibbles in the form of bread.

When you are lead to your table and find a beautiful, tempting breadbasket already laid out in anticipation of your arrival, take the opportunity to hand it back to the waitress before she leaves you.

If you think your resolve will not stand up to this type of masochistic torture, you can ask your companions (before you even get to your seat) if they would do the honors for you. This way you don't get to chicken out at the last minute.

If the waitress does a quick getaway before you've managed to laden her already burdened hands, or you and your companions chicken out of being assertive, all is not lost. You can carefully place the breadbasket somewhere else — on another table, on a clear counter, on the tray of a passing waiter…anywhere except in front of you. Or don't wash your hands for hamotzi, thereby removing the temptation in a "no way around it" manner.

While we are on the subject of bread…

Sometimes the bread will not be pure bread (shock, horror). Sometimes it will have been basted with oil or garlic butter, or come with accompanying butter pats. Now I know you're savvy enough by now to realize that butter is a big bad no-no, but what if it's served with some of that high-profile olive or vegetable oil? They're healthy, right? Well…

The scoop on oils? Basically, while it's true that butter is a saturated fat (a baddie), and olive oil is a "heart-healthy" monounsaturated fat (a goodie),[3] the bottom line is that they all contain about the same number of calories per serving. We're talking 100–125 calories per tablespoon, and that's before any of the real food.

Can't tell if the bread is pure or treated? Hold it in your hand, take a napkin, and place the bread in the center of the napkin. Gently fold the napkin around the bread and squeeze ever so slightly. Release and inspect your hand and napkin. Greasy stains? Hand sticky? Logical conclusions follow…

Don't Pass Up The 'Pas'

After scrutinizing the bread for telltale oil or butter, you might choose to base your meal around this fresh, squishy, high-carbohydrate, low-fat food.

Bread is not a bad food. It's what you put on it that either makes or breaks a diet.

Let's say that you are a bread-lover. There's no reason why you can't consider bread to be the mainstay of your meal and the rest, the extras. You can try ordering accompanying foods such as soup, salad, or vegetable-based dishes. This way you get to have your bread and eat it, too.

■ The Portion Sizes Are Too Big (Portion Sizes)

Restaurants do not make friends by serving small portions. People come there to eat. And eat lots. Often, you will be presented with twice the amount of food that you really need to eat. (Just visualize what you'd be serving for supper at home and you'll see what I mean.)

This fact can be the single most seriously damaging factor to your weight loss goals. You may justify that the food you choose conforms to all those healthy principles, but the truth is that whether you are on a low-fat, high-carb, or low-calorie diet, the calculator is on and it's adding up as you eat and eat and eat — even if it's the right type of food.

---

[3] See "Fighting Fats," page 99 for more information.

Tips

Pick An Appetizer As Your Main Course

Appetizers tend to conform to more sane portion sizing. Choose an appetizer with or without a couple of side dishes, and you have a well-orchestrated meal. Don't be scared to think laterally. Just because someone put course headings all over the menu doesn't mean you can't redefine your meal.

This option can work out to be cheaper for the credit card too.

Choose Veggies "Au Naturel"

There's no surer way to tell if the chef can cook than by choosing low-fat veggies. Cooking veggies with herbs and spices instead of drowning them in butter, cheese, or cream sauces is the hallmark of a good chef.

Try to look for veggies cooked in the following ways:

✔ In a reduced sauce (boiled down and thickened)

✔ In fat-free bouillons

✔ Grilled kebabs

✔ Pureed

✔ Steamed

✔ Low-fat stir-fry

The true flavors can permeate the palate without leaving a residue of fat on the plate of the mouth, or the plate of the restaurant.

Avoid the following types of veggie dishes:

✘ Fritters (fried)

✘ Fritto (fried)

✘ Hollandaise (sauce with butter and egg yolks)

✘ Tempura (battered and fried — double trouble)

✘ Batter-dipped

✘ Au beurre (with butter)

✘ Au gratin (with cheese sauce)

Think veggies are boring? No way. What about steamed cauliflower dusted with dill, baby peas with mint, tiny boiled onions, sugared (unbuttered) carrots, pickled beets, red cabbage, or little boiled potatoes with a crust of paprika or cumin.

Apart from creating an attractive, appetizing display, you're ingesting fewer calories, minimal fat, more fiber, and a wide range of vitamins and minerals (and you just thought you were having dinner).

Minimize The Mountainous Main Course

I once went to a restaurant with two other people, and when the main course arrived our three plates could not fit on the table at the same time. The plates were huge. The food looked like mini (or not so mini) Mount Sinais.

To avoid this dilemma, look for sane portion sizes such as:

✔ Kiddie

✔ Appetizer

✔ Luncheon

✔ Petite

✔ Regular

✔ Salad size

Avoid the following meal descriptions:

✘ Grande

✘ Jumbo

✘ Supreme

✘ King size

✘ Feast

✘ Combo

Knife-It

Even if you've managed to select a low-fat main dish, stay on the lookout for fat. Try wielding that sharp steak knife with precision to cut off all visible fat — leaving you with a truly trim yum and a truly trim tum and a smaller portion to boot.

Concoct

Try asking the waiter (there's that assertion again) to assemble a main course without the protein. Ask for extra accompanying veggies instead, and then order your protein by choosing it from the appetizer section. Have it served together with your main course. You might have to beg a bit and churn out extra smiles, but if they want your business, they'd be wise to accommodate you. Especially if you point out that this way you'll be able to order three courses instead of one, which means more profit for them.

Split It

If you are going to the restaurant with a friend who has similar tastes, why not split the main course? This way you'll still have room to order an appetizer and dessert as well.

Protein Explosion

As we said earlier, restaurants do not encourage regular customers by serving teensy weensy get-the-microscope-out size portions. Anyone who's ever set foot in a restaurant will readily surmise that the restaurant's version of a portion and that of the USDA[4] leaves a discrepancy about the size of a turnpike or two. In addition, most menus seem to be organized with the focus on protein. And this protein portion is massive.

Just to give you a real-life example of what I mean: the USDA recommends two to three protein servings per day. One serving of protein is typically your 3oz portion, visually equivalent to a deck of cards. When I went to a steakhouse restaurant, I was served a 24oz steak — about three times the size of my hand (I measured it). It was equivalent to *eight* times the recommended USDA single portion serving.

To protect ourselves against humongous portion ingestion (sounds like a disease?), it's a useful tool to store real-life versions of the recommended portions in your visual memory bank (instead of lugging your measuring cups with you — you don't want to appear obsessive, after all).

The USDA Food Guide Pyramid's serving size for most fruits and veggies is ½ cup. In visual terms, this is about the size of your fist.

A portion of rice? Think of half a cup of rice, or envision it rolled into a tennis ball.

Once you have a clear visual picture of what your body really needs, you will have a greater awareness of what proportion of food on your plate is necessary and what is (guess what) not.

Doggy Bags

Doggy bags were not invented for dogs. They were invented for dieters.

If your plate is presented to you with enough portions of a foodstuff to last you for three days, fear not. Request a doggy bag — *before* you begin. This will ensure that you only eat what you want to eat (and not what *they* want you to eat). Plus you won't have to make lunch tomorrow. Yippee.

If you can't quite see yourself pausing at the starting line by asking for the doggy bag before you start, you can always bear it in mind and ask for your meal remains to be packed up for you to take home.

Remembering that the food will not go to waste should help you limit your intake to what you feel comfortable consuming (versus forcing it down because you're paying for it anyway).

---

[4] United States Department of Agriculture, the agency responsible for providing nutritional guidelines for the public

Divide and Conquer

If the monstrous (although delicious…), mountainous, magnificent main course arrives and overtakes the table by its sheer hugeness, try dividing the plate into two sections: the part that you are prepared to eat (and would call a "normal" serving), and the part you plan on doggy-bagging. Dividing it in this way may help you in conquering the scale, too.

Pinch a Taste

Let's say that you are on familiar terms with the person dining with you (i.e., not on a date). Why not persuade your companion to order what you'd really like to have and order something healthy for yourself? Then, when your meal is served, you get to dip into your companion's plate for a *couple* of mouthfuls while filling up on your own low-calorie winner.

■ Hidden Extras

Fat is an easy way to make food taste good. It's also cheap when compared to lean meat or speciality dishes. Therefore, watch out for restaurants taking advantage of these fat facts — at your expense.

 Tips

Be a Fat Detective (No, I'm not calling you names)

Use our plan of assertion and ask how the food is prepared, what the chef adds, and whether they can offer any substitutions.

Don't be afraid to request:

✔ Fat-free or low-fat milk rather than whole milk or cream

✔ Gravy and sauces served on the side

✔ Butter-free vegetables

✔ Baked or boiled potatoes instead of french fries or fat-laden mashed potatoes

Sauces to the Sideline

Fresh crispy lettuce leaves, thinly sliced tomatoes, radishes and onion slithers, and finely grated julienne carrot strips all make attractive "best buy" choices when dining out.

However, it's best to preempt the restaurant's policy of serving the salad already dressed. We want precise control over what goes onto our salad so that we don't unwittingly undo all the good choosing that went into ordering it.

Therefore, try the following:

✔ Request a low- or non-fat dressing instead of the regular one. These days there are so many to choose from, the waitress shouldn't roll her eyes too much.

✔ Ask for the salad to be served with the dressing on the side (this means it will come in a little bowl instead of being freely poured for you). You will have greater control over how much of the dressing you want.

When you get the dressing on the side, try these tips:

- **Stab 'n' Dip**
  Stab a chunk of lettuce or tomato and dip it about ⅛ inch into the dressing. This way you use less dressing, but still get the flavor in every bite.

- **Dip 'n' Stab**
  Or try dipping the fork into the dressing first and then stabbing the salad. Minimal oil with maximized flavor.

It's worth noting that even though you might well have asked for a low-fat dressing, the calorie value might still be quite high. Therefore, it's a good idea to try out the following:

- **DIY Dressing**
  If you have asked for an oil and vinegar dressing, then request cruets (cute little bottles) of lemon juice or vinegar. Mix a teaspoon or two of the restaurant dressing with some of the vinegar or lemon juice to increase the quantity of liquid, and thus diminish the fat content in the dressing.

- **DIY Second Option**
  If all else fails and the restaurant hasn't got a low-fat dressing (or little bottles of vinegar, or any common sense…) try serving yourself one tablespoon of the prepared dressing and then giving the waitress the rest back — before she scuttles back into the kitchen. This way you have automatically limited your consumption of a potentially sky-high high-fat food (and you thought salad was "free").

Coleslaw Know-How

Thought they'd get those extra calories by you in the coleslaw? Try again.

Restaurants typically use the fattiest mayonnaise in the 'slaws *and* use a whole mayo jar per cup of cabbage (or at least it seems this way).

To reduce the amount of dressing:

✔ Try tipping the dish (holding back the cabbage with your fork) and emptying the excess liquidy mayonnaise into an empty glass. It's messy but effective (but also not something to try on a first date or at a fashionable restaurant — you do want to come again, don't you?).

If you *are* on a date (or your husband's warned you not to try your coleslaw trick because you are going somewhere fancy), there's still something you can do to thwart all that fat.

✔ Place a knife under the edge of the coleslaw plate so that the plate dips ever so slightly to the side. Now you can watch all that oil and mayonnaise swim to the lower plate side. Gently scrape the cabbage and vegetables towards the uphill side of the plate and you've got a you-can-take-me-anywhere version of the coleslaw trickle trick. This will work for any type of oily-served food. Try it. It's fun. (Besides, it makes for interesting table conversation....)

The "Red Sauce Rule"

A tomato-based sauce on pasta or chicken is less fattening than a cream-based white one.

■ There's Just Too Many Courses

It's not written anywhere that you *have* to eat every course on the menu. Many people will choose to skip the appetizer, stick with the main course, and only make a decision to have the dessert when they know for sure their waistband button isn't going to pop. You can too.

 Tips

Be Creative

They're making it fresh especially for you anyway, so there's no reason why you can't choose some of what goes into it or onto it, and leave out what you don't want.

Let's take the example of pizza and see what we can do to make a potentially high-fat food into a good low-fat choice instead:

✔ Ask for low-fat/fat-free cheese (there's even low-fat Mozzarella available nowadays);

✔ Skip the cheese and ask for extra tomato sauce;

✔ Substitute other low-fat protein foods such as (pareve) salami or pepperoni for the high-fat cheese;

✔ Ask for extra veggies/toppings (such as broccoli, mushrooms, onions, tomatoes, or olives);

✔ Only order one slice and substitute the other slice you would have ordered with a plain bread bun (even if you still have the french fries, you've just knocked off over 200 calories from your total).

Beware The Buffet

If we're talking about too many courses, when it comes to a buffet bar, we're talking about one massive course — without end.

Look at the entire table before putting one morsel on the plate. This way you won't fill your plate up with everything you pass.

Delay Dessert

I know that little waiter is standing at your right elbow, pen at the ready, waiting to jot down everything you say, but try not to order dessert until after the main course.

This way you will be able to ask your stomach if it truly has any room left inside to house something sweet, instead of signing a contract forcing you to have that chocolate sundae just because you thought you'd manage it at the start of the meal.

It doesn't take very long to prepare dessert. So if you do want to have it after your main course, it isn't going to take forever to come.

Sharing, Sharing

Presumably you are not dining alone. Be kind to yourself and your companion: Choose a treat and split it. Shared company. Shared calories. Shared enjoyment.

Free Coffee

Or you can opt for a sweetened fat-free coffee. Can't stand coffee? Have a diet soda (it's also free).

 Extra Tip

Become A Regular

If you do dine out frequently, consider becoming a regular at one place. That way, the waiters, waitresses, and kitchen get to know you and what you like. They can draw your attention to new diet-friendly dishes and won't be surprised by the requests of this assertive man or woman. Plus, they will be able to preempt your requests and will be more likely to acquiesce to them even during busy times (if they've done it before, they can do it again).

Conclusion

Dining out can be a fun, enjoyable, positive experience. You don't have to break your diet in order to enjoy yourself. A little forethought, a little assertiveness, and a little lateral thinking might be all it takes to eat right when eating out.

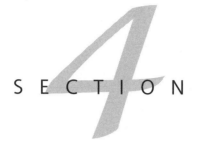

SECTION 4

Runner's Cramp — Oh No, I've Hit A Plateau

You've been nibbling on carrot sticks and wolfing down every imaginable permutation of vegetable soup. White, refined breads and crackers have been replaced by their sun-tanned, brown, whole-wheat equivalents. You've lost weight, which is great, but now your motivation is sluggish. You feel fed up, bored, and disenchanted.

Know that you are not alone. This scenario is sooooo common. The boredom kind of creeps up on you and can be a catalyst to spur you off track when you were really doing so well. Dieting can sometimes be a long journey. That makes it all the more important to enjoy the tour and keep the cogs of motivation well greased.

Let's look at some of the things you can do to give yourself that much needed sense of renewed motivation, invigoration, and focus.

We've divided this section into two. Chapter 12 has suggestions on how to reawaken an apathetic mind-set: "I just don't care any more. I can't be bothered to continue." Chapter 13 contains suggestions on how to recharge a sluggish body that refuses to part with its excess pounds anymore.

Let's start with the mind and then tackle the body...

Chapter 12

—◆◆◆—

Re-Motivation

Lose Weight

It's not usually the weight-losing regulars who find their motivation flagging. A good one to two pounds off at the scale each week is perhaps the most powerful weight-loss motivator there is. Each week's mini-success gives you the sense of accomplishment that is so important in propelling you toward your goal. You feel you worked for it, deserved it, and got it.

If your weight loss slumps (like the rest of you) and you find yourself either staying the same, losing half a pound, or putting it on, then you get frustrated that your goal seems further away and altogether less attainable.

Therefore, capitalize on the awareness that weight loss usually follows weight loss. Your immediate goal to re-motivate yourself is to try your hardest to actually see some weight coming off.

Review Your Reasons

Right at the starting, line I suggested you write down a list of the reasons why you want to lose weight (see "Focusing on Yourself," page 47).

> *Hang in there, this chapter should re-energize your worn out willpower.*

This list was to serve as a springboard into your dieting campaign. Now is a great time to remind yourself of all those reasons and reignite your sagging enthusiasm. Maybe reviewing this list will bring new reasons to light, reasons that will help you tune in to the fact that you have so much to gain by continuing.

Sometimes we feel like we are plodding on and on, not really knowing where we're going. Reviewing this list should remind us of where we are going and why the journey is worthwhile.

Lax Versus Exact

It's human nature to want to cut corners. We're busy. We want to skip the attention to detail and make our lives easy. That's why, several months into dieting, you might find yourself not quite as strict and regimented as you were right at the outset.

Aim for a rerun of your first week on the program. Try adopting the following measures to reenact Week One:

✔ Quit estimating, get the scale out;

✔ Total all those points/calories/treats that need to be tallied;

✔ Plan your menus;

✔ Stock up on fruits and veggies, low-calorie snacks and tempting diet drinks, etc.

✔ Reread the diet book.

Fill Out a Food Diary

You'll feel the renewed consciousness that the attention to detail a food diary provides, and you're more likely to lose weight. Weight loss is in itself a powerful motivating force (as we mentioned earlier).

Monitor Your Weight Loss

If losing weight is the number one motivator, then watching the weight come off must follow straight behind as the number two motivator.

There are several different ways to monitor your weight loss. The more ways you monitor it, the more motivated you are likely to feel.

Written Pound-Loss

This is your basic how-much-I-lost-this-week record. Add a column for the cumulative total amount lost for an additional boost (see Figure below). If you belong to a Group, your leader will probably have one of these for you. Ask her to show it to you and feel the surge of pride. You are definitely moving in the right direction.

Figure: An Example Of How To Track The Pounds Coming Off

Week Number	Date	Weight (lbs)	Loss (lbs)	Total Weight Lost (lbs)
1	Jan 1	200		
2	Jan 8	197	3	3
3	Jan 15	195	2	5

Recorded Inch-Loss

Have you made your "Pinch an Inch" chart? (See "Pinch an Inch," page 107.) If not, it's never too late to start. If you have, examine it and then go find the clothes that fit you perfectly on the day you made that chart. Put them on and see those numbers come to life. I bet you can pinch an inch (or near enough) on every part of your garment's arms, waist, thighs, etc. Now who wants to give up after all that success?

Plotted Pounds-Lost

Seeing a visual representation, such as a graph, is a powerful motivator in creating curves in all the right places…So make a graph of your weight loss and show yourself, "Hey, I'm on the way!"

Photograph

Take out that photograph you took right at the beginning of your diet (see "Smile, Please," page 107 — you didn't skip that chapter, did you?) and any subsequent photographs you took (at every fifteen-pound loss interval) and now go look in the mirror. See the difference? And you want to stop now???

Variety — the Spice of Life

Dieting has to stay fresh. If you become bored, it only means that you are bored with the types of food you are eating.

Try out new foods. Try out new recipes. Exchange Shabbos salads with a friend who is also dieting. Keep your eyes open for low-calorie, quick, and easy frozen meals for the odd emergency occasion. The key is to stay on top of the diet by being creative and not allowing mildew to set in. The golden rule: If your husband's not jealous of your plate, you're not doing it right!

Build Up a Stockpile

No, not of all those odd socks, although I'm sure they're piling up anyway…but of *different* low-calorie snacks, so that you can always have something interesting to nibble on.

Surround Yourself with Success

There's nothing like reading success stories to inspire us. Reading about how someone lost fifty pounds and achieved her goal translates into "she did it, and so can I."

Even if you can't get your hands on some inspiring reading material, you can try to find someone who is a real-life, flesh-and-blood personification of a dieting success story. Doesn't matter if you've never been introduced formally. Just pick up the phone, tell her where you are coming from, and ask away. You might come away not just with renewed inspiration, but with a new friend as well.

Use Your External Support

(See "Chapter 5: Tips on Enlisting External Support.")

Reenlisting the support, encouragement, and love of your nearest and dearest may help steer you back on course, re-motivate you, and give you the sense that you are not fighting this battle all alone.

Sometimes just verbalizing your reservations helps clarify and minimize the issues.

Failing motivation doesn't have to be earthshattering to be worth mentioning to your Diet Group leader. She will be able to empathize, encourage, and offer solutions.

Make Sure You Are Rewarding Yourself

Rewards pull and push us through the tough times and are such positive, easy, powerful steps in increasing a sense of personal achievement, that it seems a shame not to use them.

Whenever I ask a floundering dieter whether she is rewarding herself, invariably the answer is no. It might take a little creative energy to contemplate the reward that is right for you, but it's time well spent. Anyone who has taken rewarding herself seriously will tell you how effective it is as a motivational tool. And how simple.

It may take a degree of energy (and self-control), but I hereby entreat you to flick to page 51, to reread the full rendition about rewards.

Complying with Complacency

Complacency can be a real pitfall.

Perhaps you've had a week of overdoing it with extra treats and nibblies, but you've still lost weight the next week. You may think you've "gotten away with it" and that you can do it again the next week, but you can't do it too often or it will slow down your weight loss.

Our bodies are not predictable machines. They can often fluctuate in weight readings. It doesn't always follow that too much food one week automatically shows up on the scale right away. It might take a couple of weeks for the truth to come out. But there's no escaping the harsh realities — the scales don't lie.

There's only one way to go, and that's forward.

Change Diet

If you see that your motivation is low and that your dieting plan is not going the way you would like, it might mean that you need to reassess.

Maybe your lifestyle has changed and your current diet is difficult to follow under these circumstances. Maybe you would be happier on a diet that requires you to count points/calories a little less and allow free reign a little more on fruit or other food groups.

Changing your diet can give you a motivational boost because:
- It's new (and therefore it'll be exciting);
- It forces you to undertake a new way of eating (and limits boredom);
- It will be easier to maintain, given its compatibility with your current lifestyle.

If you are changing diets, maybe you can change Diet Groups too. You'll make new friends and feel supported while you undertake your new venture.

Learn To Learn

Learning about weight loss, nutrition, and healthy living can be very inspiring. You may develop an appreciation and understanding of the whys and hows. For example, when you understand more about the benefits of a high-fiber diet, you will be more likely to make sure that you increase your fiber intake.

Get Back on Track

If your plateau is only a recent setback, a week or two old, and it's really due to you falling off the diet track, then read this next bit of inspiration and try again.

Imagine opening the door one morning to find Interflora handing you the most exquisite, huge bouquet of flowers and orchids. They are simply stunning — in all imaginable colors and hues. There's only one thing wrong with the bouquet: There is one flower right in the middle that is a dried out, lackluster, ugly weed. What do you do? Do you throw out the whole bunch of flowers just because the perfection of its beauty is spoiled? Or do you pluck it out, throw it away, and again create a perfectly beautiful bouquet?

When you have let yourself go, it's all too easy to fall prey to the temptation of abandoning the rigors of dieting. You feel you've broken the spell and can jump off the bandwagon with gusto. That's a big mistake.

One bad day doesn't have to become a week. One bad week doesn't have to become a month. Don't let it. Pick out the weed and focus on the beauty. Pick yourself up from where you landed and continue forwards.

Conclusion

Most successful dieters have gone through tough times. What has kept them going is their keen motivation. They really wanted to reach their goal.

The race is never an easy one. We are always up against tough competition — i.e., ourselves. The way to victory is paved with many stumbling blocks. **The winner is not the one who never falls, but the one who can fall and pick herself up again and again, time after time.**

Always keep two things crystal clear in your mind and you'll also be a winner: number one — where you have come from (you never want to go back), and number two — what life is going to be like on the other side of the finishing line, in the winner's circle.

You can do it. Keep going. Give it another shot. Get back in the race and I'll see you at your victory party.

Chapter 13

—— ◆ ◆ ◆ ——

Blasting The Plateau

*N*ow that we've handled the mind, let's take on that stubborn body of ours.

You're up and running on your chosen diet and you have experienced the sweet joy of seeing the pounds come off week after week. With a Cheshire cat grin on your face, you know that if you work hard, you will see dividends on the scales. In fact, you come to expect a loss each week.

So when a time comes when there's no change, and you can't think of an obvious reason for it (that blow-out wedding was two weeks ago, not this week…), it can come as a shock. Even though you know your reaction is out of proportion, you might feel a cocktail of negative emotions: disappointed, angry, cheated, or defiant — all of which can be damaging to your long-term slimming campaign.

Few of us would give up after just one week with no weight loss. But what if it lasts for longer? And what if the blip in your progress turns into the dreaded "plateau?" (A plateau is simply three weeks or longer without a weight loss.)

Getting stuck at a plateau can de-motivate the most motivated of us. Sure, we all know when we overindulge we see more bulge, but what about when we didn't overdo things? We think, "All that hard work — and for nothing…. What's the point in trying if I am not getting the results I

stuck in a rut? Here comes the dieting tow truck.

want?" This can herald the beginning of the end. Our knee-jerk reaction may be to blow off the whole thing and drown our sorrows in the cookie jar.

This plateau is more common in two types of people: Those who have been dieting for a while (longer than two months), and those who are within fourteen pounds of their hoped-for target weight. When we realize this, we understand how truly sad and pitiful it is that a person gives up at this point.

All that hard work goes down the drain,
So close to the finish — oh, what a shame.

Here are a few tips designed to help you get the scale moving down and your motivation moving up.

All Change

I have never seen any scientific literature proving what I am about to say. All I can tell you is that I have personally seen it proven time and time again.

Our bodies get used to the types of food we eat. They get smug and cozy and decide not to shift those pounds. They get stuck in a food routine when we end up eating the same kind of planned meals.

Many successful dieters tend to stick with tried and tested meals, possibly the ones that they started off with and that have been proven to work. Familiarity makes life easier, so the status quo remains. The same two pieces of whole-wheat toast for breakfast every day...

But the truth is, when your body gets used to your routine, it slows down its pound-shedding process and you begin to plateau. It's then that your sluggish body needs a wake-up call.

One way to do this is to make a conscious decision to change the foods you eat. For example, if you have Bran Flakes for breakfast every day, you should try having Shredded Wheat one day, toast the next, Weetabix the next, etc. If you always have a tuna sandwich and soup for lunch, you could try having an open chicken sandwich or a baked potato and salad.

Not very scientific, but it works.

Time for More Change

Another way to shake your body out of a metabolic slumber is to change the times of day that you eat.

So instead of having breakfast at 8:30am, you can try having a coffee at 8:30am and holding out till 10am for the cereal. Why not continue by making lunch at a different time too?

We get into habits and may find ourselves taking our eating cues from the clock rather than from our tummies. Challenge yourself to eat only when you are hungry.

See "Eating by the Clock," page 71.

Yet More Change

And if you're ready for more change still…try changing the quantities of what you eat. So, instead of having two bowls of Shredded Wheat for breakfast, try having one now and one later. Think in terms of small and often throughout the day, instead of big and seldom.

Choose Your Fruits and Veggies Wisely

No, I'm not telling you to make sure the tomatoes aren't squishy or the mangos aren't bruised. I speak of higher levels of discernment.

Presuming that you've chosen a nutritious, well-balanced, sensible program, then it follows that fruits and vegetables will be playing a prominent role in your menu planning.

Although it's true that fruits and veggies will give you beneficial nutrients and minerals, etc., they also provide fiber and calories. Some have more than others. Therefore, it makes sense that if you are trying to kick-start yourself out of a plateau, you want to double check that you are choosing those fruits and veggies that will provide above the norm amounts of fiber and slightly below the norm in terms of calories. This means skipping certain favorites that have potentially higher calories mouthful by mouthful.

Veggies to avoid when you're on a plateau-busting campaign are: potatoes, if used as a vegetable instead of as a starch; peas (garden, petit pois, etc.); and corn/corn on the cob (although not baby corn).

Fruit to avoid during this self-imposed exile are: bananas, grapes, jambu fruit, jujube, lychees, mangoes, mangosteen, physalis, sharon fruit, and ugli fruit.

This list is tucked away inside this chapter and not blasted over the front cover because choosing only "booster" options for now and forever will mean you lose out on the variety, flavor, texture, nutrition, and enjoyment of these other delicious fruits and veggies. That would be a shame. It would also be boring. So, use this list as a temporary selection and when that plateau is broken, raid the grocery store for them once again.

Eat Enough

Did you know that there is a concept of eating too little? I know it might seem logical that the fewer calories you consume, the faster the weight will come off. But that only works up till a point.

Once you eat less than 1,000 calories a day, your body goes into "starvation mode" (and so do you). Your body doesn't know whether you are stranded on a dessert island with only a palm tree for company or that you're just dieting to get into that nice black dress for Cousin Sarah's wedding. This means that its life-preserving mechanisms will kick in as soon as its calorie thermometer reads low. Basically, this results in your body trying to conserve every calorie it can get. Sluggish system, low metabolism, and, yep, weight plateau ensue.

And surprisingly enough, you don't even have to be depriving yourself of a massive quantity of calories to start hitting a status quo. If you eat 300–400 calories a day less than you are supposed to, you could find yourself frustratingly stranded at an even-Steven weight. Your body will desperately hold on tight to every calorie it can get. (If you want to find out how many calories your body needs per day to maintain its current weight, see page 378.)

I had one client who came to me in despair. She claimed she had been dieting for years and had never lost her last fourteen pounds. I analyzed what she had been eating and saw right away that she was eating far too little. It was hard for her to accept this, but I urged her to increase her calorie intake for the next two weeks and see whether she had begun to lose by the third. (I gave her the two weeks to give her body a chance to boost her metabolism again.) And what do you know? The weight started coming off and I had one happy customer. Incidentally, she went on to lose those fourteen pounds that had been sticking around for years.

Make Fiber Your Friend

Over this plateau-breaking period, make a conscious effort to base your menus around high-fiber foods. Try out some new fiber-rich options so that you're changing the types of foods you're eating as well (see above). The fiber will fill you up faster and for longer on fewer calories. A neat trick that should help kick-start your weight loss again.

Remember to make sure you drink plenty while you're on the fiber rampage and have a peek at Appendix 2, to see a list of high-fiber foods.

Exercise Your Exercise Options

Exercise burns up calories. (See "The Equation," page 17.) Exercising more burns up more calories. Therefore, when you hit a plateau, try focusing on the cardio-vascular, huffy-puffy types of exercise to "jog" your weight loss.

In practical terms, this means walking a little further or a little faster this week, or trying out a new form of aerobics. Maybe your dieting stagnation is affecting your exercise regime — don't let it. Any activity that increases your energy output will be beneficial, both psychologically and physically.

Drink

Just this week a client asked me, "Is it true that water helps you to lose weight?" (See "Drinking Flushes Away Excess Calories," page 393.) Even though water is not magic, if you don't drink enough, you will tend to become constipated and your system will become sluggish.

Fed up with the same old drinks? Now is the time to try out whatever your friends are drinking. Ask them for a slurp or two to see if you like it. A new low-cal drink will also give your diet an extra zap that will freshen up a stale menu.

Limit Freebies

There are all kinds of popular diets out there that promote an unlimited consumption of certain types of foods. If you are on one of these diets — especially one that promotes unlimited carbohydrates or proteins (as opposed to unlimited fruits and vegetables) — maybe it's time to put a self-imposed limit on them to help get the scale moving again.

I have had clients come to me with a look of horror on their faces when I suggest they cut back on the amount of free pasta they were consuming. "But it's freeeeee!" they complain. Yes, but if you are having bowl number three just because it's free, and not because you are hungry, then those "free" calories become excess and your body reads "surplus to demand."

I, myself, once tried a diet that only restricted my fat intake. It was great. I had loads of homemade fresh bread, as much fruit as I wanted, and bowlfuls of pasta. I really enjoyed myself, but I didn't lose an ounce. When I worked out the calories involved, I discovered that I was not creating the necessary deficit to justify any weight loss. Hence my plateau — and one frustrated dieter.

Limiting your freebies isn't a life-sentence, just a plateau-blasting strategy. When weight loss resumes, you can try gradually increasing the intake of all those freebies again. For those who mean business, turn to Appendix 3, and work out how many calories you really need each day to break even (note, not even to lose weight). Then go figure out how many calories you are having each day. You might be amazed…

A Change is As Good As a Rest

If all else fails, instead of getting frustrated and veering off your chosen diet's track, try enforcing a lifestyle change and change your diet.

The different types and quantities of foods will automatically give you a sense of increased variety and pleasure. The newness might be just what your body needs to pick it up out of its complacency.

Conclusion

These ten tried and tested ways to get the stubborn scale moving again are a great plan of attack. They focus on the practical measures you can take to shake yourself out of plateau-land and back into the realm of success.

But remember, the main point is to summon up the energy, creativity, and focus for a short-term, three-week (at the most), plateau-busting, super-dieting, kick-start period. It's not a life sentence or even a long-term one. It's short, powerful, and successful. And when you've broken through and made it to the finishing line, you can come join me in the next section, where we'll let you in on the secrets of how to remain a lifetime member of the winner's circle.

Keep Going – Exercise

So far, we have been focusing on the issues of dieting and calorie control. Now it's time to focus on a brand new topic that also happens to be one of my personal hobbyhorses: exercise. Not only do I do it, I teach it, learn it (live it, breathe it, eat it), and love it.

I have found that most people will agree that exercise is good for you. When pressed for a reason (or hundred) they will quite readily mention words such as "heart, weight loss, health," etc. What they don't fully realize is that half an hour of exercise can have a mighty ripple effect into the rest of their day (read: life).

I have seen people quite literally blossom before my very eyes. Each week they arrive still carrying the burdens of their responsibilities. When we begin, they loosen up, and their attention becomes focused on what they are doing right now, not on what they have yet to do. They let go of their worries, their aggravations, their bills. They are living in the present and are enjoying the now. Our days are made up of many minutes of nows. It's up to us how we spend them. Is thirty minutes so heavy a price to pay to spread splashes of happiness into the other fifteen waking hours? (I know, I know, I also don't get eight hours of sleep a night, but somebody who reads this book must.)

Like money in the bank, the investment reaps dividends (long-term *and* short-term). But if you don't even put any money in the bank, then you are, indeed, paying a heavy price.

This section discusses exercise in say-it-like-it-is terms without the confusing jargon. It clarifies such issues as:

- Exercise — Why bother?
- Which exercises do what?
- What's an exercise class all about anyway?
- Do's and don'ts of exercise.
- Exercise tips.
- Debunking fitness myths.

When you've finished this section, you're likely to rediscover the simple joys of using your body for what it does best — moving and loving it.

Chapter 14

— ◆ ◆ ◆ —

Exercise – Why Bother?

Knowledge is empowering. Understanding the reasons why exercise is good for you should not only educate you, but it should also help to motivate you to finally take exercise seriously (although you're still allowed to smile…).

Let's find out exactly why exercise is a worthy reason to get off the sofa.

150 Reasons To Exercise

Just in case your aversion to exercise is working overtime, it is worth considering the following points as you ponder the reasons listed below.

✔ Not every exercise will apply to every reason.

✔ Not every reason is for everyone. Just because you nod your head vigorously at only forty reasons, don't be tempted to boo-hiss exercise because you didn't get to check off every *single* reason.

✔ Some reasons will scare the living daylights out of you. Some will make you think. Some will make you laugh. All are, nevertheless, reasons worthy of consideration.

✔ There are 150 reasons listed below (I told you this was my hobby-horse). So for now, I'll allow you to snuggle yourself comfortably on the sofa until your mind and heart begin to tell you otherwise…

> *I really had more than 150 reasons to exercise, but 150 is a nice, round number.*

Talking Heart To Heart

1. **It's good for your heart.** You increase the amount of blood the heart pumps with each beat. Basically, your heart becomes more effective as a blood pumper, sending that much-needed oxygen left, right, and center — all over your body.

2. **You reduce your risk of developing high blood pressure.** Too-high blood pressure increases the risk of horrible things like strokes and heart attacks. (You also end up taking yucky medicine and getting headaches.)

3. **If you *do* have high blood pressure, you will help to keep it under control.** Exercise will help to minimize the negative effects of a diagnosed condition of high blood pressure.

4. **You increase your cholesterol good guys (HDL[1]).** Not all cholesterol clogs your arteries and makes you susceptible to heart disease. Some cholesterol is good for us.

5. **You lower your cholesterol bad guys (LDL[2]).** Too much of this artery-clogging stuff can restrict the flow of blood, leading to possible strokes, heart attacks, and death. Ugh. (I told you they were bad guys.)

6. **You reduce your risk of Coronary Heart Disease — the Western World's number one killer.** Don't tell me you haven't heard that one before. People who don't exercise are as likely to develop heart disease as people who smoke.

7. **You reduce your risk of having a stroke,** the brother and close relation to Mr. Heart Attack.

8. **You lower your resting heart rate.** This means that you are putting less strain and wear and tear on your heart when you are not exercising.

9. **You reduce the chances of an irregular beat.** We want a boom-petty-boom, not a boom-petty-petty-boom. An irregular beat, apart from making you feel like you are having a mini heart attack, means that the blood is not being pumped efficiently.

10. **You improve your circulation.** Blood will go with the flow and will reach all those extremities like fingertips and toes.

11. **You reduce the thickness of the blood.** Who wants gunky blood? Icky-icky. Thinner blood is easier on the arteries.

12. **You increase your volume of blood plasma.** Regular exercise increases the liquid component in the blood. This reduces the risk of developing dangerous clots.

13. **You slow your panic-sounding heartbeat when you run up the stairs.** It gets easier to get the things you forgot the first time.

14. **You increase your chances of surviving a heart attack.** Which we hope you won't get, but we'd all quite like to live to see 120 (even if we are attacked along the way, G-d forbid.)

---

[1] HDL: High Density Lipoproteins
[2] LDL: Low Density Lipoproteins

15. **You can ease the pain of varicose veins.** The walls of varicose veins have been stretched, allowing blood to pool in the legs. Exercise helps relieve the resulting swelling and aching because the contraction of calf muscles causes blood to shoot upward.

16. **You will increase your ability to supply blood flow to the skin for cooling.** Just as a dog needs to pant to cool down, we need to cool ourselves down by making sure the hot blood rises to the large surface area of the skin so that the colder external environment can cool us. Especially good for hot-heads, hot-tempers, hot-blooded males…

Better for Diabetics

17. **You're less likely to *get* diabetes.** Staying fit can drastically reduce your chances of developing type 2 (non-insulin dependent) diabetes by lowering blood sugar and blood fat levels. And if you already have diabetes? Guess what? Exercise can help control the symptoms. Told you this was good stuff.

18. **You can help reduce the amount of insulin required to control your blood sugar levels if you are a type 1 (insulin dependent) diabetic.** More good news for diabetics.

19. **You increase your tissues' responsiveness to the actions of insulin, helping you to better control your blood sugar.** This is getting exciting.

Inside Out (Internal Organs, Lungs, Intestines, and Stuff)

20. **You improve your breathing.** In other words, with each breath you get more of the wonderful stuff called oxygen. In terms of real-life benefits, your breathing becomes less labored.

21. **You reduce your risk of developing colon cancer.** Exercise increases the efficiency of the whole body — bones, muscles, heart, and yes, even the bowel. Moderate daily exercise, such as an hour-long walk or a half-hour jog, may reduce your colon cancer risk by as much as half.

22. **You may reduce the risk of developing breast cancer.** Although the evidence isn't conclusive, research suggests that physically active women are less prone to breast cancer than women who don't work out.

23. **You improve your respiratory muscle strength and endurance.** This is particularly important for asthmatics.

24. **You are less likely to need gallbladder surgery.** Doctors have known for years that obesity increases the risk of gallstones, but now research has shown that a sedentary lifestyle is another contributive factor.

25. **You are less likely to be constipated.** Exercise improves the rate at which harmful waste matter travels through the system.

26. **You improve your gastrointestinal and digestive functions.** Exercise kinda gets things moving along all around.

27. **You improve the function of your immune system.** You are less likely to experience all those coughs and colds, unlike Mrs. Couch (aaaasheeew) Potato. Bless you.

28. **You will build up your tolerance to lactic acid.** It's lactic acid, a natural body toxin, that stops you from continuing your 100-yard dash for the bus that pulls away without you. It also stops you from performing limitless strenuous repetitive actions that seem to beg you to stop (stuff like hedge-cutting and climbing lots of stairs).

Body Bits (Bones, Muscle, Cartilage, etc.)

29. **You will increase the density and strength of your bones.** Bones are not just something that are buried with you when your time is up. Bones are made up of living matter. They respond to the demands made on them and will become stronger if they need to.

30. **You will reduce your risk of developing osteoporosis (brittle bone disease[3]).** This nasty condition keeps rearing its ugly head in the media and health journals. That's because it's serious (see the frown). Brittle bones can break easily and can signal the onset of immobility and infirmity. Research has now shown that exercise is a highly effective tool in preventing osteoporosis.

31. **You can slow down the rate of joint degeneration if you suffer from osteoarthritis.** This means less pain in the long run. (Get it? "Long run...")

32. **You can help to retard bone loss as you age.** Since it's downhill after thirty (both men and women start losing bone mass between ages thirty and forty, together with their keys, their glasses, their pens...), we want to glide the gradient gently versus falling off the cliff edge. Not only can lifting weights stop the decline, but in some cases weightlifting can reverse it. Weight-bearing activities like walking and running also help keep your bones strong.

33. **You will increase the density and strength of ligaments and tendons.** These are the bits that keep the bones and muscles strung together. We want our ligaments and tendons to be strong like elastic, not to snap with a crack.

34. **You will increase the thickness of the cartilage in your joints.** This is good because the joint cartilage can erode and cause us to suffer pain and difficulty in movement. And we don't want that to happen, do we?

35. **You will improve and maintain your level of joint flexibility.** Bending those knees to pick up Shnocky's favorite toy becomes a whole new experience — void of moans and groans.

36. **Flexibility improves your quality of life.** You'll be able to reach your back to give yourself a good, long scratch, instead of jumping up and down against the side of the door.

37. **You'll get strong muscles.** Not only will your muscles gain definition, but you get to pick up Shnocky without flinching.

---

[3] See page 294.

38. **You will increase your levels of muscular endurance.** You will be able to lift Shnocky up and hold him for hours on end (or at least until he stops crying).

39. **You will increase the thickness and number of fibers within each muscle, thereby improving your aerobic capabilities.** You will be able to push the stroller quickly for longer without getting out of breath.

40. **You will increase your muscle glycogen levels.** Glycogen is a form of energy for the muscles. With a bountiful supply we are ready…steady…fire…go.

Oops-A-Daisy Injury (Prevention and Recovery)

41. **You will be better protected against injury during your day.** Having strong bones, strong heart, strong lungs, strong joints, strong ligaments, and strong tendons will make you —what? You guessed it — strong. In other words, you'll be less likely to suffer all those horrible things that not-strong people get (like a pulled muscle or a torn ligament that sends them home from a shopping spree before they've even had a chance to whip out their credit card).

42. **You are more likely to recover faster from an accident.** If you are involved in a car crash or serious accident (G-d forbid), the fitter you are, the higher your chances are of recovering fully and quickly.

43. **You are less likely to develop lower back problems.** Let's make that shoulder, upper, middle, and lower back problems. So many backaches are the result of poor posture. Research shows that having strong abdominal and back muscles is a highly effective preventative measure to counteract those immobilizing aches and pains.

44. **You can help to alleviate back pain.** If all this talk about posture is news to you and finds you holding your lower back with a grimace on your face, all is not lost. Many potential candidates for back surgery have successfully avoided surgery through a regimen of exercise, and have even improved their condition until they became pain-free. It's worth considering exercise as a potential antidote before reaching the operating table.

45. **You are less likely to injure yourself by spontaneously jumping off the chair to play rough and tumble with the kids.** Having strong and flexible muscles can help you avoid that nasty hamstring pull that sends you back to the chair while you miss all the fun. Think I'm repeating myself? Perish the thought. No, this is not the same as No. 41. There, we were talking about injuries incurred on a day-to-day basis. Here, we're talking rapid, awkward movements that result in a piercing scream.

46. **You are less likely to develop carpal tunnel syndrome.** Strengthening the wrist, arm, and hand muscles can make you less prone to this painful condition of the wrist that is common among people who are involved in repetitive-motion tasks (like typing).

Weight Loss Wonders

47. **You will increase your chances of losing weight.** By burning up calories through exercise you burn off pounds (even if you are not on a diet[4]).

48. **You are more likely to maintain your weight loss, unlike when dieting alone, where you are more likely to regain lost weight.** Studies show that people who lose weight by dieting alone regain it within one to three years — but that's because they don't exercise. In a study conducted on those who successfully lost weight *and* exercised, ninety-five percent kept it off.

49. **You will reduce your overall amount of body fat.** We want to replace excess body fat with muscle or zap it into oblivion. Yes, dieting shifts pounds. But much of that lost weight will be muscle, not fat. Some exercise classes are advertised as "Fat-Busters." Now you know why.

50. **You can reduce your level of abdominal obesity.** Not only will your skirts close more easily, but you will diminish the scientifically proven and significant health risk factors (heart disease) associated with carrying an excess fat surplus around the midriff.

51. **You will burn off excess calories.** If you overindulged in that mini chocolate bar, you can eradicate your misdemeanor on the exercise bike.

52. **You will protect yourself against creeping obesity.** No, I'm not talking about a 300-pound giant on his hands and knees who is following you as fast as he can. I'm talking about the slow-but-steady weight gain that can occur as you get older (and move less).

53. **You will decrease your appetite.** This only works short-term. Sorry.

54. **You will help to increase your resting metabolic rate.** This means you'll need more calories just to do…nothing.[5]

55. **You will help to maintain your resting metabolic rate.** Since this is such a great way to spend calories, we want to hold onto it long-term (let's make that forever).

56. **You are less likely to overeat.** After working hard to achieve your ideal shape and ease of movement, it's easier to withstand the temptation of seconds of hot chocolate fudge cake when you know how heavy and gunky you'll feel afterwards. (Well, maybe some will find it easier…)

---

[4] See "The Equation," page 18.
[5] See page 295.

Mirror, Mirror on the Wall, Who's the Fairest of Us All? (Appearance)

57. **You will look younger.** Acting younger will make you look younger. (You can take your thumb out your mouth now.)

58. **You will improve your physical appearance.** It will become a pleasure to meet yourself in the mirror.

59. **You will tone up and firm up all those hidden parts.** Baggy sweaters hiding flabby contours? Exercise soon puts things right.

60. **Your clothes will fit you better.** You'll work your waist away as you waste away.

61. **You will regain your pre-pregnancy figure more quickly.** There's nothing like exercise to re-sculpt the body back into shape.

The Feel-Good Factor

62. **You will gain confidence that will spill over to the rest of your life.** Ran a mile? Did ten push-ups? Swam fifteen minutes non-stop? The sense of accomplishment that comes from succeeding in these areas may give you the confidence to make that presentation to your most important client, or help you muster up the confidence to take on a new challenge.

63. **You will feel younger.** Having more energy gives you an unmistakable vibrant vitality usually found only in young people.

64. **You will learn the art of teamwork.** That is, if you never learned it in school. There's nothing like a game of volleyball or basketball to give you a refresher course.

65. **You will reduce your anxiety levels.** Exercise can be extremely therapeutic. Besides, when you're working out, you haven't got time to worry.

66. **You will handle your stress more effectively.** If you can't bash, punch, or kick the person who's stressing you out, then why not go and let out your aggravations in the gym? More than 150 studies prove it: Regular exercise makes you less tense and better able to cope with events that might otherwise transform you into Mr. Hyde.

67. **You will improve your mood.** Exercise increases the feel-good hormones called endorphins. Because the endorphin rush is so commonly experienced after exercise, it has been nicknamed "runner's high." It's been scientifically proven that exercise can put you in a good mood. Both aerobic and weight-training sessions seem to offer this boost.

68. **You can alleviate depression.** Research clearly shows that exercise can help clinically depressed men and women of all ages. Depression breeds apathy. Exercise can help to break the vicious cycle.

69. **You feel happier over the long-term.** Not only does a single workout make you feel better, but regular exercisers enjoy long-term psychological benefits.

70. **You can improve your pain tolerance.** Clinics in chronic pain management strongly encourage their patients to utilize exercise as an effective method in counteracting their condition.

71. **You have fewer tension headaches.** People who have chronic tension headaches have reported feeling better after they workout.

72. **You will get warm.** Raising your heartbeat automatically means that heat will be created in the process. So, if you are feeling the chill factor of winter, exchange your thermal undies for your exercise kit and feel the warmth permeate.

73. **(On the other hand…) You improve your tolerance to heat.** You are less likely to get hot and bothered when you are sunbathing in the Bahamas (or is that why you went?).

74. **You will increase your ability to adapt to cold environments.** You increase the efficiency of your body's internal thermostat.

Living it Up (Quality of Life)

75. **You will be able to consume greater quantities of food and still maintain a calorie balance.** The more you exercise, the more energy you need. Food provides us with that energy. Seconds of pasta, anyone?

76. **You are more likely to maintain an independent lifestyle.** We're not talking about taking dad's car without asking, or moving from home to share an apartment. We're talking about older people who will be less likely to fracture a bone in a fall and need long-term help.

77. **You will be able to respond better to emergencies.** Not the toddler tantrum kind of emergency; we're talking about being able to sprint for help — and still have some breath leftover to call 911.

78. **You lessen the symptoms of PMS.** Exercise may reduce the bloating, lower back pain, headaches, and anxiety that often accompany premenstrual syndrome.

79. **You ease symptoms of menopause.** Highly active menopausal women experience fewer hot flashes than their sedentary counterparts. They also experience a mood boost after an aerobic workout.

80. **You're more useful around the house.** No need to ask Dad to help you with that stuck pickle jar, or to help shift the mattress to the guest room — Mighty Mom is here.

81. **You will enjoy the snow more.** Instead of wrapping up layer upon layer in an effort to gloss over those other hiding layers, you may be more inclined to try sledding, skating, or skiing (otherwise known as trying to walk to the shops in winter instead of taking the car), or even snowball fighting with the kids.

82. **You increase your chances of an easier birth experience.** You'll do less huffing and puffing, and will find it easier to position yourself correctly.

83. **You may give birth more quickly.** Research suggests that fit women have labors one-third shorter than women who don't exercise (although research is not conclusive).

84. **You can make it easier to stop smoking.** Anyone *not* read the billboards recently? Just for the record: Smoking kills.

85. **You gain perspective.** You notice a lot more about your neighborhood when you walk, jog, or bike around it than when you whiz by at thirty miles per hour concentrating on the traffic lights, the cars, and rush hour. Who wants life to whiz by us? We want to live life and experience its simple pleasures.

86. **You will enjoy your retirement more.** No, there's nothing wrong with Scrabble or playing bridge. It's just that the options become endless when movement is involved. How about golf, gardening, bowling, or going for that walk with the grandchildren instead of staying home?

87. **You can relieve arthritis pain.** Not only can arthritis patients safely participate in exercise programs, but they are often rewarded for their efforts with pain relief and increased mobility.

88. **You will have oodles more energy to meet the demands of daily life.** So many people think exercise drains your energy, whereas quite the opposite is true. So long as you are working at a level appropriate to your fitness levels (and not at the level of the jumping jack in the leotard who stands in front of you) exercise *gives* you energy. (You're only sitting there shaking your head at me in total disbelief because you've never tried it.)

89. **You will improve your balance.** You'll be able to stand on one leg while you get the stone out of your other shoe — without toppling over onto the pavement.

90. **You will improve your coordination in exercise.** When the instructor tells you to move your legs this way and your arms that way, you will go to the top of the class.

91. **You will improve your overall coordination.** You will be able to pat your head and rub your tummy at the same time…you'll be able to dance at a wedding like a pro…you'll be able to rock the baby chair on the floor with one foot while you talk on the phone and make a challah dough at the same time. The opportunities are endless…

92. **You will help to improve conditions such as dyslexia and dyspraxia.** Improving hand-eye coordination, alternate limb movements, and multi-tasking can help people with these conditions. Exercise can often require a person to do two things at once (i.e., march and move your arms); hence it can provide a useful corrective therapy.

93. **You improve your posture.** You will be able to, "Walk tall, walk straight, and look the world right in the eye…." Not only will walking, standing, or sitting correctly make you look slimmer and taller (shoulders back yet?), but you will incur many health benefits such as being able to breathe deeply (told you that you needed your shoulders back…) and avoiding (ouch) back pain.

94. **You are likely to perform better in school.** Compared to sedentary girls, active girls have better grades and are more likely to succeed academically.

95. **You can improve your athletic performance.** Want to swim with the kids this summer, instead of just watching them?

96. **You will find new ways to reward/treat yourself.** Instead of going for a pizza and french fries lunch, you might try that new dance class or opt for a thirty-minute appointment at the health spa. This way you won't be undoing all the hard work you have put into yourself and you still get to have a great time.

97. **You will be able to move fast.** You will be able to outrun Shnocky as he makes a quick getaway.

98. **You will be able to continue moving for longer.** You'll be able to run all the way to the park with him instead of dragging behind.

99. **You will increase your travel options.** Instead of going to the countryside to sit in a deck chair, you can consider going canoeing in Colorado, skiing in Switzerland, hiking in the Himalayas, or bicycling through Budapest.

100. **You can satisfy your competitive urges.** Playing golf can channel all those competitive energies. Likewise when you try to beat the clock.

101. **You will have more stamina.** You will endure the rigors of Pesach cleaning, mowing the lawn, and shoe shopping for longer.

102. **You may become more creative.** That's not surprising. Many people come up with their best ideas while on the treadmill.

103. **You will increase your overall health.** They don't say "hale and hearty" for nothing.

104. **You will stay supple and stretchy.** Don't worry, you won't end up looking like an elastic band — but you might get to feel like one, and that's not such a bad thing. Want to reach that purse from the backseat? Need to pick up Shnocky's shoes for the umpteenth time? As little as five minutes of stretching a day helps you keep your muscles loose and helps you stay agile.

105. **You will increase your quality of life.** Being able to move more freely, faster, and for longer means living more fully. You will be able to experience the sweet and simple joys in life, without the huffing, puffing, moans, and groans — unless, of course, you take your teenager with you.

106. **You will have more options for family togetherness.** Instead of watching your wedding video from ten years ago while sitting in the living room, how about kicking a ball around or playing tag with the family?

107. **You can catch up on your reading.** Bored on the exercise bike? Utilize this time with a two-for-one occupation.

108. **You can listen to a tape.** This one is especially effective at getting you to stay on the exercise bike longer — so that you can hear the end of the lecture/story/song.

109. **You will sleep better.** Sedentary people turned exercise-aholics boost the amount of time they spend in slow-wave sleep (the type of sleep that is restorative). They are also less likely to wake up in the night, before the alarm clock brrrrrrings them to life.

110. **You can feel more relaxed.** Some less rigorous classes, like Pilates, Yoga, or Stretch-'n'-Tone, can especially help to calm your mind and improve your lung capacity. All that deep breathing is enough to unwind the most wound up of workers.

111. **You will increase your circle of friends.** You will make new friends at the gym or class. Relationships can flourish with all sorts of people whom you wouldn't normally meet.

112. **You will stay connected with those who are close to you.** Dragging teenage daughter to gym class, going for a walk with the elusive husband, and biking with a friend are all good ways of catching up with the important people in our lives.

113. **You will have fun.** Once you find the type of exercise that you enjoy, whether it's step, aerobics, aqua fit, or hiking with the boys, you stop thinking of exercise as a drag and start looking forward to lacing up your sneakers. Exercise becomes like it used to be at recess time in school — a time to stop being serious and just get out and have fun.

114. **You will be able to reward yourself with some well-deserved pampering.** Most decent gyms have a sauna. Some even have solariums, Jacuzzis, and massages. What better way to give yourself a pat on the back than by giving yourself some luxury body-time?

115. **You will improve your self-esteem.** You are giving yourself the message that you are important enough to look after.

Spiritual Reasoning

116. **It's a mitzvah to guard your health.** Being the right weight for your height and exercising regularly will become additional merits. Don't know about you, but I could sure do with some. Conversely, we may be held accountable for the years we knocked off our allotment by not taking precautions against disease and premature death.

117. **It's a mitzvah to serve G-d with joy.** We need a healthy sense of self-esteem to be truly happy. Exercise may be just the thing we need to build a sense of accomplishment and self-worth into our life.

118. **It's a mitzvah to feel joy with all the good that the Al-mighty has given us.** Being in pain, being depressed, and having a low self-esteem are all obstacles to fulfilling this mitzvah properly. As we have mentioned, exercise may be just the thing to help.

119. **It's a mitzvah to look good for your husband.** He's not going to tell you, so I'll do it for him. He prefers you to be fit (and slim) rather than fat (and grim).

120. **It's a mitzvah to look after the gift you received from G-d.** Just like a father would be happy to see his son playing nicely with the expensive electric train set he just gave him for a present (and not bashing it up, throwing it around, or jumping on it), so too, will our Father "upstairs" get nachas if we look after the gift He so lovingly gave us to use every day and every night.

121. **It's easier to serve G-d if your body is working well.** If you have a health imped-iment or are stuck in a hospital bed, it's much harder to do His bidding (or any-one else's for that matter).

This is our last section on the benefits of exercise. I saved this one for last because, although all the reasons are true and (I hope) persuasive, many of them are unusual, previously undiscovered, funny, and, well, kind of cute (if I do say so myself). Get ready for a giggle.

Perks of the Job (Side Benefits)

122. **You will increase your own body appreciation.** Instead of just wearing your body automatically, you will begin to enjoy the way it sorta fits.

123. **You will improve your knowledge in health issues.** You will find out what an elliptical trainer is (not a personal trainer who has fits), what a gluteus maximus is (not a planet), and what a hamstring stretch is (don't worry, it's kosher).

124. **You will learn a lot about your body.** When you perform certain exercises, you will become intimately acquainted with your muscles and the actions they per-form for you. You will live, learn, and feel that you use your quadricep muscles (front thigh) to squat down and your gluteus maximus (buttock muscles) to squat up (when you go to pick up Shnocky's pacifier from the floor).

125. **You're more likely to live a long life.** In an eight-year study of more than 20,000 men, those who were lean but unfit had twice the risk of death as fit, lean men. Even *fat* men who were fit had a lower death rate than those who were lean but unfit. The same goes for women.

126. **You will have a greater appreciation for the physical exertion of others.** You don't understand how hard it is to tread water for five minutes until you've done it yourself. Then, when you say "Wow!" to Shnocky, you'll really mean it.

127. **Your family will become more exercise-conscious.** There's nothing like the power of example to get everyone wanting to follow in your footsteps. You'll be helping your children grow up healthy and strong and they will (we hope) develop good lifetime habits. This is especially important in an age in which childhood obesity is at an all-time high.

128. **You will improve your memory.** In a six-month study of previously sedentary men and women ages sixty to seventy-five, those who walked three times a week scored twenty-five percent better on memory and judgment tasks, such as recalling schedules and quickly differentiating between vowels and conso-nants.

129. **You can increase your mental alertness.** Alert body, alert mind.

130. **You will have more job opportunities.** You can't be a Hatzolah volunteer, a gym teacher, or a gofer (someone who goes for this and goes for that) if you flunk the physical.

131. **You're likely to perform better on the job.** What with physical prowess, increased self-esteem, mental alertness, and stamina, is it any wonder that you'll be more productive?

132. **You will reduce the number of workdays you miss due to illness.** Your boss will be happy to have you around.

133. **You will incur fewer health care and medical expenses.** Ill health means more trips to the doctor, more medication, and more prescriptions. Put them together and what have you got? Less money.

134. **You save money.** OK, after you've bought some trendy exercise gear…Just think of all those emergency measures you take when you are ill: oven fries and pareve sausages, more housecleaning help, and extra babysitting expenses, to name just a few.

135. **You save the country money.** Perhaps saving the president a cool few thousand dollars isn't as high on your list as saving your own skin, but just consider that in America alone, obesity-related diseases cost the nation $100 billion a year.

136. **You will get some cool stuff.** If you run a national marathon or take part in a charity gala event, you will probably get a memento of the occasion — be it a trendy T-shirt, mug, or sweatband.

137. **You will be able to have a shower in peace.** If you stay at the gym for a shower, there won't be anyone to "Moooooooommy" you outside the bathroom door.

138. **You will discover abilities you never knew you had.** Chances are you will have a natural ability for some type of movement — whether it's running, aerobics, or dancing. But you won't know until you try.

139. **You have an excuse to go shopping.** You can buy an endless number of nifty sports gadgets — like heart rate monitors (in watch or armband form), resistance bands, dumbbells, sweatbands, new thick sports socks, and a decent water bottle (instead of Shnocky's leftover soda bottle that leaks).

140. **You can encourage your unfit friends to become more fit.** When Friend Fraidy hears that you have started doing something constructive about becoming more fit, she'll want to get on the bandwagon too. Maybe you can set up a regular rendezvous — just the two of you.

141. **You get to be alone.** There are so many ways to exercise all by your lonesome. If you live amidst a continuous tumult, this may provide you with some precious (guilt-free) time for yourself.

142. **You get to rest your aching feet.** Not all exercise involves standing on your feet. How about trying an aqua class, weight machines in the gym, a rowing machine (no, not the argumentative kind), a stretch and tone class, or the good ole stationary exercise bike?

143. **You will calm your conscience.** Been meaning to join the gym since last summer? Been thinking about going swimming with the girls but somehow didn't get around to it? Stop your conscience dead in its tracks — do something about your resolutions.

144. **You will reap tangible rewards.** Stick to it — even if just for a couple of weeks, and you will see how quickly you improve. Whereas a set of ten reps (repetitions) may have been five more than you felt comfortable with last month, this month it's a breeze.

145. **You will become more efficient.** How else are you going to manage to shop, cook, clean, bake, pick up the kids, go to the doctor, make supper, *and* fit in an hour at the gym?

146. **You might create new career opportunities.** Maybe the exercise bug will bite you so thoroughly that you'll want to share it with others and become an exercise instructor yourself. (Don't laugh, it happened to me.) Maybe going to the pool again after a fifteen-year hiatus will inspire you to become a lifeguard or swimming teacher.

147. **You'll become more interesting.** It'll give you something extra to share with your spouse at suppertime. ("I met Fraidy at the gym and she told me…")

148. **You'll be able to laugh better.** With all that increased lung capacity, expanded chest cavity, and endurance training, you'll be able to giggle, guffaw, snigger, snortle, chuckle, titter, and hoot for hours on end. (She who laughs last…is the fit lady).

149. **You will have another reason to use those sneakers you bought especially for Tisha B'Av.** If your sneakers are sitting in the closet getting dusty waiting for their twice-a-year appearance, why not give them another *raison d' être*?

150. **You'll get out of the house.** This is my all-time favorite reason (that's why I saved it for last). It's so refreshing to see beyond our familiar four walls, to air out, to meet people, to use a different part of our brain (and not just for thinking, "What's for lunch? What time is that appointment? Where's the Scotch tape?"). I have had people come up to me after an exercise class and remark, "Thank you so much — that was such a tonic for me."

If you want my honest opinion about exercise — yes, it's true that the physical benefits are tremendous, but I would argue that the psychological benefits even surpass them. Don't believe me? Go on. I dare you. Prove me wrong and get mooooooooooving!

Now, if 150 reasons aren't enough to persuade you that it's about time you started taking exercise seriously, I figure you must be super-glued to the sofa. With so many benefits to your health, mind, work, and finances — can you afford not to start exercising?

I can just hear you saying it's all well and good to be charged with an energetic impetus to begin this new and exciting venture, but which exercises do what? How often should I do them, and for how long? What's the best way to access exercise? What's an exercise class about anyway? Are there any do's and don'ts for exercise? What tips will help me get the most out of the exercise I choose to do?

You've got so many questions — good. Keep turning the pages (good finger exercise) and let's see if we can start answering some of them.

Chapter 15

—— ◆ ◆ ◆ ——

Which Exercises Do What?

*T*here are different types of fitness. That sounds like a simple enough statement. The issue becomes more complex, however, when we don't know which type of fitness is a good "fit," and which type of exercise will give us the benefits we desire.

So let's demystify all the jargon and try to understand exactly what we have to do to achieve the results we want.

There are four basic forms of exercise that will render fitness in each area (there *are* other forms, too, but we'll stick to the most common ones). Our levels of fitness (and competency) depend upon which form of exercise we choose to do:

- Aerobics;
- Stretching;
- Strength training;
- Mind-Body.

In each area, we want to know exactly what that type of exercise is; what it's supposed to accomplish; how it accomplishes it; and which classes (or alternatives) will offer that type of exercise. Hold on to your hats while we take a whirlwind tour through each area.

Do you want to know which exercises help for which parts of the body? Then read on.

Aerobics

What is Aerobics?

Aerobic exercise is any repetitive motion that involves the body's larger muscles (arms, legs, etc.), performed at an intensity that challenges the heart and lungs.

"Aerobic" literally means "with air." When we exercise in the manner described above, remaining in constant motion for an extended period of time, our bodies need extra oxygen (air) to cope. The harder we exercise, the more oxygen we need (just like a car needs more gas when zooming along the highway at seventy miles per hour than when it's stuck at a standstill in traffic).

We get this extra oxygen by breathing harder (faster and more fully) — fondly called huffing and puffing. This, in turn, makes our lungs work harder. Therefore, aerobic exercise is really a workout designed, quite literally, to work the lungs (and thereby improve their efficiency).

But that's not all. You may hear exercise-minded people using the words "aerobics" and "cardio" interchangeably. That's because they *are* interchangeable. "Cardio" is a term that is tossed about by all those people who seem to know what they're talking about. ("My gym has some amazing, hi-tech cardio equipment.") It's colloquial for "cardiovascular" and can sometimes be abbreviated to a simple "CV." "Cardio" literally means "for your heart," because it refers to the kind of exercise that strengthens your heart.

At the same time as our lungs are working harder to take in all that oxygen, our hearts are pumping harder to get all that new oxygen (now residing in the bloodstream) all around the body.

So, in effect, aerobics/cardiovascular exercises are those exercises that give both the lungs and the heart a really good workout.

Why Should I Do Aerobic Exercise?

Improving the efficiency of our lungs and heart are two bumper reasons that should persuade anyone with a heart and two lungs to start this type of exercise. But there are oodles of "real-life" reasons (where you can actually see and measure the benefits of this type of exercise) that should further propel you into motion. Ready for an "oodle" or two?

- You will be able to walk quickly/jog more easily (without getting out of breath);
- You will recover more quickly from physical exertion (like running for the bus);
- You will increase your energy levels;
- You will de-stress and relieve tension;

- You will access your fat-burning energy system to help burn up calories and speed up weight loss;
- You will improve the body's metabolic efficiency;
- You will get a "mood-boost" (from all those happy endorphins roaming around the body);
- You will lower your blood pressure;
- You will reduce the risk of heart disease (including strokes and attacks);
- You will increase your chances of living longer.

Although some exercises will primarily give you a great aerobic workout, they can also carry additional benefits. Walking briskly will also make your bones stronger, because you will be performing a "weight-bearing" exercise. (No, this is not an excuse to put on weight.) This simply means that the legs have to accommodate the body's weight, which, in turn, acts as a bone-strengthening[1] force. In more practical "so – what?" terms, these types of exercise help to prevent the dreaded bone disease called "osteoporosis"[2] that's so prevalent in older ladies.

How Do You Work Aerobically?

Well, you do have to huff and puff a bit (but not enough to blow the house down…). If you're working at a mild, strolling-through-the-park level, your heart won't be benefiting much. They don't call it "working out" for nothing. However, you also don't have to jump around as though you were allergic to the force of gravity either. Somewhere between the two lies a happy medium.

Practically speaking, there are three factors involved in order to improve your aerobic fitness: **F**requency, **I**ntensity, and **T**ime. These conveniently spell out "**FIT**" so you can remember them.

Frequency

Ideally, we have to work our heart and lungs effectively three to five times a week to improve our aerobic capacity.

Intensity

You have to work at sixty to eighty percent of your Maximum Heart Rate. That's the official jargon for breathing so hard that you can still talk but you can't sing. (At least it'll give you a good excuse as to why you're singing off-key.)

Time

The recommended period of time you have to work in order to see improvement is twenty to sixty minutes. (Thirty is OK if your blood pressure went up at the mention of a sixty-minute workout).

---

[1] See page 272, #29.
[2] See later, page 294.

However, see later, "I have to exercise for thirty consecutive minutes in order to benefit," page 337.

Irregular, mild exercise such as golf or window-shopping is, unfortunately, ineffective in developing levels of aerobic fitness (although they might improve your mood). There's no escaping the facts. You have to move if you want to move better.

A Word About Impact

If you go to an aerobics class, chances are that you will hear the terms "low impact" and "high impact" thrown around quite freely (that's because the words don't cost anything). "Low impact" means that you are performing the steps with at least one foot in contact with the floor at all times. "High impact" means that both feet are off the floor at the same time for a split second or two. If that sounds confusing, just think of low impact as walking it through, and high impact as jogging/jumping it through.

Note that aerobic exercise does *not* have to be performed by jumping around in order to be effective. In fact, if you are very heavy, it is inadvisable to overexert yourself in this way. (Jumping around when overweight is not just overly stressful for your heart; it also increases your risk of injury.) The most important level for you to work at is the one that is comfortable for you — where you feel like you are working but not like you are in a medieval torture chamber.

In addition, if you suffer from a weak pelvic floor[3], stay with the low-impact options. Your already weakened pelvic floor won't take too kindly to all that extra jumping.

Warning

Although the instructor might be the most motivating specimen of humanity and makes leaping through the air look as easy as a hyperactive frog, don't be mislead by her encouragement and overwork yourself. This means that if you feel you are working at a comfortable, relatively demanding rate and would feel uncomfortable or in pain from working any harder, stick with the level that works well for you. There is no such concept as a necessity of pain to feel that you are working sufficiently hard. Remember, *"If pain, no gain."* See also, later, page 290.

Different Types of Aerobic Exercises

There are all sorts of classes and equipment that will render an aerobic workout. It doesn't have to be advertised as an aerobics class (although that is the most obvious one). Your heart doesn't care much whether you went to a studio class, used the treadmill, or chased after the kids for three blocks with their forgotten lunchboxes. Your heart will thank you either way (and it's not a bad idea to stay on his good side).

Below is a list of a few alternatives:

✔ Walking briskly;

✔ Jogging;

✔ Running;

---

[3] See page 333.

✔ Jumping rope;

✔ Bicycling (or exercise bicycling);

✔ Spinning;[4]

✔ Swimming (note: not including shmoozing in the shallow end);

✔ Dancing;

✔ Ice skating (continuously);

✔ Skiing (note: *not* including chair lifts);

✔ Stair climbing;[5]

✔ Step classes;[6]

✔ Tennis;[7]

✔ Badminton;

✔ Hiking;

✔ Volleyball;[8]

✔ Aquafit classes;

✔ Gardening (if it's a big mess and you're feeling enthusiastic);

✔ Washing the car (with enthusiasm);

✔ Vacuuming (if you're in a hurry and have a large floor space of carpet that'll take you twenty to thirty minutes).

Stretching

The second type of exercise on our list is stretching. Unfortunately, stretching doesn't usually get headlines or even much of a mention, but it should. It's overlooked, neglected, and abused, probably because it doesn't help you lose weight or build muscle. Although it's usually the first thing to go when we're under pressure for time, it's such a worthwhile investment that we've done stretching a favor and given it its very own, well-deserved headline.

What is Stretching?

Although there are various forms of stretching, we're going to focus on the most common form — traditional stretching. Basically, stretching the muscle is the opposite of contracting the muscle. Whereas a contraction will make the muscle tight (and short), stretching will "loosen" (and lengthen) it. Start thinking of your body as an elastic band and you get the idea.

---

[4] A group session conducted with the whole group performing exercises on stationary exercise bikes. See later, page 309.

[5] We're referring to the Stair Climber machines in the gym that ensure a constant workout — not the stairs that you use to get up to the bedroom and down again in five seconds flat.

[6] Another form of group exercise focused on choreography up, down, and around exercise steps. See later, page 306.

[7] Tennis (and badminton) count as an aerobic workout only when your movement is constant. This will usually occur only when a person is fairly fit and plays against a similarly fit (or even fitter) opponent.

[8] Volleyball will only qualify as an aerobic workout if your fellow team members (and you) play a good, fast-moving game. Spending more time bending over, retrieving the ball, or watching it bash into the net just doesn't qualify.

Why Should I Stretch?

 You will improve your flexibility.

Stretching is the way to go in order to maintain (and improve) your flexibility. What is flexibility? It's how far and how easily you can move your joints. We need to be flexible because we want to be able to move more freely. Certain positions become more accessible (and less dangerous). We can bend to tie our shoelace (without groaning); we can reach the sugar from the top shelf (without having to grow four inches); we can bend properly in prayer; we can twist around to pass a drink to someone in the backseat of the car…

As we get older, our tendons (the tissues that connect muscle to bone) begin to shorten and tighten. This restricts our flexibility. Our movements become slower and more inhibited. We don't stand up like a soldier (ram-rod straight) anymore (did we ever?). We walk more stiffly and with a shorter stride. We find it harder to go up and down the curb or to bend over to kiss little Shnocky. Without stretching, we become a prisoner in our own body.

 You will improve your posture.

Flexibility is pivotal to good posture. When your front neck muscles are tight, your head drops forward. When your chest and shoulders are constricted, your shoulders round (and your breathing becomes restricted). When your lower back, rear thigh, and hip muscles are tight, your back develops an exaggerated curve (which puts a strain on the rest of the body). All indicate a hunchback in the making, and all are bad news.

 You may reduce back pain.

Poor posture is closely associated with back pain and can be effectively improved by stretching out the muscles in the lower back and rear thighs.

☺ **You can correct muscle imbalances.**

"So what?" you may ask. Well, muscles work in pairs, rather like a Mr. and Mrs. When one is working, the other is relaxing, and when one is weak, the other needs to be strong (when one yells, the other just listens…).

A typical condition is the rear thigh muscles being too tight and weak. The opposing muscle group (i.e., the partner in the pair — or, the Mr. versus the Mrs.), is the front thigh muscles, which are typically strong but would be relied upon more heavily than they should be, in order to counteract the weaker muscles' inadequacies.

There may be no glaringly noticeable repercussions, but our gait may become imbalanced — albeit in subtle ways. You may have a short stride or too high a bounce in your step. Such muscle imbalances can eventually lead to injuries such as pulled muscles. They can also be a contributing factor to clumsiness — not only might you trip and end up as an embarrassed mess on the pavement, but you might also injure yourself. Both unpleasant.

☺ You can reduce muscle soreness after strenuous activity.

Most classes finish with (excuse the "exercise lingo"...) "the-cooldown-'n'-stretch" (see "A Word About Stretching," page 311), because stretching out the worked muscles may reduce potential discomfort. The kind the world knows as "Charley Horse," which sounds friendlier than it feels.

☺ You can reduce your risk of injury.

Not only will it be easier to reach and bend, but if you don't stay flexible, you are much more likely to pull a muscle. Ever reached for your purse in the backseat of the car and felt something (ow!) "go," snap, or twinge?

Another common scenario for a good stretch is during the warm-up of any exercise or sports class, or, for example, before a tennis match or a swimming race. This is because a warm muscle that is adequately stretched may be able to cope better with the upcoming workload, than a cold muscle would.

☺ You will be able to relax — both mentally and physically.

Our bodies need to stretch (hope you got the message). But a wonderful, automatic outcome of taking the time to stretch properly (you just can't rush a stretch) is that you will become more relaxed. Think about it. We run and rush our way through the day. Our thoughts are quick-fire, our actions staccato. Here we have the opportunity to really breathe (when was the last time you breathed deeply?) and center ourselves. Stretching forces us to slow down, to calm down, and to let go of all that built-up tension that we carry around with us during our day. Apart from doing something good for your body, you also get to enjoy the benefits of relaxation.

☺ You can look and feel great.

Flexible people can move more freely, stand taller (good posture), and look more confident. Just compare such a person to the mental picture of a really old hunchbacked woman shuffling down the street with a walking stick. (Prevention is better than cure.) Not only is stretching good for you, but it also helps you feel good. It's just much harder to continue being in a bad mood after a good stretch. It somehow ignites that magic feeling of re-energizing the mind and body simultaneously.

How Do I Stretch?

✔ **Make sure your body is physically warm before you stretch any muscle.**
Our muscles are just like a rubber band. A warm rubber band has greater elasticity than a cold rubber band — which can easily snap. Not only do you end up with no rubber band if you stretch when cold, but you also end up in bed with a pulled muscle.

For this reason, stretching is definitely *not* the thing to do first thing on a chilly morning (however enthusiastically charged you may be after reading all this). Nor is it the sensible thing to do immediately upon arriving at the park for your daily jog. Warm up first and then go right ahead.

✔ **Move into each stretch gradually.**
Beginners, be warned: If you watch the instructor wrap spaghetti-like arms and legs around while you wonder how the Dickens she did that, don't try to keep pace before she changes position again. Rather than jerking your limbs into position (and risk getting hurt), just watch and take notes for next week.

✔ **Hold each stretch for eight to thirty[9] seconds.**
Once you find yourself in a comfortable stretch position, hold it or gradually deepen the stretch by extending the movement just a touch. Keep your position static (that means you are still), not bouncing. **If you "bounce" the stretch, you risk tearing a muscle.** (This is a worldwide mistake — especially with "macho" men).

✔ **Stretch often — daily is best.**
Maximum results for maximum effort. Besides, stretching doesn't take much effort (certainly not compared to all that huffing and puffing of aerobics that we spoke about earlier). Can't manage every day? (What do you mean, you've got other things to do?) Then stretching whenever you can is better than not at all. (Think: "I don't want to become a rusty car" to get you going.)

✔ **Feel the tension in the stretch.**
There should be a pleasant, mild tension in the muscle. There should never be any sharp or severe pain in any body part when stretching. Everyone has different levels of flexibility, so don't be tempted to compete with the girl in front of you, or you could end up the loser in more ways than one. **Just as "no pain, no gain" isn't an adage applicable to aerobics, it's also not applicable to stretching (let's make that universal — it's totally inapplicable to all things exercise).**[10]

✔ **Breeeeeeeathe.**
Because stretches can last anywhere between eight and thirty seconds, you'll feel more comfortable if you remember to breathe. Because stretching does not require immense effort, it's not as important *when* you breathe as *that* you breathe. As you hold each stretch, take two deep breaths. Inhaling in this way not only injects your muscles with oxygen (always a good idea), but also aids relaxation (ahhh, that's better...). (Besides, if you turn blue, you'll probably clash with your T-shirt...)

---

[9] A shorter span of time (eight to twenty seconds) is for those stretches designed to maintain your levels of flexibility. Stretches designed to improve your levels of flexibility require a longer time span (twenty to thirty seconds).
[10] See "Going for 'The Burn' Is the Way to Go," page 340.

Just for the record, in clear-cut terms, let's go through the FIT steps:

Frequency

Ideally, we should stretch every day. If you can't manage this daily small pleasure, try doing upper body one day and lower body the next. It doesn't have to take long to render long-lasting benefits.

Intensity

Go for ease with a slight feeling of resistance. Never go beyond what is comfortable for you. There's no way to race your way into a flexible body. It'll take time. Enjoy the journey — stretching is a real winner in terms of helping to instill a sense of calm and centeredness.

Time

Different stretches can take different lengths of time to be effective. As a general rule, eight- to twenty-second stretches will maintain your levels of flexibility (called, not surprisingly, "maintenance stretches"), whereas a stretch lasting twenty to thirty seconds will improve your flexibility (these are called "developmental stretches").

How long till you see results? Five minutes daily, and you'll see an improvement after ten days, a significant improvement after twenty days, and a new range of movement (and a new you) after thirty days.

Different Stretching Classes

If you want to improve your flexibility, try these activities:

- ✔ Following a step-by-step stretch 'n' tone exercise book[11] to take you through your paces (this way you get all the benefits without the stress of finding a babysitter);
- ✔ Swimming;
- ✔ Yoga.[12]

The less active you are in your day (computer job, anyone?) the more likely you are to need to improve your flexibility. Muscles that are not stretched become shorter and tighter until you are not able to stretch them even if you wanted to. So next time you're in the armchair reading a bedtime story to the kids, why not sit on the floor and stretch out a muscle or two at the same time? (I'm all in favor of two-for-one activities.) Better yet, find a quiet corner and turn on some relaxing music or work in time to your own breathing. (Remember to lock the door and have earplugs available before you start.)

---

[11] In order to ascertain that the exercises are safe and effective, it is best to verify that the person writing the book is properly qualified. This information is either on the inside flap or in the blurb "about the author."

[12] See the end of this chapter for further elaboration.

Strength Training

The next type of fitness on our list is strength training. Don't be too quick to flick the page, thinking you don't ever want to beef your muscles up to look like a world-class weight-lifting champion. Of course you don't. But not all strength training is designed with that in mind. There are a whole lot of reasons why becoming stronger is good news for all of us — right from youngsters to great-grannies, and everyone in between.

What is Strength Training?

Strength training has numerous aliases. It is also known as "weight lifting," "weight training," "resistance training," "body conditioning," "body toning," and "body sculpting," to name just a few favorites. We're going to stick to "strength training" so the various names won't confuse us.

Muscles and bones need to work (hard) in order to improve their capacity to be strong. In technical jargon, this is called "overloading." Just like you won't learn "bon" French if you never get past your first ten vocabulary words, our muscles and bones need to be used if they are to shape-up and strengthen-up.

Getting the body accustomed to being used in this way can be achieved in a number of ways. Hence, there is lots of confusion about which class, gym, equipment, or routine is best. Let's get down to brass tacks and define each route to strength.

⟟ Weight Machines

When you go into a gym and feel like you're inside the garage of a cables-and-pullies-minded weirdo, don't be intimidated. At first glance you might quietly wonder (since you don't want to seem ignorant), "Where do I sit?" "What do I push?" or "Will I ever get out of here alive?" Fear not. Gyms make big money on you returning (and returning and returning), so it's definitely in their best interests to keep you alive. Besides, weight machines are really quite simple once you get the hang of them.

Basically, gym machines typically focus on one muscle group (in fitness jargon, they "isolate" the muscle) and provide an effective position for you to pull, push, or resist a force or weight. You might pull on handlebars attached to weights. You might have to push your outer thighs against a resistance. You might have to squeeze your elbows together in front of you while holding onto something that resists doing what you want it to do (no, not Shnocky this time). All these machines are designed to improve the strength in each particular muscle group.

Gym machines are ideal for beginners because they are quite safe. They are also effective and time efficient (you won't have to adjust a barbell[13] with different weights for each exercise). They do not generally require a high level of competence in coordination and, once you are familiar with the different machines, you can pick and choose which body parts to work on at your own time and pace.

---

[13] See the following paragraph.

⚐ Free Weights

When they offer you free weights at the gym, don't think they're giving you a going-home present. Free weights are simply bars with weight plates on each end. The long bars are called "barbells" and the short bars are called "dumbbells." You'll need two hands to pick up a barbell, but only one to pick up a dumbbell.

Free weights are more versatile than machines. You can use the same barbell in different ways to work different muscles. They are also more portable than a five-ton, screwed-to-the-floor gym machine. The drawback, however, is that you *do* have to know what you are doing. Technique is important in avoiding potential injury.

⚐ Tubes and Bands

An exercise tube will look something like a thin rubber tire your seven-year-old kid found in the back lane, but the exercise-variety usually comes in bright colors. Sometimes they have handles attached to aid a strong grip. Exercise bands are long, flat strips of rubbery elastic (or elasticy rubber…), also in different colors — each color is indicative of a different level of difficulty.

Tubes and bands have several advantages: They are even more portable than the previous two types of equipment (getting itchy feet to go anywhere, by any chance?), and they take up zero space in the already-bursting suitcase. They are also your cheapest bet, costing about $5–$15 for two. The most glaring disadvantage: Unless you have been instructed in some technically correct classes, you might just end up using them as belts to hold your skirt up.

⚐ Your Body

Your own body can also function as a pretty effective tool in strength training. You can lift it, pull it, push it, twist it, and curl it into all different positions to fight the force of gravity and give you some serious weight to lift. Just think of all those push-ups, leg-lifts, and sit-ups, and you'll get the picture.

The advantage of using your body to strength train is that you always have it with you. (Yes, it's your most portable option.) The workout you receive is effective and you can perform your routine anyplace, any day, anytime.

Why Should I Do Strength Training?

☺ You'll stay strong for everyday living.

Let's get really frightening: People who don't exercise lose thirty to forty percent of their strength by age sixty-five. That means they won't be able to carry a heavy bag of groceries or lift Shnocky onto the swing. These inadequacies are not the result of natural aging; they are the result of neglect. If you haven't been taking care of your muscles, they won't be around to take care of you when you need them.

Since I don't want to get too scary, now is a good point to tell you that strength is one of the easiest physical abilities to retain. You can do more about stopping strength-loss than you can about stopping hair-loss, hearing-loss, or memory-loss. (That should inspire you, by the way.)

There's simply so much more to enjoy in life once you are strong, like closing the overstuffed suitcase (essentials only, of course), or being able to carry the groceries all the way to the car.

☺ You will keep your bones healthy.

Yep, we're going to mention it again. Osteoporosis. It's a killer. And I don't think I'm exaggerating. Basically, osteoporosis is a disease of severe bone loss that causes 1.5 million fractures a year in the Western World alone, mostly in the wrist, hip, and back. Roughly half of those people who break their hips never regain their natural gait. In addition, many of these fractures lead to fatal complications. Just imagine your bones being like chalk — porous and fragile. When bones are weak like this, they are so easily broken that they don't even need a fall to crack them. Simply bending over or coughing too hard can do the job instead.

It doesn't have to be this way. We all start out with the ingredients for strong, dense bones. All it takes is a little awareness (and strength training) to increase your bones' strength and to arrest (and even improve) this serious condition. Bones are made up of living matter. They can become stronger. We only have to ask them to.

☺ You can prevent injuries.

Apart from ending up in the hospital with a broken bone because of osteoporosis, you might end up at the same address (G-d forbid) because of being generally more susceptible to injuries. Slip off the curb? Weak ankle equals sprained ankle. Bending over to pick up the shopping? Weak back equals pain. The list goes on. When your muscles are strong, you're less injury prone. You have a greater sense of balance, sure-footedness, and resilience to life's rough and tumbles.

☺ You look better.

Although we can't selectively zap off fat, we can shape, tighten, firm-up, and lift-up our bodies. We can focus on a particular area and reshape it through strength training.

In addition, strengthening your muscles will improve your posture, which in turn will give you a slimmer, more elongated appearance (as well as 101 other health benefits) — all without necessarily losing an ounce.

☺   **You speed up your metabolism.**

When we talk about metabolism, we are talking about the minimum number of calories needed to maintain vital functions like breathing and keeping the heart beating.

Briefly, a more muscular, lean (low in fat) body will need more calories just to exist than his fat counterpart (who might even weigh the same but whose muscle-to-fat ratio is very different). Muscle needs more calories than fat just to sit on the couch doing nothing. (This means you get to enjoy more food for less work.)

Let's add that if you don't strength train, your metabolism will slow down every year as your muscles slowly waste away. The result? Extra poundage — even if you are eating the same as you always did.

An additional note for dieters: You need to build up your muscles, as dieting can zap off precious muscle as well as fat. If you lift weights while dieting, you can build up your muscles *and* raise your metabolic rate at the same time as losing weight. Neat.

How Do I Perform Strength Training?

Before we discuss this question, we have to spend a moment clarifying two terms that are crucial to all things strength-training: rep and set (clue: they're not dog names). "Rep" is short for repetition. It is one complete motion of an exercise. For example, take a sit-up: When you have lifted your head and shoulders up and then lowered them back down again, you have completed one rep. A "set" is a group of consecutive repetitions. For example, you might say (brag?), "I did two sets of eight reps today." This means you did the exercise eight times, rested, and then repeated it. (It also means you're a clever girl.)

Remember that cute anagram for improving a particular type of fitness — FIT: Frequency, Intensity, and Time? Well, here it is again…

Frequency

Working each muscle two or three times a week is your best option. Try to schedule days of rest before working on a particular muscle group again. Muscles need a day or two to recover, rebuild, and end up stronger, instead of being prone to overuse-injuries. In practical terms, this means you could work the upper body on Sundays, Tuesdays, and Thursdays, and the lower body on Mondays, Wednesdays, and Fridays.

Intensity

To improve your general strength so that everyday tasks become a cinch (like moving furniture or shovelling snow), aim to do eight to fifteen reps per set. In umph-and-groan terms, you need to lift a weight heavy enough to feel that the last rep in a set is a struggle (but not impossible).

This means that if you are new to weight training, start off with lighter weights, and when you feel yourself managing the exercises with ease, gradually add more weight to make it harder (no, it's not supposed to be easy).

To see improvement, you'll need to work each muscle to "fatigue." This means that when you feel the muscle complain about its workload, you know you've done enough. As everyone has different levels of fitness, this is difficult to quantify globally. Your best course is to listen to your own body (and don't worry about Mighty Mom in the corner pumping ten pound weights for half an hour).

Start off performing one set — concentrating on correct form and technique (think "quality, not quantity"). After two to four weeks of training, you might want to add another set for each muscle group so that you feel truly challenged.

Beginners should rest about ninety seconds between sets to give their muscles adequate time to recover. As you get into better shape, you'll need to rest less (maybe only thirty seconds) before your muscles feel ready (eager and begging...) for another set.

Time

It should take you a full two seconds to lift a weight and two to four seconds to lower it. Note the built-in warning device with barbell weights: Lifting it faster than two seconds will usually mean noisier. This is because the weights will probably clank and clink. This noise is alerting you to the fact that you'll be relying on momentum, rather than muscle power, to execute the rep. Slow and steady is the name of the game if you want your muscles to truly work the way they are intended.

Different Strength Training Classes/Activities

- BLT (Bottoms, Legs, and Tummies) classes;
- Body Conditioning classes;
- Body Pump;
- Gym equipment;
- Weightlifting;
- Dynaband/Tubing/Resistance work.

Mind-Body Exercise

Now that we have covered the three basic areas of fitness (aerobic exercise, stretching, and strength training), it's time to address an area that isn't quite so easily pigeonholed. That's because it sometimes incorporates more than one of these fitness areas, or none of them. Some may argue that this area has a definite identity crisis, but I like to think of it in terms of a smorgasbord. A little of this, a little of that, and what have you got? Variety, satisfaction, and, of course, fun.

What is Mind-Body Exercise?

Although we in the West have traditionally viewed exercise as being of the purely physical, grit-your-teeth-and-bear-it-or-you-won't-get-any-results variety, those enlightened folks in the East have maintained for centuries that exercise is also beneficial to the mind.

The advent of greater global communication has enabled nations to learn from each other. Hence the last ten years have seen a veritable explosion in classes such as Yoga, Tai Chi, and Pilates (no, not the guys who fly the planes. I know you're wondering how on earth to pronounce it, so here goes: it's "pih-lah-tees" — not "pie-lates").

Mind-Body exercise is difficult to define. Some may consider it an alternative way to reduce stress and pain. Others may view it as a tool to center themselves emotionally and spiritually. Still others will use it to complement their other traditional exercise programs because of the physical dividends. For example, Yoga demands intense concentration, good posture, and a focusing on several muscle groups at once. These all render tangible benefits.

Why Should I Do Mind-Body Exercises?

 Variety

One of the benefits of Mind-Body exercise is that you can substitute these workouts for your regular exercise class when you feel like a change — be it of routine, intensity, or style. You still get to go home feeling absolved of the guilt that not doing any exercise at all brings — plus you stand to benefit both physically and mentally.

Although these Mind-Body classes are distinctly different from your average mainstay class, the same muscles are still getting a workout.

 Relaxation

Who couldn't do with a little relaxation after a hard day? Getting back in touch with your body's natural rhythms might be just what you need to become more calm and at peace with the world around you.

 Breathe

Most people only remember to breathe deeply when their bodies force them to yawn, or when they sigh deeply with exasperation at their children for being so…childish.

Breathing deeply is not only calming but also revitalizes you because of the increased supply of oxygen to the blood, organs, and brain.

Some Mind-Body classes will give you plenty of opportunity to breathe deeply. Just be careful not to fall asleep on your mat.

Body Consciousness

Sometimes, traditional exercises force us to focus so hard on improving our body's functionality that we lose focus on where it is actually holding.

Mind-Body classes are great for getting in tune with your own body and discovering new ways to wear it, move it, and enjoy it.

 Deeper Muscles

Some classes will require you to focus on internal muscles that you didn't even know you had — and can now be grateful that you do.

Many people think the only way to condition their abdominal muscles is to do a zillion crunches (sit-ups). Although a correctly performed crunch will work some of the abdominal muscles, just try out a first-class Pilates class and see if your other, inner abs, aren't worked out in a very deep and meaningful way.

 Balance

We're all supposed to have learned how to balance as a toddler, and we are expected to just continue balancing throughout our lives. However, increasing our sense and ability to balance can help us to avoid injury (fall off the chair/ladder/step lately?).

In addition, an increased sense of balance can help us appear more graceful, poised, and self-assured.

 Flexibility

Instead of rushing through the warm-up or cool-down stretches one-two-three, as in a traditional aerobics class, you perform the stretches in a mind-body class as though you have all the time in the world (or at least until the hour's up).

This can mean that your levels of flexibility will greatly improve (instead of merely being maintained without improvement if performed for only a few seconds at a shot — as we mentioned above in the Stretching section).

 Attention

Most Mind-Body classes have a limit to the number of participants that the instructor will admit. This is to ensure that each participant gets the individual attention that she needs to perform the exercise correctly and safely.

If you like small, intimate classes, this might be just the thing for you. (Plus, you stand to discover a new friend or two.)

How Do I Access the Benefits of a Mind-Body Exercise?

Whichever way you view them, access to these alternative-style classes has never been easier. Health clubs, local fitness gyms, and exercise studios world-wide are offering them as staples on their menu — right beside your aerobics, stretch 'n' tone, and body-building classes. You can even hire personal trainers well versed in these areas.

Frequency

If you are using this type of class to augment an already effective schedule of exercise, then going once or twice a week will complement it beautifully.

If this more gentle type of exercise is your main staple, then you will have to go to a class two or three times a week to see (and feel) its benefits.

Intensity

More than with any other discipline, it's important not to ignore your body's warning system. If you feel pain or awkwardness from a move, you should immediately stop, watch the instructor, listen carefully, and only perform the exercise at a level you feel comfortable performing.

There's no point in exerting intensity into an exercise performed with poor technique (unless you *want* a bad back…). Technique is everything in these classes.

Some Mind-Body classes are conducted with either gentle "wafty" music, or no music at all. This way, participants will work to the rhythm of their own breathing and at their own level (as opposed to working either to the beat of the music or in sync with the instructor). As this is highly individual, there are no external universal guidelines for intensity.

Time

Although each class is typically an hour in length, the benefits of performing thirty minutes of such types of exercise are also substantial (just remember to warm up first).

Different Types of Mind-Body Classes

✔ **Yoga**

Characteristically, Yoga involves the body in a series of different poses that are held for anything from a few seconds to a few minutes. These moves are designed to blend flexibility, strength, and mind-body awareness.

Beginners should definitely go for a "Beginner's" Yoga class, as the more advanced classes can require you to impersonate your three-year-old's spiral straw (although they don't require you to be see-through). Besides, who wants to look like a crisp stick of celery next to a bunch of bendy-spaghetti-legs? There are many forms of Yoga; however, most include the same fundamental poses while varying the breathing and length of time the poses are held.

✔ Pilates

Pilates moves are designed to work your main muscle groups — abs, lower back, thighs, and backside. Unlike typical gym equipment, which requires you to work on one or two specific muscles at a time, Pilates will require you to engage the whole body. If you merely watch a Pilates class you won't see much action (I know someone who fell asleep while watching a class), but if you are taking part in a class, you may be surprised at how hard some of the easy-looking exercises actually are.

The focus of a Pilates class is on good posture and body mechanics, and developing strength, flexibility, muscular endurance, coordination, and balance (phew, and you thought you were taking the easier option).

Perseverance is a must, as it may take time to tune into this alternative form and mindset.

Pilates classes are not recommended for those who are unfit, or who are prone to back injuries. If you don't fall into either of these categories, and you want to give Pilates a shot, find a course for beginners. This way you can learn the exercise techniques correctly. Ideally there should be no more than fifteen participants in a class. This enables the instructor to properly supervise each individual.

✔ Tai Chi (Pronounced: "tie-chee")

This ancient Chinese martial art (non-combatant — don't worry, no black eyes) involves lots of slow-motion movements, deep breathing, and concentration.

The slow movements are beautiful to watch and calming to perform. Plus, there's very limited risk of injury.

The slow, soft, flowing movements emphasize precision and force, not sheer physical brute strength. Although normally Tai Chi won't develop as much strength as Yoga or Pilates, some stances do require high levels of muscle power.

This brings us to the end of our four areas of fitness. Each area offers its own unique benefits and life-enhancers. All it takes is a little effort and a little perseverance, and you stand to gain so much. It's time to stop complaining and wishing you could be fitter (usually while you shmooze on the phone sitting at the kitchen table), and actually go and do something about it instead. If I offered you a healthy, strong, flexible, conditioned body to step into tomorrow morning when you wake up, would you say no? I *am* offering it — you only have to go and get it.

Chapter 16

—— ◆ ◆ ◆ ——

What's An Exercise Class All About?

This chapter will give you an inside view at what makes an exercise class tick.

Now that we understand what each type of exercise does, we stand on the threshold of yet more uncharted territory. We may even feel suitably inspired to pack a gym bag and head out for an exercise class. But what can we expect when we get there? What will we have to do during the class?

Knowing what to expect can go a long way in reducing the sense of intimidation that can often accompany a novice on her way. This, in turn, will hopefully inspire her to venture forth and try out a new experience or two.

So let's start at the very beginning, with a component that will wiggle its way to the forefront of most, if not all, conventional exercise classes.

The Warm-Up

Rochel slept past the third snooze on her alarm, sprang out of bed like a striking cobra, grabbed her sneakers, and headed out for her morning jog without the fuss of warming up. What happened to her? Perhaps a sprained ankle, a pulled muscle, strained ligament, minor pain, or some discomfort, or maybe she got by without anything going seriously wrong *this* time. But if she keeps it up, over the long run, she won't come out a winner. Her joints will suffer, potentially causing premature arthritis, and one day she probably will end up with some sort of sprain, strain, and/or pain — shame.

So what was she missing? A warm-up.

The warm-up not only serves to prevent such unpleasantness, but it also helps to ease your way into the exercise session. Just like you warm up a cold car before you take it for a drive, you need to do the same service for your body. Just as a car needs preparation in order to go from a resting state to active motion, so too, your body needs the necessary time to adjust. The warm-up gets the blood flowing to our heart and muscles much like gas makes its way through the reverberating engine. (We take care of our car 'cause it cost us a year's worth of paychecks; we should take care of our body because it's priceless. Besides, spare parts are hard to come by these days.)

What is a Warm-Up?

Typically, warm-up movements start off gentle, low in intensity, and controlled, gaining momentum as they go.

They make their way through the body like a shopping list. Each muscle group and major joint is prepared to be used (i.e., the neck, shoulders, arm to shoulder joint, spine, legs, etc., all go through their paces). This increases the flexibility of the joints and connective tissue.

After going through some easy-to-do motions for a few minutes, the intensity should pick up. This increase in effort is designed to literally warm the body up, which helps to prevent injury (remember the elastic band — warm and stretchy, or cold and...snap?).

For example, one might start with a small, single, side-to-side step that will progress into a larger step, followed by the addition of simultaneous arm movements, etc. In addition to warming up (and having fun) this process of beginning with small movements before larger ones lubricates the joints (for the car analogy, read: greases the wheels). This makes it easier (and safer) to move your limbs.

Next, the instructor may introduce a number of static (you are standing still now) stretches. As the heart rate will automatically drop slightly because you are not moving as much during these stretches, you'll probably finish warming up with more huffy-puffy moves to prepare your heart for the aerobic component. Your heart rate will be raised gently so that it is better prepared to deal with the upcoming workload.

A warm-up possesses many endearing qualities. As we have mentioned, it loosens the joints, stretches the muscles, and physically warms and prepares the body for its upcoming workout. But that's not all it does: The warm-up also psyches up the mind for the ensuing exercise session (all at no extra cost). In this way, it will be ready for the following, more complex steps.

For example, when we are about to embark on an action-packed aerobics class, the warm-up should take us through some of the more basic moves on which the planned choreography is based. This puts our minds in the right frame of reference for the ensuing activities. In technical jargon, we are preparing the neuromuscular transmitters. In real terms, we're getting into it.

The warm-up can take anywhere between five and fifteen minutes. Why the discrepancy? Well, fit people take less time to warm up (although they do still need to warm up), as do younger people. Yep, you got it. That means that if you are unfit and/or old, it's going to take you a few minutes longer to get that body into gear.

This is important to realize, because when you go to a certain class because it's convenient (your babysitter can only manage to arrive at 8pm) rather than because it's aimed at your particular fitness level, you might want to take an extra few minutes warming up before stunning them all with your performance.

A Stitch in Time Saves Nine

It's true that if you are a born show-off, you're going to have to wait about ten minutes before you can truly strut your stuff. But I have seen plenty of born show-offs skip the warm-up only to come to an untimely end — doubled over with a stitch. What happened?

Well, if a body needs ten minutes (or so) to warm up and it doesn't get them, it will complain (just like the kid who doesn't get the candy). Placing high demands on an unprepared body will mean that Mr. Body will need lots of oxygen — and quick. Sometimes he simply won't be able to get enough of it or get it quickly enough to continue his inspired contortions. Basically, the car runs out of gas.

So when you go to a class and everyone's doing seemingly boring marches and low, little, innocuous knee bends, you should too.

Going it Alone

It's a breeze going to a studio class and just doing what the instructor says, but what if you're all alone or are in a non-warm-up-friendly environment? What do you do then?

For those who are into DIY (Do It Yourself: not the hammer-and-nail variety, but the stay-at-home-to-exercise variety), here are a few extra points to consider before you pound the ceiling of the room below you:

- ✔ The general idea is to start out easy, move slowly, and build up your speed gradually. (Sorry, but as yet they haven't invented any shortcuts.)
- ✔ Do remember to breathe (just in case you were planning not to) and listen to your body. This means that if you feel breathlessness, discomfort, or pain, back off and either stop or reduce the intensity of what you are doing.
- ✔ Under no circumstances should you skip the warm-up because you're short of time (we're all short of time and we all need to warm up).
- ✔ Make sure you move your body through a full *range of motion*. This means you can't yawn your way through the movements. Your limbs should be controlled and gently taken to their furthest point. Start with shoulder rolls, proceed to larger arm rolls, and then take it into a full arm-length, sweeping, extended circle.

✔ Mimic the workout of whichever form of exercise you're preparing to do. This means going through the motions that you are about to do as part of the exercise routine, but doing them without any resistance (i.e., no weights/bars till the real meat and potatoes), and at a low intensity. And remember, you should be feeling generally warm before you start any strenuous stuff.

✔ When you are warm, you can stretch out whichever major muscles you are planning to use in your workout.

Just to get into the swing of things, here are three specific activities and some suggestions to ensure you warm-up adequately for each.

Doing acrobatics in seminary? Preparing for a show? Go through a mini, easy, fun routine before you start. Make sure you feel warm before you start the real spellbinding tricks, and make sure to go through some serious stretching, too. Practice your technique at the same time as warming up — try performing sloooow perfect somersaults forwards and back, then stretch up, sideways, twist, etc. The better prepared your body is before you start all that tumbling about, the better chance you'll have to make it to the show instead of nursing an injury on the sidelines.

Going for a jog? If you live in a stair-filled house, you can get suitably warm and ready just by going up and down the stairs for five minutes (you'll also be preparing your front and back thigh muscles if your jog is up/downhill). If you live in a single-story apartment, you can either start your route gently and gradually build up, or you can warm-up inside by performing on-the-spot moves such as knee lifts, kicks, and side taps. Don't forget to stretch (especially the leg muscles that you are about to activate), and you're up and running. Literally.

Planning to play tennis? Mimic the motions first, without the racket. Swing forwards and back, low and easy. Walk around the court to raise the heart rate. Introduce a few squats or lunges (you're going to do some serious lunging for that ball, remember). If you don't have your very own ball boys, practice reaching down to the ground (knees bent, legs wide, chest lifted, versus dropping your shoulders forward and bending at the hips). This way you are less likely to pull a muscle or develop a backache from picking up all those missed (cough, cough) balls.

So, the next time you go through the warm-up motions, know that you are not wasting your time by doing seemingly simple movements. The warm-up may well be your best investment of the day. Sometimes it's the simple things in life that are the most significant.

The Class

Now that we're all stretched out and warm as toast, let's focus on the different types of classes and what we can expect from each. I like to think of this part in terms of the filling in the sandwich. The warm-up and cooldown are the slices of bread because they're on either side of the real stuff. The actual type of class is the exciting variable or filling, which makes the exercise sandwich a truly nourishing, satisfying experience. Hmm, sounds good already…

Aerobic Classes

All aerobic classes are based around the "aerobic peak." No, you won't be taking a detour from the studio to Mount Everest, but you may well feel that you're struggling uphill. And that's exactly the point. We want to work our heart and lungs hard enough to make them stronger. Too easy is no good (although it may feel good at the time), and working too hard will thwart endurance (you'll end up sitting it out with a stitch) and can be dangerous.

Dangerous? I hear you ask. Put it this way: An unqualified instructor once held an unofficial class in a community hall and worked the participants too hard too quickly and then reduced the intensity too abruptly. One participant blacked out and hit her head on the edge of a table and, gulp…how shall we say this?…is no longer here to tell the tale. A true story. So I think the word *dangerous* is apt, even if unpleasant.

If I would plot the "aerobic peak" on a graph, it would look like a mini Mount Sinai. The idea is to start off gradually, pick up intensity, and then safely reduce that intensity until we're back to square one. This is the blueprint upon which all aerobic-based classes are designed.

Variety comes into play in all the different ways that we can climb this peak without ever stepping foot amidst the Himalayas.

Below is an at-a-glance list of some of the more common exercise classes (sandwich fillers) and the ways in which they differ from each other.

High and low impact aerobics

Aerobics has come a long way from the leggings and hype of the 1970s and '80s. It has moved away from its initial trendy, fashion statement image and has become a standard (as well as diverse and exciting) exercise staple.

A typical high-low (as they're sometimes called) aerobics class will incorporate a traditional dance-inspired routine set to music. With low impact, you always have one foot on the floor — you don't do any jumping or hopping. High impact moves at a slower pace, but you jump around a lot. High-low combines the two types of routines.

You'll enjoy movements such as kicking, jumping, squatting, and brisk marching/jogging. These moves may sound simple, but once you add coordinating arm movements, then your brain, as well as your brawn, has something to work on.

When you begin a typical aerobics class, you will stand facing the instructor in rows, about two feet apart. She will call out the name of each movement-change a second or so before its performance. This is called "cueing." It'll only take a couple of weeks to learn the lingo of "grapevines, heel digs, swings, or spotty dogs." (These are staple aerobic steps even though they may sound like you're touring a garden).

The instructor will stand at the front of the class, providing a mirror image for you to follow. She might turn her back towards you intermittently — not because she doesn't like the look of you, but because sometimes it's easier to mimic certain moves from that position.

She might also turn the whole class a quarter turn of the room and instruct from the new frontline. Most good instructors will incorporate some type of turn. This is in order to give participants, other than the front row, more focus. As newcomers or inexperienced exercisers tend to cower at the back, this is a great teaching tactic to ensure that those who need the extra attention get it. Besides, facing a different wall, even if it is the same color, can make a nice change.

Aerobics classes invariably involve some form of choreography (dance-like routines). Sometimes this may be very simple and repetitive, and sometimes you'll wonder if your feet are connected to your brain. Variations on the more basic aerobic classes are classes advertised as "Jazzercise" (a class incorporating jazz dance moves), "Salsa Aerobics" (a class with a distinctly Latin American flavor), or "Exercise to Music" (alternating between typical dance moves and traditional aerobic moves).

Less common, although fun, are "Funk" and "Hip Hop" (note: not Hopscotch) classes, where you dance to funky music with offbeat, choreographed dance moves.

Step Aerobics

Although you may argue you don't need to go to a Steps class to keep you fit because you go up and down the stairs all day anyway, I'll bet you don't get up to all these creative permutations when you're at home.

If you imagine a rectangular piece of plastic measuring 43" long × 16" wide × 4" high, you have a picture of a typical exercise step. The step is adjustable, so if you want to work harder, you can increase the step height and tone the leg muscles at the same time as working your CVS (no, not "*chas v'shalom*,"[1] but "cardiovascular system").

---

[1] G-d forbid.

Although you might think that you'll work harder staying at home trotting up and down your stairs because your typical home stair measures 7" high (as opposed to the step's 4"), you'll be surprised how effective the repetitive motion of up-step, down-step feels, even at a lower height (just talk to your quads[2] the next morning and you'll know what I mean).

Before I went to my first Step class I thought Step would be boring. I mean, how exciting can it be to go up and down for an hour? This was, of course, one of my many life mistakes.

While Step classes by definition involve up-step, down-step foot patterns, they can incorporate other exciting moves including knee lifts, squats, turn-arounds, and taps to the step board, in addition to performing moves on the short end of the step, around the step, and to the side of the step. All these creative permutations are performed in time to the music.

While the choreography for Step can range from simple to complex, variables such as directional changes or tempo alterations can make Step so extremely exciting and so dance-like that you'll feel like you're auditioning for a Broadway musical. Classes also naturally develop strength in the muscles of the front and back thigh as well as the gluteals.[3] This makes it a great 2-for-1 activity.

Caution: **Never use a step so high that your knee is higher than your hip when you step up.** This contributes to knee injuries.

Another word of warning: As soon as you turn a quarter turn in a Step class, the instructor is no longer as visible and you're on your own (you might feel like Mommy just let go of your hand). That's why it's a good idea to position yourself in the middle of the group, so that you'll always have someone in front of you to follow.

Box Aerobics (also known as Boxercise)

Box aerobics classes incorporate boxing techniques (not necessarily with the punching bag) with aerobic dance to give you a great cardiovascular workout and help improve your balance, coordination, and agility.

These classes typically look easier than they feel. There can be a certain gracefulness to the movements, although at first glance they may appear to be somewhat masculine or aggressive (but you *don't* actually hit anyone).

With correct technique and form, this class also strengthens the inner abdominal muscles, which must be in a state of contraction to execute many of the punch-like movements. So, while you think you are there to exercise your heart and lungs, your abs get a workout as an extra bonus.

Note that this class does not instruct you in self-defense or in combatant skills, and therefore should not be treated as such.

---

[2] Front thigh muscles.
[3] Muscles of the backside.

Water Aerobics

Water aerobics classes do traditional aerobics moves in waist-to-neck-high water. Sometimes the classes use webbed gloves to make the workouts harder.

Because water is twelve to fourteen times thicker than air and offers resistance in every direction, these classes can give you great muscle tone. The downside is that you just don't get to burn as many calories as you do on land.

Anyone can enjoy water aerobics; however, because water is a naturally more buoyant, gentle medium, the intensity of the workout is sometimes lacking.

Water aerobics is particularly good for anyone who has or is recovering from injuries. It's also ideal for pregnant women, older people, people with multiple sclerosis, osteoporosis, or any degenerative disease, because moving through the water is much easier on the body's joints.

Circuit

Imagine an exercise version of musical chairs and you've got a circuit class. Basically, it's a fast-paced class in which you do one exercise for anywhere between thirty seconds to five minutes and then move on to another exercise. It's all-change when the instructor shouts, "Time!" and everyone moves to the next station.

There are many different ways to set up a circuit class. Some classes will have large cards (and the relevant equipment) dotted around the outskirts of the room. Each card will tell you what to do at each workstation (e.g., "Sit-ups" or "Forward lunges," etc.). The cards may also have stick figures to illustrate the moves (note: you will not become a stick figure even if you do perform each move), and may provide brief points to correct technique. For example, "Sit-ups" might list points such as "Elbows to either side of head; breathe out as you come up, in as you go down," etc.

Of course, you can't compare the number of calories burned by reading the cards to actually doing the exercise, so try not to dwell too long over the small print.

Some classes intersperse aerobic activities (like stepping or jumping jacks) in between each workout station. This way you go from muscle conditioning workouts (like using weights) to aerobic activities and back again.

Although circuits are fast and fun (you usually go around each station in pairs, so you get to be friendly), they are not quite as effective as either a stand-alone aerobics or muscle conditioning class. Consider the circuit class as a general makeover (but remember to put your lipstick on afterwards).

Spinning (also known as Power Pacing and Reebok Studio Cycling)

This class has recently become extremely popular, especially in the United States. Imagine a room full of stationary exercise bikes and a group of women sitting on the bikes either reducing or increasing the tension in the wheels. Add an instructor who helps you work truly hard by verbalizing visual images ("We're going up a really steep hill…it's not much longer now…"), and you have spinning.

Spinning is an intense class, great for an aerobic workout and particularly good for people who have problems with general weight-bearing exercise (i.e., when their legs carry their bodies). It's also a great thigh and calf strengthener, although those with weak/injured/recovering knees should take care.

Caution: Ask your instructor to help you adjust the height of the handlebars, the height of the seat, and the distance of the seat from the handlebars. You're going to be working really hard and become intimately acquainted with the bike over the hour, so it's wise to make sure you're safe and comfortable.

Body Sculpting (also known as Body Conditioning/BLT)

As we mentioned earlier, this is a non-aerobic muscle toning class. Most classes will use some form of additional resistance, be it in terms of body bars, dumbbells, or exercise bands. Typically, you perform weight-training moves in a class setting.

Although there are many more types of exercise classes, they are less common and therefore not quite as widely accessible as the ones we have covered. However, don't let that stop you from trying out an unusual-sounding class. If you don't like surprises, you can always call first to check out whether it's going to be something you'd enjoy.

This brings us to the last slice of bread in our exercise sandwich. We've munched and crunched our way through the warm-up and the exercise main course. Now it's time to finish up, cool down, and check out.

The Cooldown

I've often seen people skip this part of the exercise session, grabbing their bags and dashing out of the studio, which I think is such a shame. In a way, the cooldown represents a pleasant pat on the back. You've done all the hard work, you've huffed and puffed like a dragon, or worked out muscles you didn't know you had, and now you are being released from all that effort with a calming, centering cooldown. It's like having a dessert of non-dairy ice cream after steak and fries. Cool and sweet and represents a closure.

Remember our non-hiking "aerobic peak?" Well, the downhill slope on the graph represents the aerobic cooldown. As with most downhill journeys, the descent is an easy ride. Although enjoyment might be reason enough to embark on this pleasure-filled coasting, there are also some serious reasons why it's a good idea to stay around and cool down.

At the end of an exercise session, especially a vigorous cardiovascular workout, your body needs time to readjust back to its normal mode. Your accelerated heart rate needs time to fall back to its gentle thumpity-thump versus its boompity-boom. Reserving time to cool your body down helps maintain the blood flow to your heart, which can prevent a cardiac disturbance. From the side of safety, we should always try to allow the heart rate and flow of blood to and from the heart to decrease gradually — no one (including Mr. Heart) likes the shock of a cold-turkey (sudden stop) scenario.

How To Cool Down

How do we cool down safely and effectively? Well, it's the upside-down version of the warm-up. After a strenuous aerobic-based session, we can slow down the heart rate by doing the same activity we just did, but at a much slower pace. A simple, no-frills walk around the room for a few minutes will also do the trick.

Whichever way you choose to return to your normal state, you should make sure you don't stop dead in your tracks and drop to the floor in a relieved pile of "phew, glad that's over" fatigue. Although it's tempting to do just that, you may cause painful muscle contractions and pooling of the blood in your lower extremities. The blood would therefore potentially leave the upper extremities, and the heart, gasping for blood — which may lead to fainting.

It's worth noting that the fitter one is, the faster it takes for the heart rate to return to normal (ever raced for the bus and found your heart still racing even though you had already reached the bus stop?). This is because conditioned, exercise-loving individuals have better control of temperature and blood flow, and also have better stress hormone regulation.

For example, an experienced runner might only need a couple of minutes to return her heart rate back to its automatic-cruise-control state, but a beginner might take up to ten minutes to be able to breathe like a regular human being again. In addition, how long you spend cooling down will also depend upon how strenuous your workout was. A cooldown will typically take anything between five to ten minutes.

Therefore, if you're new to exercise and still find your heartbeat performing thudding summersaults during the cooldown (and beyond), know that this will improve the more efficient your CV system becomes (i.e., the fitter you get). The most important thing is to keep moving and lower the intensity gradually.

No matter how fit you are, when you are trying to cool down, concentrate on your breathing. Try taking slower breaths. Make them long and deep, focusing on inhaling and exhaling from the diaphragm instead of short, shallow breathing from the chest. This way you help to lower your raised heart rate, and at the same time you ensure an adequate amount of oxygen is being pumped around the body.

Make sure you're breathing normally and feel relatively calm before you jump into a hot shower or bath — after all, you don't want to faint under such embarrassing circumstances.

A Word About Stretching (Well, Maybe a Few Words...)

Many cooldowns entail some stationary stretching. Our body's muscles have been put through their paces and have contracted with the effort. It's good exercise practice to undo that tension through stretching. The body is warm and conditions are ideal for this relaxing aid to realignment and flexibility. Besides, the truth is that after all that exertion, it feels really good (mentally and physically) to stretch it all out again.

In addition, some fitness professionals maintain that stretching out properly after an intense workout will prevent waking up the next day feeling as though your muscles have been through a 16th century torture chamber.

While it is normal to wake up feeling a *little* achy and bruised after your first few workouts, you shouldn't feel *so* bad that you can't get out of bed or walk up the stairs. This discomfort is usually at its worst about forty-eight hours after a workout and is technically called "Delayed Onset Muscle Soreness" or "DOMS," although it sometimes prefers to use its nickname "Charley Horse."

This slight discomfort is nothing to worry about (at least not compared to the bills). Almost everyone experiences some degree of soreness after their first workout or five, even if they are careful. This is because your muscles are complaining about (and getting used to) the extra workload you just gave them.

So, if you have just participated in a body-toning class, you can expect that the cooldown will focus on stretching those muscle groups that you have focused on. If you have been playing tennis, you'll be looking to stretch out your biceps, shoulders, upper back, and leg muscles. If you have been to a Step class, you'll need to focus on stretching out the rear thigh (hamstring) muscles as well as the gluteals and front thigh (quadriceps) muscles. Even if you have just gone for a jog, you should stretch out your calf muscles.

Cooldown stretches can be performed standing, sitting, or lying down. It's common for the instructor to instruct the stretch routine as a continuation of the last exercise. Therefore, if you have just finished a Step class and are standing, you will probably perform the relevant stretches in a standing position; if you went to a body-toning class and the last exercise left you lying supine (and sublime?) on the mat, you might continue the stretches in a horizontal position.

Now that we've made such a nutritious exercise sandwich, all it takes to fully enjoy its tastes, textures, and diversities is to go and take a bite. So, bon appetit — but before you go ahead and enjoy, there are a few pertinent do's and don'ts to consider that should help you digest your "meal."

Chapter 17

—◆◆◆—

Do's And Don'ts Of Exercise

Eating

- Don't eat just before exercising.
- Don't exercise on an empty stomach.
- Do eat two to three hours before exercising.

It doesn't make any sense to eat just before you exercise. Blood that would normally be used in digestion is diverted to the exercising muscles to help you lift that weight or move those legs. This slows down digestion, and increases discomfort and the risk of a stitch.

Conversely, it's also not advisable to exercise if you have not eaten for a long time. Your low blood sugar levels may cause a fatigued feeling (beyond the normal "I only went to bed last night at three" fatigue). So when *can* you eat? You should feel fine if you have something to eat two to three hours before you begin your workout.

Another skull-and-crossbones warning: A high simple-sugar intake (sodas, chocolate bars, cookies, etc.) less than forty-five minutes before exercise will cause low blood sugar (hypoglycemia) and you will find the workout veeeeeeery difficult (yes, even more than usual).

This chapter should help you enjoy your workout more.

Drinking

- Do drink water at least ten minutes before class.
- Do drink during the class.

Maintaining your fluid intake before and during exercise is important, especially when the environment you are working out in (whether it be a studio or outdoors) reaches temperatures of over seventy-seven degrees Fahrenheit.

Whenever we work out, we lose body water through perspiration. We need to drink more (either before, during, or after a class) in order to replace our levels of fluid.

If it's hot, make sure you have a cup of water to drink at least ten minutes before the class starts. If you drink small amounts of water two or three times during a one-hour class, it will help you cope with the heat. A small cup (6oz) every twenty minutes is usually enough.

It's worth noting that when it is hot, the blood is shunted out to the skin and heat is lost through sweat evaporation. This is the body's natural air conditioner to help keep you cool. Consequently, less blood is available for transporting oxygen to exercising muscles. So if you don't drink to cool down (instead of all that blood shunting), you might not feel so dandy.

Nausea

- Do reduce the intensity of the workout to reduce feelings of nausea.
- Don't overdo it if you haven't been regularly working out.
- Don't eat right before exercising.

Vigorous exercise by people not used to exercising may cause nausea and even vomiting (although vomiting is not so common). It may be due to a reduced oxygen supply to the stomach and intestines when blood is redistributed to the skin and muscles during exercise.

If you're not used to exercising, your lower cardiovascular efficiency cannot cope with your body's need to cool itself (blood to the skin surface to sweat out the heat, see "Drinking" above) *and* exercise (blood to the muscles), so more than usual amounts of blood may be taken away from the digestive system.

If you're experiencing these icky feelings of sickness and nausea, apart from not eating directly before exercise (see above), you might need to reduce the intensity at which you are working. Remember, slow and steady wins the race.

Insomnia

- Do exercise regularly for sound sleep.
- Don't exercise less than two hours before bedtime.

If you've ever headed out for the Land of Nod and you've ended up in the backwaters of insomnia, you'll know just how frustrating this can be.

It's even more frustrating to try to improve the healthfulness of your lifestyle by exercising, only to find that it leaves you more drained and tired (due to insomnia) than when you first started.

Insomnia is most prevalent in beginners who exercise too vigorously, especially close to bedtime. It is not advisable to exercise within two hours of going to bed because it takes approximately two hours for the physiological and neurological stimulation of exercise to subside. (In plain English, that means your body and brain are turbo-charged). This may last even longer in the unconditioned exerciser.

If all that sounds like a yawn-boring drag, the good news is that people who exercise regularly tend to sleep more soundly (when they get there) than those who don't exercise.

Physical Conditions

- Do get your doctor's consent if you have a medical condition.
- Do tell the instructor about any health issues affected by exercise.

Although you might feel hale and hearty, there are some health conditions (e.g., heart/lung disease or conditions, blood pressure irregularities, being under/over-weight, previous surgery, bad knees, arthritis, pregnancy, asthma, etc.) that necessitate a doctor's consent before embarking on a fitness campaign.

Don't be surprised if you have to sign a written consent form before a class. This form is designed to give the instructor any necessary information about your health to allow her to take it into account during the class and accommodate you accordingly. For example, she may recommend that you perform the routine without the high intensity of jumping or jogging.

You also might have forgotten that your blood pressure reading was high the last time you visited the doctor, or that you had knee surgery a year and a half ago. The instructor is not being nosy — she needs to know these things for your benefit.

In the event that no form was requested, it's still wise to inform the instructor of any condition you think is important before the lesson begins. Don't be shy; she's there to help take care of you.

Shmoozing

- Don't talk to friends during class.

Although this one doesn't technically come with a government health warning banner, it's still a big no-no. In terms of exercise etiquette, it's just plain rude to talk to your friend during a class.

It might feel like you are invisible (losing yourself amongst the throngs of humanity) but you are very, very visible — not just to the instructor, but to those participants who want to hear every cue, instruction, and teaching point. It's distracting, it's irritating, and it's just plain old rude (to the instructor). So save it for the natural breaks or book a walk 'n' talk with your friend on the way home.

Armed with all this information, I know you are ready to step into the studio knowing exactly what to expect. You want to leave your intimidation at the door and look forward to the new, stimulating, and invigorating medium of the exercise class. But before we let you grab your sneakers, water bottle, and towel and go for it, here are some tips that should make your exercise experience that much more enjoyable, successful, and productive.

Chapter 18

— ◆ ◆ ◆ —

Exercise Tips

*R*ather than having your exercise journey hampered with hiccups (like false starts, running out of gas, etc.), let's discuss some practical, hands-on tips to ensure that the road to fitness is as smooth and trouble-free as possible. These tips are designed to help not only the newcomer to exercise, but anyone who has never gotten a lot out of exercise before or who could do with getting more out of exercise now.

Since a large percentage of newcomers to exercise quit within eight weeks, it helps to heed the following tips to try to ensure that you'll be one of those who live (with exercise) happily ever after.

Get the most out of your workout: Try these well-tested tips.

Benefits Are Sure (When You Endure)

If you've neglected your body for years, don't expect it to feel revitalized in hours, or even days. Exercise is a serious commitment, especially if you want to see long-term benefits. You can only expect these benefits when you've exerted some real effort over an extended period of time. (For example, after several weeks of aerobic exercise, you should have the nice surprise of being able to catch up with Shnocky to give him his forgotten pencil case — without feeling asphyxiated or exhausted.)

Unfortunately, exercise only works while you are doing it. That means that good intentions don't count. *Doing* it works. *Thinking* about it while cozy on the sofa doesn't. Therefore, if your sofa has had a magical, magnetic pull on you for a few weeks, you'll find it that much harder to start up again.

No Pain, No Gain

I know I've always maintained that "no pain, no gain" isn't true, but tell me this isn't painful: When that soft armchair envelops you and it's time to extract your totally relaxed frame up and out of it in order to pound, pummel, and push that same gravity-drawn, relaxed body, doesn't that hurt? Point to ponder to help you out…it'll only take a second for you to extricate yourself out of that comfort zone, whereas the benefits will last much longer.

Tune in To Yourself

People come in all shapes and sizes. They also progress at different rates. Just make peace with yourself and only compete against the one and only you — not your neighbor who runs through the neighborhood every night for an hour. Be happy that you go for your Monday night brisk walks with your buddy and enjoy it, guilt free. Don't diminish your own accomplishments by looking over your shoulder at what others are doing. *If you're doing great, take the time to feel great.*

Falling Off the Bandwagon

Don't be too hard on yourself if you fall off the exercise bandwagon for a few days or even weeks. When you can manage, just climb right back on. Accept the lapse and move forward. You've got the rest of your life to get this right.

Staying Motivated

Admittedly, there are those who are addicted to exercise and remain so focused and motivated that it makes them look almost obsessive. But most of us fall into the category of preferring an easy, comfortable, healthy life without all that movement. No one likes hard work. We just like the results that hard work brings. If I didn't believe in (and experience) some serious benefits resulting from working out, I'd be quite happy to hit the snooze button and roll over.

Some skeptics will complain that exercise is boring. Although we will discuss this later (see "Exercise Is Boring," page 338), let's whisk up one or two other ways that we can motivate ourselves out of bed and into the gym.

Do Less

For the first few months, do less than you think you can. It will keep you coming back for more while also helping you avoid injury.

Log it

Keep a log of all your exercising, inside the house and out. Include the ten minutes on your stationary bike in your bedroom, all those half laps in the swimming pool and the hour-long aerobics class you attend. It'll serve to motivate you further when you see it all written down, and you'll be inspired to exercise because you know you are keeping a record of your movements.

Work Out with a Friend

If you're having trouble getting out of bed every day to go for that promised early morning jog, or, more realistically, getting out of the house in the evening for that aerobics class down the road, try pairing up with a friend to get you both there. There's nothing like guilt to get you moving, especially at dawn ("This bed is so delicious…but she'll be waiting for me, I can't let her down…") or at nighttime ("I would rather go to bed, but I promised"). Besides, it's so much more fun to work out with company than to rely on our own battery power.

Keep Your Goals in Sight — Literally

Place your exercise goals where you can see them. Maybe you'll put them up on the inside of your gym locker, on your computer's screensaver, or on the inside door of the cookie cupboard. Wherever you put them, when they are in sight, they are more likely to be in mind.

Train for an Event

If there's a gala swim, marathon run, or even a walk that's been organized to raise money for charity, sign up. You'll get to shape up, have a goal to work towards, raise money for charity, and feel truly smug at the end. The minute you agree to join, you'll have a new sense of purpose. The feeling of accomplishment you'll get from completing the event and raising all that money is like nothing else.

One Olympic medalist is quoted as having said, "If I wasn't training for the Olympics, I probably wouldn't even work out." Training for an event works wonders for sagging motivation.

No organized event for you to join? Well, don't you think it's a good idea to get one started?

Keep Yourself Entertained

Once you combine exercise with other guilty pleasures, you'll feel the time fly and will soon be looking forward to the next workout. Listening to music or a light lecture while you jog might just inspire you to go around the block an extra time to hear the end of the tape. Saving a gripping read for the exercise bike will also help you anticipate the session.

The Right Gear

Starting a class in first gear as opposed to reverse is always a good idea, but there's gear and then there's gear…

Clothing

While it's true that the leisure industry has its own fashion standards, rules, and regs, we don't have to go *that* far to get the most out of what exercise has to offer.

Comfort comes high on the list of dress priorities. Don't pull on that old T-shirt that itches on every seam (nor the one that's too tight, nor the one that makes you too hot…) and expect to enjoy your workout.

Although fashion is not our goal in this context, we can still look and feel good. What kind of continued motivation will you experience if you wear your husband's old, baggy pajamas? Juxtapose them with a new, flattering, loose, stylish, and special-for-exercise t-shirt that you simply love, and maybe you'll be that little bit more inspired to come again (and again, and again…).

Similarly, if you choose to wear exercise clothes with holes in them, ripped seams, old stains, missing buttons (I've seen it all…), where's the sense of self-worth? Forget about honoring exercise, what about honoring yourself? You're worth it. And what you're doing is worth it. See "Chapter 2: Are You Ready? Correct Attitudes, Take Pride in How You Diet." It applies to exercise as well.

Extra Tip: Try laying out the next day's workout clothes every night before going to bed. It helps to get you into a motivated mode, besides an organized mode.

Water Bottles

We've already mentioned how important it is to drink when exercising, so it's a good idea to invest in a special no-cup-involved drinking bottle. The sports bottles that have the pull-out, push-in spout are ideal (no spills). Whatever type of exercise you're going to go for, you'll need a drink.

If you're going for a jog, why not invest in a special belt with a pouch for the bottle, designed so that you can run more comfortably, with your hands free? They're not expensive and you might even want to take it on vacation when you see how great they are. They are available in sports shops or sportswear catalogues.

Watches

Although you'll probably be taking your watch with you anyway to keep an eye on what time you need to be back home, a watch with a stopwatch capability is a useful gadget to have around when exercising.

When you time your session, either on your walk or in a class, you can compete against yourself for extra motivation. Week one might entail a fifteen-minute walk (or walking through the routine for fifteen minutes), week two might see you progress to twenty minutes, etc. By the time you get to week six, you might choose to walk for ten minutes, jog for twenty, walk for ten. Having your progress monitored so easily and immediately can be very satisfying.

Using the stopwatch display on your watch also means that instead of *feeling* like you must have been on the go for at least half an hour (it was only ten minutes…), you'll *know* whether you deserve your coffee break or not.

Footwear

Ever been to a wedding in uncomfortable, high heeled shoes? Did you enjoy dancing with the bride? Mmm, couldn't wait to sit down, right? Well, I don't know about you, but I know that I, for one, don't go far in fancy footwear — certainly not much further than the first aid box for a bandage for that blister.

If we want to go far on this exercise jaunt, we have to make sure we're snug as a bug and treat our feet properly.

A surgeon wouldn't dream of operating with a blunt or dirty scalpel; a professional carpenter wouldn't build a bookcase with a toy saw and hammer; and we shouldn't go out to exercise without the right workout equipment.

Cycling isn't going to be much fun if you're using your kid brother's old clanger with broken gears and an uncomfortable seat (we're being polite). Walking isn't going to be comfortable (or safe) in trendy, non-supportive pumps or sandals. And we can't do aerobics in our slippers or canvas sneakers.

It doesn't have to set you back two paychecks to invest in the right equipment for your chosen activity. But the right equipment might mean the difference between success and failure, or enjoyment and torture.

I had one girl come to an aerobics class wearing her skirt, shirt, sweater, and canvas sneakers. She wasn't very inspired because, "Aerobics makes me hot and makes my feet ache." I advised her to take her sweater off and invest in proper sneakers and voila, she changed her tune to, "Aerobics is great!"

Since footwear is so important to many exercises, let's look at a few points to help us choose our shoes.

Choosing The Right Sports Shoe

I'll be the first to agree that it can be overwhelming to go into a sports shoe shop these days. There are shoes in every color, specific to every sport, with all sorts of technical jargon requiring a degree in body biomechanics. Let's cut through all that and get down to the real stuff of what exactly we should be looking for when choosing a pair of sneakers.

✔ **Buy the right shoe for your sport**

If running is your thing, then you need a "running shoe" (they're actually called that). If aerobics is your forté, then you need a "cross trainer" (no, not a grumpy exercise dictator). This means a shoe designed for running will not be suitable for high-low workouts. "Why?" you may ask. "Surely aerobics needs the cushioning you get in a running shoe?" Yes, they do need the impact technology (cushioning so you can jump), but they need lateral support as well, for all those side steps and grapevines. In other words, runners' feet are moving forward (unless they're six-year-old smart aleck boys) and aerobics' feet move sideways and so need lateral support.

A cross trainer is appropriate if you dabble in a variety of sports, from walking one day, biking the next, and lifting weights the next. But if you spend a lot of time doing one type of activity, do yourself and your feet a favor and buy a shoe that's specific to that sport.

✔ **Make sure it fits**

Sounds like Cinderella? (Well, you don't want to be the ugly stepsister, do you?) It's very easy to be swayed by fashion and new trends (and forceful salesmen), but remember, your feet must come first. Fit is the key to comfort and injury reduction.

Forget about all this "breaking in" business. Make sure the shoes feel comfortable from the moment you put them on. What qualities are you looking for? You want a shoe that allows for movement of the toes, supports the arch, and allows for easy heel-toe action (i.e., heel strikes floor first followed by toes) with cushioning to absorb the force, which leads us to the next step…(hey, that's cute, get it?…"step"…)

✔ **Picking the shoe**

Go prepared by either wearing or taking along a pair of sports socks that you would normally wear to work out in, plus a second pair of thin socks and a pair of dark sunglasses.

Put on both pairs of socks when you try on both shoes. This mimics the foot's expansion when you exercise and gives a more realistic sensation of what you'll feel like during a workout. Put on the sunglasses and lace up the sneakers properly (even if that means undoing all those horrible weird lace patterns). Now put the shoes through their paces. So it's 3…2…1…Grapevine to the right, to the left, forward march, side squat, etc. Now you see why you need the sunglasses.

A little inflexibility in the shoe is acceptable, but *no* discomfort or pressure is allowed. The slightest bit of pressure means that you need to try on a different shoe.

As this process may take some patience, make sure you have scheduled enough time in the sports shop to try on several shoes, in order to make sure you are selecting the right pair for you.

✔ **Cost**

Even though your sneakers might cost more than your Shabbos shoes, consider them an investment. Beneath all those stripes and flashy colors is some serious technical engineering designed to protect your feet, ankles, and joints. Go for a brand name so that you can rely on the quality. You can try looking for brand names in discount stores. Or, once you know which sneaker suits you (and you've stopped growing), you can look for your sneakers on sale in the shops, online, or in sports catalogues.

One thing's for sure. An expensive pair of sneakers will cost you less than a trip to the orthopedist.

✔ **Regular testing**

Once you have chosen the right sneaker for you, do a regular inspection, like the one done on your car, to see if it's road-worthy. You must look for *wear* and *tear*. The first place to check is the insoles, followed by the outside of the shoe.

If the insoles are losing shape or look deformed, or if you can see any splitting or stretching on the sides of the shoes, it's time to take your sunglasses on another expedition.

Try not to look negatively at buying a new pair ("Oh dear, this is going to set me back a buck or two…"). Rather, consider it a victory; you've been exercising to the point that you need another pair of sneakers. You get nachas when the family polishes off that delicious pot roast even though you're left with the dishes: The dirty dishes, void of remnants, attest to your successful cooking. Enjoy nachas from your old sneakers, too: The worn out sneakers similarly attest to your successful exercise campaign.

Lacing

Although your mother probably gave you an excellent lesson in how to lace up those pretty booties when you were five, she might not have shown you one or two extra permutations that can go a long way in making your sneakers as comfortable as your old slippers (see diagrams below).

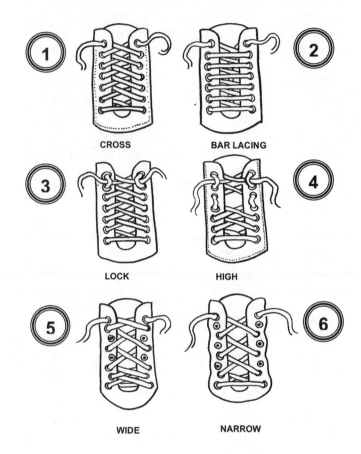

1. *Cross Lacing*

   Holds the foot firmly in position (important for lateral movements). The disadvantage: It can put an uncomfortable amount of pressure on the top of the foot if the laces are pulled too tight.

2. *Bar Lacing*

   Places less pressure on the top of the foot. The disadvantage: the laces can stretch, which reduces stability.

3. *Lock Lacing*

    Using an extra twist at the top holes, this method allows for expansion during exercise. Take each end of the lace back inside the shoe through the hole above it and form a loop. Lace through the opposite loop and pull towards the ankle to tighten.

4. *High Insteps*

    If your foot has a naturally high instep, this lacing might relieve some of the pressure typical to conventional lacing. Lace around the peak of the instep using cross lacing (see No. 1) below the instep and lock lacing (see No. 3) above it. This will eliminate pressure on the top of the foot.

5. *Wide Feet*[1]

    Use lines of holes that are furthest apart (across the shoe's width) to make the shoe fitting wider.

6. *Narrow Feet*

    Use the holes that are nearest together to give a narrower fitting.

Motivated? Check. Water bottles? Check. Comfy sneakers? Check. Well then, you're up and running...

---

[1] Occasionally sneakers will have holes/eyelets forming a zig-zag line on either side. We refer to this type of sneaker in diagrams 5 and 6.

Chapter 19

◆ ◆ ◆

Debunking Fitness Myths

(Yes, "debunking" is in the dictionary)

*A*s I have said before, there's literally mega-giga-whopping-bytes worth of information on exercise and fitness. But I reckon there's nearly as much misinformation out there as well. By this I mean all those old wives' tales that we have unwittingly swallowed but never stopped to scrutinize. Just because this false information got itself into print doesn't mean it's fact, tried, tested, and airtight (unless, of course, it appears in this book). This misinformation can give exercise a bad name and can act as a powerful, even misleading, deterrent. So let's see if there is any truth to all those hitherto sworn-by beliefs and myths.

Who Needs Exercise?

Exercise is a Modern Invention for the Bored — My Grandmother Managed Very Well Without it — I Can Too (You'd Be Amazed By the Myths I've Heard…).

We live very sedentary lives in this hi-tech generation. Technology has catered to each and every lazy whim. We have cars to shuttle us from A to B so we don't have to walk. We have escalators and elevators to take us up and down so we don't have to use the staircase. And we have every modern convenience to help us in the home — right from food processors (we don't have to stir anymore), to washing machines (want to walk to the

> *I can't tell you how many times I have heard or read these fitness myths. It's time the truth was told.*

local river?), to remote control handsets for the stereo (so we don't have to get up to turn it on/off). Let's face it: We really are lazy lumps.

Even at work we don't move. We sit on swivel chairs at the workstation and command our environment with the touch of a button.

All this does not bode well for our bodies. If we are to function optimally, we must look after our bodies. Part of this prescription is to keep them moving. In a generation where life has become so much easier for us on a physical level, we have to make a more conscious effort to put our bodies through their paces. That's where the explosion of exercise comes from. We have had to create a contrived environment to help enable us to exercise, whereas Great-Grandmother Gertrude didn't have to.

Secondly, I don't think there are many people these days who would qualify as bored — they are too busy being stressed (and could do with more time, not less. How ironic that we've got more timesaving conveniences and yet less time...). Although the exercise industry is closely associated with the leisure and pleasure industries, they differ in that exercise is a prerequisite for a healthy life, whereas the leisure and pleasure industries are not.

Exercise is Not for Me. I'm Too Old.

Are you too old to breathe? Are you too old to smile? You'll soon experience the sweet joys of better breathing (and better smiling) once you start to move.

Joking apart, exercise is crucial to the mature (we'll skip the title "old") individual. **If you don't use it, you lose it**. If you never have to stretch past the dinner plate (for the salt), you end up not being able to stretch even when you want to. Ditto for walking, lifting, carrying, etc. In extreme circumstances, the elderly become quite literally frightened to move. This can be the unfortunate precursor to immobility and premature death — not that I want to scare you (OK, maybe just a bit). Let's put it another way: Getting old does not have to be synonymous with moving less.

I know a fitness instructor who has been teaching exercise for over forty-five years. She must be in her early seventies (as her white hair testifies). She moves better than some of her class participants a fraction of her age, she is the picture of health, and she knocks years off her appearance — not because she has the perfect figure (she hasn't), but because her movements are those of a twenty-year-old woman.

One of my regular class participants is a wonderful, sprightly great-grandmother in her late seventies who stands beside ladies a quarter of her age. I'm convinced her youthful attitude (she's got plenty of "get up and go") is keeping her young (not to mention healthy).

Exercise is Not for Me. I'm Too Fat.

Fat people can be fit people. When I was in America, I once saw an exercise video with about eight ladies in the studio. One of them was, excuse me, absolutely huge. I couldn't help but think to myself how distasteful it was to produce a video focusing on how inadequately this woman was going to perform the routine. It turned out that she was the instructor. Not only did she perform the routine, but she did a superb job. She executed neatly choreographed steps at high impact (basically she jumped around a lot), was light on her feet, and never got out of breath once. Needless to say, I cast my preconceptions in the nearest garbage can and humbly watched the rest of the video. (By the way, take a look at page 334 later in this chapter, where we discuss what exercise can and can't do, and you'll understand why so many instructors may be fit, but they sure aren't all thin).

So, if it's true that fat people can be fit people, the question remains, what exactly is stopping fat people from exercising?

Danger

So long as Plump Penina has her doctor's permission (she'll probably have his insistence, encouragement, and his blessing), and she works at her own level and does not strain herself excessively, there is absolutely no reason why she won't be able to enjoy the benefits of exercise as much as her skinny sister. It'll not only help her lose those unwanted pounds, but it will also help to improve her self-image.

Embarrassment

Most fat people carry around not just extra pounds, but also heavy psychological baggage too. They feel self-conscious at the best of times — let alone in a gym or studio among size six exercise-aholics. However, all is not doom and gloom. Penina could persuade a fellow fuller-figure female (say that one quickly) to go along with her so that neither of them feels out of place. And they could stand at the back of the class in order to feel less conspicuous. But they should take it from me (an instructor who can see everyone) that no one is paying attention to them anyway, as they are all busy concentrating on the instructor and on getting it right themselves.

Alternatively, Penina could begin her exercise program on her own. I'm sure she's been for a walk before in her life. Now all she needs to do is change the gear: from gear one (pleasant stroll) to gear two (brisk gait). And she still gets to do the shopping. She could invest in an exercise bike, stepper, or treadmill. All of these measures might help her gain confidence — both in terms of her movements and her confidence in exercising. When she has tasted the sweet joys of accomplishment on her own, she will be less inhibited to join the social setting if she wants to. The difference here is that it will be *her* choice whether or not she goes. She will not feel a victim of her circumstances.

Exercise is Not for Me. I'm Too Skinny.

I know, your heart is having a hard time bleeding for her, so if you want to skip this one, feel free. Skinnies, stay with me.

Although it's true that exercise (especially aerobic exercise) will help burn off calories (which you might not want to do if you are *so* skinny), it also builds muscle mass, which most really skinny people seem to lack. Not only does a Skinny Minnie need muscle mass (to be stronger, to cushion the body, etc.), but she also needs to develop and maintain other areas of fitness — such as flexibility, stamina, strength, and cardiovascular endurance. Hey, you might be skinny, but you still need to run for the bus if you're late.

I Can't Exercise. I've Never Done it Before.

Live in England by any chance? I don't know what it is about the English mentality (although I do find it quite comfortable most of the time); while the mentality can boast some real winning characteristics, a sense of adventure is not one of them.

"He who has never tried and failed has never truly succeeded." Can't remember where I got that one from, but it's good.

If we never choose to go beyond our comfort zone, we never grow, be it in the spiritual realm (this is getting holy) or in the physical (ah, that's more comfortable). Just because you've never been a mother/grandmother before, doesn't mean to say you won't make a perfectly good one. Just because you've never lifted anything heavier than a can of baked beans out of the shopping bag doesn't mean you won't enjoy the benefits of lifting weights (and becoming stronger).

There's a book with a great title (although I confess I haven't read the book yet). It's called *Feel the Fear and Do It Anyway*. Why is this such a great title? Because we all have fears; it's how we handle them that either makes us or breaks us. Nothing ventured, nothing gained. You could be denying yourself the amazing benefits of good health (not to mention one of life's rainbow colors of pleasure) by staying put instead of facing the challenge and meeting it like a real winner.

By the way, in case you didn't gather, I don't classify never-having- done-it-before as a valid excuse.

I Can't Exercise Because I Get Dizzy.

Dizziness may be caused by insufficient oxygen to the brain. It can occur through overexertion, exercising in very hot conditions, or because of low blood pressure. People who regularly suffer from low blood pressure should consult their doctor, although exercise will often aid the stabilization of blood pressure.

In the case of becoming dizzy because of overexertion, it is important to remember to maintain a comfortable level of intensity; only increase the workload gradually, over a period of weeks or months, as the initial level of intensity becomes too easy.

Too many people work too hard too soon. To become overweight or unfit has taken many years of inactivity that cannot be rectified in one or two blasts of frenzied aerobic exercise.

Another way to prevent becoming dizzy is by exercising in cool, open environments with good air circulation. If you still find you are getting dizzy during a session, you should stop immediately, sit or lie down, and breathe deeply in a slow, normal rhythm until the dizziness subsides.

I Can't Exercise Because it's Too Expensive.

True, joining an upscale exercise studio can set you back a few paychecks, but joining a studio is not the only way to exercise. Many women's gyms, Young Israel centers, etc. provide exactly the same services as a posh 'n' polished, plush exercise studio, but at a fraction of the cost — plus in some cases, you don't have to take out a monthly or yearly membership.

You can try out different classes on a casual basis and see which one you enjoy the most. If you don't want to go to a local gym (or you don't have access to one), you can always hire a qualified exercise instructor to give private lessons (ask your doctor, local gym, or in-shape friends to recommend some names) and split the cost with a few other exercise-conscious friends.

In addition, this is as good a place as any to mention that it doesn't cost to walk (unless it's along Fifth Avenue and you've $100 spare). We may have water bills, gas bills, and electricity bills, but so far we haven't got a walking bill. Let's take advantage before it's too late.

I Can't Exercise Because I Am Pregnant.

A generation ago, pregnancy was viewed more like an illness than a condition. Bedrest, no strain, and taking it easy were the prescription. Nowadays, research reveals that (so long as you have the OK from your doctor) there is no reason why you can't be pregnant and work out at the same time. Of course, we have to be sensible. We don't want to go bananas at this time and try to set a new world record for the high jump (no matter how excited you are to be pregnant).

Not only is moderate exercise safe for baby, but it's also good for mom. Pregnant exercisers experience fewer aches and pains, an increased sense of self-esteem, have more energy, and higher levels of stamina and endurance.

Is it safe to exercise in pregnancy if you are not already in shape? So long as you go easy on yourself and listen to your body (and your doctor and your qualified ante/postnatal instructor[1]), you get the green light. Of course, if you have had any complications or past medical history, a medical opinion is an even bigger must. Otherwise, try viewing it as a training ground for a lifelong marathon of nachas.

---

[1] As opposed to your local *haimishe* friend who runs an exercise class but is not thoroughly qualified in this area.

I Can't Exercise Because I've Just Had a Baby.

Although I have seen new mothers rush from their hospital bed straight to the grocery store with a day-old baby, I think it's worth clarifying what is good and wise in terms of postnatal exercise.

There are four main considerations when thinking about exercising with babe in arms (yes, you *can* put the babe down while you exercise...):

✔ **You are not as fit as you were.**

Even if you did exercise throughout your pregnancy, your movements were automatically hindered by the change in your body shape. It can take time to reacquaint yourself with the subsequent shift of balance. Considering that little babies usually take up a good portion of Mommy's time after their arrival, it is fair to assume that Mommy won't have seen the inside of a gym for a while. All this adds up to the fact that you are probably quite deconditioned (I thought that was more polite than saying "out of shape").

Practical implications? You will need to take it really easy at the start of your fitness campaign. Consider yourself a beginner and take it from there (even if you know what the instructor is going to do next). Build up your levels gradually and listen to your body. If it complains, take the easier option.

✔ **Hormones.**

During pregnancy and after (even if you are not nursing), the body has an elevated level of the hormone relaxin. This has enabled the body to accommodate the extra shape and weight. It allows the joints a little extra leeway, and therefore you will find yourself rather more flexible than you were before gestation. The levels of relaxin remain elevated as long as you are nursing (but if you are not nursing, they automatically stabilize after about six months).

Practical implications? You will be able to squat deeper, bend further, and stretch higher because of the effects of these hormones on the body. Extra care should be taken not to overstretch or take the body beyond its natural range of movement. A properly qualified ante/postnatal instructor will be able to design a safe program that takes these factors into account.

✔ **Bridging the Ab-Gap.**

Due to all that stretching during pregnancy, the two sheets of tummy muscle (from the bottom of the ribs to the pelvis) will sometimes take time to get back together again. (By the way, this gap is not influenced by body fat.)

Practical implications? You should only take part in abdominal exercises once you know how big this gap is and therefore at what level it is safe for you to work. In order to ascertain the gap's size, your qualified ante/postnatal instructor (or doctor) will perform a quick, painless "rec-check" (Rectus Abdominus check) by feeling the tummy muscles' position.

Working at a level that is inappropriate for your own abdominal muscles can put undue pressure on an area that is not ready for such intensity. Having a gap larger than a ¾ of an inch diameter may mean that you should work at an easier level, i.e., performing pelvic tilts rather than full abdominal crunches.

Although it might mean asking the doctor for an extra couple of minutes at your postnatal examination, or asking your instructor to check you before the lesson, it's a couple of minutes well spent in effectively safeguarding your health.

✔ **The Checkup.**
Before resuming any exercise class or gym sessions, it is essential that you have a clean bill of health from your doctor. He is going to know whether your type of delivery excludes you from certain exercises/lifting/pressure. He will check out any medication that you might be taking that may necessitate postponing your return to exercise and will be responsible for giving you a once-over exam. He has your best interests at heart and is definitely worth visiting after about six weeks (besides, he's probably missed you).

I Can't Exercise Because I Suffer From Stress Incontinence.

The first sign of stress incontinence is a small leakage of urine when coughing, laughing, lifting heavy objects, or bouncing up and down during exercise. It may be caused by a defect or weakness in the urethral sphincter (bladder exit), or by a weak pelvic floor that is unable to counter the inside abdominal pressure built up during repetitious bouncy exercise. This condition is more common in women who have had at least one baby, as the muscle tone automatically deteriorates during pregnancy.

Prevention and cure of this condition are one and the same. Five pelvic floor contractions (a.k.a. Kegel's exercises), ten times per day (or more), will help to strengthen the pelvic floor muscles. These exercises can be done at any time of day (while waiting for a bus, standing at the kitchen sink, or on the phone — and no one even has to notice you doing them). Physical therapists with a special interest in obstetrics will gladly help you learn how to perform these exercises correctly, as will any well-qualified ante/postnatal instructor.

A diagnosed weak pelvic floor does not automatically mean that you have to give up exercise. It just means that while making a concerted effort to strengthen these muscles, you may also feel more comfortable performing non-jumping cardiovascular exercise (such as brisk walks/exercise bike/treadmill/stepper, etc.). See further page 286.

Now that we have covered who can and can't exercise, it's time to turn our attention to what exercise can or can't do for us. If we start an exercise program expecting unrealistic results, we have failed before we have even begun. And that's depressing. Let's see what we can realistically expect from our newfound pleasure.

What Exercise Can and Can't Do

I Need To Lose Weight, Therefore I Need To Exercise (Read: Without Dieting).

I wish I had a dollar for every person I have met who thinks this way, 'cause then I'd be rich.

Let's set the record straight on this one, once and for all. If you are in a hurry to lose those extra pounds (ever met anyone *not* in a hurry?), go on a diet versus relying on exercise. Why? Well, get the calculators out (do you remember where you put it down last time we did this?) and we'll do some math.

It takes a deficit of 3,500 calories (or a good kick to the bathroom scales) to lose one pound. That's a daily deficit of roughly 500 calories over a seven-day week. On a diet, you can reach that goal by cutting back your portion sizes by one-third at dinner, and eating an apple instead of a slice of apple pie for dessert. To burn that number of calories through exercise, however, you'll need to jog for an hour (note: this means non-stop jogging — not strolling, stopping, and starting…). To get that magic pound off in a week, you'll need to jog every single day (7 × 500 = 3,500) come rain, hail, your mother-in-law visiting, or a headache from all this math.

If losing weight is your most pressing concern, dieting is the surest and fastest route to follow. It's just so much quicker in the short-run to take a few less bites, than it is to burn the weight off through all that time-consuming huffing and puffing. A few seconds of restraint versus hours of sweat.

I don't want to be unfair to Exercise, but I'm sure he won't mind me saying that he's a great aid to the dieting treadmill even if he's not the number one choice when he's going it alone. Besides, he's got so many other qualifications to his name (we already mentioned 150 of them), that his ego can still remain intact.

It is worth noting that dieters often end up losing both fat *and* muscle tissue when they shed their pounds, which is not the ideal goal of healthy weight loss. Exercise can counteract these negative effects quite markedly. By increasing physical activity, you'll burn fat *and* build muscle tissue.

However, and here's more ammunition to inflate Exercise's ego: Exercise may well be your best bet if you are committed to losing weight *and* keeping it off for good.

Why? Well, sometimes people on diets can feel negative about all the "don't do's," whereas people who exercise may actually begin to enjoy the lifestyle change of being more physically active. Over time, they are more likely to stick with exercise than with dieting — and they are therefore more likely to maintain their weight loss. It's a twenty-four hour unrelenting battle against willpower on one hand (this is not an excuse to blow an existing diet if you're on one — it isn't), versus a three-times-a-week struggle (to overcome your laziness) against the armchair on the other.

An additional word or two on this topic is in order, since so many people are confused by all that's written, spoken, or inferred about the subject. The most effective way to lose weight is with a *combination* of both dieting and exercising. But, a lot of people may feel overwhelmed at the thought of changing everything — diet, lifestyle, routine, etc. See "Avoiding False Starts," page 54. If so, focus on what you want most now (weight loss or fitness benefits) and give it your best shot. When you are at ease in your newfound lifestyle and have achieved a comfortable status quo, you can introduce further changes — without the stress.

I Don't Need To Go To a Gym Or Exercise Class — I'm on the Move All Day.

This one usually comes from the grandmas. They are under the mistaken impression that baking all day (we're not even talking about all that tasting...), answering the phone/door, and doing the laundry automatically exempts them from exercise because they are "on the go/moving" all the time. If this were true, no one would have thought to invent the gym. Unfortunately, the fitness benefits incurred when only minimally engaged in activity (like stirring the batter) are usually negligible.

When we are trying to increase our aerobic fitness levels (so we don't huff and puff when we walk uphill or run for the bus), we need to raise the heart rate to a level where it's working quite hard for a continuous time period (at least ten minutes). Going shopping and stopping to shmooze with the locals, sadly, does not qualify (I also wish it did). Neither does walking up and down stairs carrying baskets of laundry. True, you might feel like you are working extremely hard, but you are not improving your levels of fitness (unless you are doing this activity strenuously and for an extended period — read: after Tisha B'Av).

Same principle holds true for building muscle strength/tone. Sure, you're working hard when you lift that ten-pound sack of potatoes onto the counter, but you are not working the muscles consistently or sufficiently enough to render significant improvements.

In real terms, this means that although you feel you are on a domestic merry-go-round and may well feel exhausted before falling into bed at night, you won't find it any easier to do the same amount of work tomorrow, next week, or next month.

I Was Really Fit Three Months Ago. Now That I Want To Start Exercising Again, I'm Going To Continue From Where I Left Off.

Oh no, you're not. Three months might not be long enough for you to forget the joys of being super-fit, but it's plenty long enough for your body to forget. Unfortunate though it may be, the benefits of exercise are not eternal. Just as your fitness levels improve with time, so do they (sigh) deteriorate with time. You just can't put fitness in the freezer.

Don't think that ultra-fit people such as aerobics instructors are exempt from the inevitable downward spiral. We're still human. I can feel the pinch when returning to giving classes after only a three-week break. It's just that drop harder to talk my way through jumping jacks and shuttle runs. The answer? Back to the grindstone…

A word of warning is due here. If you do expect to pick up from where you left off, you may run the risk of experiencing the discomfort of a stitch or breathlessness, which may stop you from continuing with the rest of the class. You may also run the risk of overexerting yourself and therefore making yourself vulnerable to injuries. If you remember that you performed eight sets of eight repetitions without breaking a sweat before, you might be inclined to push yourself beyond your body's comfort zone in an effort to dispel the horrible truth: You're going to have to start again almost from scratch. So take it slow and easy and build up gradually. (Oh, and when they invent the exercise pill, please let me know).

Exercise Will Cure All Aches and Pains.

While exercise purports terrific physical benefits to our bodies, it is not the cure-all for all pain. If your body experiences pain, that is the beginning of a warning system designed to wake you up to paying closer attention to that particular body part. (E.g., an earache heralds an infection in need of antibiotics, not more jumping jacks.)

Some exercises may even make the pain worse. Consider a knee injury, not yet healed. Jumping around the studio may well be a great idea for the rest of your body, but Mr. Kneecap may resent the strain. This increased workload may indeed impede recovery as well as potentially exacerbate the problem.

However, exercises specifically designed by physical therapists and medical practitioners are not the same as the exercises performed to increase general levels of fitness. These therapeutic exercises can therefore be extremely beneficial in terms of strengthening the muscles surrounding the injury and in terms of being generally restorative.

Exercising Once a Week is Useless.

I have been asked, "Is exercising once a week futile?" in different forms many times. Let me ask you a question first: Are you asking me whether you gain any fitness benefits from exercising once a week, or are you telling me that this is your excuse not to exercise at all? We'll address the first case scenario and leave the second case scenario protagonist to ponder her levels of honesty.

The answer to this myth is four-fold:

    ✔ If you go to a class (or devote a chunk of time specifically to exercise, be it at home or in a gym, etc.) you are exerting yourself to invest in yourself. This consciousness will permeate the rest of your week. For example, you may choose to use the subway stairs instead of the escalator because you are more exercise conscious and because you want to maximize the benefits incurred from your specified exercise session.

✔ The rate of progress (in anything, actually, but with particular reference to exercise) directly correlates to the amount of energy you are willing to invest into something. This means that, yes, you will accrue fitness benefits, but your progress may be slower than if you exercised three times a week.

✔ Once you have committed yourself to a once-a-week formal exercise session, it is easier to augment it with other, less formal sessions during your week. For example, if you go swimming on Sunday, maybe you can go for a brisk walk to the park on Tuesday, and do some floorwork (next to the bed on a double-folded towel) on Thursday.

✔ If you do decide to spend an hour a week on exercising more formally, you are heading in the right direction. You never know, you might somehow be able to eventually squeeze another session into your week, thereby doubling up on the benefits. It usually requires more energy to embark on a new project than it does to augment an existing one. I say, go for it.

Exercising Once a Week is Enough.

Just in case you're looking all smug and comfy after having been told that your weekly session is definitely *not* useless, that doesn't mean that it's your best option.

Recently there has been a vast amount of research designed to clarify just how long we should work out, how often, how hard, and in which particular exercise discipline.

We have already discussed different types of exercise, how long/how often they should be performed, etc. We can say that one is better than none; however, three is more than three times better than one (did you catch all those numbers?).

I Have To Exercise for Thirty Consecutive Minutes in Order To Benefit.

Three ten-minute sessions of aerobic exercise burn as many calories and provide *nearly* the same health benefits as one thirty-minute session.

This is worth knowing. Why? Because if you've only got a forty-five minute lunch break, you can exercise for ten minutes and still have over half an hour to munch (just don't forget to do your two other ten-minute workouts, i.e., one in the morning before work, and one after work).

If I Stop Exercising, My Muscles Will Turn To Fat.

No, they won't. They'll just shrink. Fat and muscles are two different entities; you can't turn one into the other (although you can increase the size of either).

By Focusing on Abdominal Exercises I Will Get Rid of My Excess Midriff.

We can't tell fat where to go (although we'd like to). And even an exercise instructor who is consuming calories beyond her needs will find that her body will decide exactly where it is going to store all that fat — regardless of how loudly she protests. This is why you see some fat instructors. Exercise is not a foolproof recipe for the perfect body.

It's also worth knowing that most abdominal exercises aim to strengthen, tone, and condition the abdominal muscles — and are not necessarily aiming to obliterate them.

Now that we have defined more clearly what exercise can and can't do, it's time to address those myths that pertain to the exercise session itself. If you feel the noose tightening around your neck as the degree of accountability increases, remember that one way to shake it free is to step into an exercise class and try it out...

The Class/Session Itself

Exercise is Boring.

(See "Staying Motivated," page 318, for other tips on this topic.)

It's boring only if you are. There are so many different types of exercises you can perform that it's almost overwhelming. However, if you have been going to the same class for some time, I think we'd all agree you might get a little bored in the process.

If you are getting tired of aerobics, try something else for a while and come back when you are fresh. There is nothing worse than persisting with an exercise class when you are finding it a chore. Besides, it may eventually turn you off aerobics forever. Therefore, make a long-term investment and keep yourself interested in the exercises you are doing, or find a new fun exercise-activity for a while. Only return to your aerobics class when you have fresh enthusiasm.

Although some people thrive on routine, most of us need a bit of variety to stay motivated. For this reason, you might want to try cross-training (no, not shouting at your two-year-old son when he hits the baby...). Cross-training means mixing up your workouts. You can try swimming on Monday, an aerobics class on Wednesday, and exercise biking on Friday. Or, you can vary the pace or intensity — walking fast along the flat track one day, walking uphill another, or walking on pavement/grass/sand. You can also try varying the equipment you are using for an extra pizzazz. One day you can use weight machines, the next day free weights, and the next, resistance bands. You get the same results, plus the bonus of being excited about your workout.

You can also try to focus on different aspects of fitness. One day could be stretch and relaxation, the next a brisk walk to town and back, and another day you might enjoy a body-conditioning class.

If you're working out in your house, maybe it's time to consider getting out of the house (at least for one session a week) to give you the boost you need. This doesn't have to be a formal class; you can go for a brisk walk, jog, or swim — either on your own, or with company.

If the reason you are finding a particular class boring is because the instructor has forgotten the meaning of the words "smile," "humor," and "fun," maybe it's time to change class. Don't let a stale instructor diminish your right to have fun.

Whatever your situation, there's no excuse for boredom.

I Can Only Join a Gym If I've Got the Latest Gear.[2]

So many people are self-conscious when it comes to how they look — even more so when it's a question of how they look during an exercise class. Maybe it's the studio mirror glaring the truth of our image back to us. Maybe it's the newness of the exercise experience. Whatever the reason, the truth is that there's no uniform you have to be worried about conforming to.

The older we get, the more we realize that people are not as interested in us as we once imagined. This is just as true inside the gym as it is outside the gym — so don't worry about your gym clothes meeting high-fashion standards.

I Can't Go To an Aerobics Class Because I Won't Be Able To Follow All the Moves (and Therefore I Won't Benefit).

This is a two-for-one myth (the type you buy on sale).

Number one: There's a natural learning curve inherent within any newly acquired skill. True, at first you might get your lefts and rights mixed up and your feet might feel like they're not attached to the rest of your body. But you'll be surprised by how quickly you'll pick up the step names and moves. On average, it only takes a complete beginner three sessions to pick up all the basics and to feel at ease in the class (and that's a generous estimate).

That's number one taken care of — you will manage to master the steps, it just might take a week or two of perseverance. An additional point: If you have a really good instructor, she will break down the more complicated steps into their basic components and will constantly offer easier alternatives to more complex moves.

Number two: It works the heart just as hard to move two steps to the right as it does to do a fancy step-behind-step-together (grapevine) right. If fancy footwork is not your forté, don't worry, your heart doesn't know the difference. It just knows it's still getting its money's worth by coming to the class anyway.

---

[2] If you choose to wear a skirt, it is advisable for it to be flared and reach only to knee-level. This is to ensure your safety (i.e., to avoid tripping or falling) and so that the instructor can see your knee alignment.

I'm Really Fit So I Can't Go To a Regular (Easy) Aerobics Class.

If the instructor spends most of her time explaining and not performing, I would agree with you. However, in the event that the class is termed "easy" or "beginner's" because she only offers non-jumping (low impact) moves and automatically performs the exercise at a beginner's level herself, then I think you can still stand to gain in terms of your own fitness benefits once you take the following into account:

✔ Even if the warm-up seems designer-made for tortoises, don't skip it, literally and figuratively. Don't miss it out *and* don't jump/skip your way through it either. (See "The Warm-Up," page 301, for more about the importance of the warm up.) Your body needs to acclimate to the increased workload you are about to place on it, so give it a chance to get used to the idea.

✔ There are tons of high-impact options, where both feet are off the floor at a given moment (don't worry, you will come down again). You can perform these high-impact options at the same time as your instructor performs the low-impact moves. This way, you can end up with a workout appropriate for your fitness level. For example, if she marches in place, you can opt to jog. If you are super-fit, then you have probably been to classes before and know the high-impact moves very well. It's up to you to take them as an option. (Likewise when using weights: Just because everyone else is using three-pound hand weights, doesn't mean you can't go ahead and perform the same exercise with an increased resistance, i.e., by using five-pound weights).

An additional word of advice for the exercise mavin: If you haven't been to the class before but know in advance that it is considered "easy," stay in the back. Why? Well, for two reasons. One, you don't want to intimidate the other participants, who are probably mostly beginners. And two, the instructor herself might feel slighted or thrown off-guard to have a jumping jack in her class. It always pays to bear other people's sensitivities in mind.

Going for "the Burn" is the Way To Go.

Definitely. Straight out the door — quickly. Going for "the burn" does not mean burning down the house, the meat, or yourself in the oven. It's the uncomfortable sensation experienced by the muscles after they have been worked beyond their comfort zone. They resist further exertion by providing a mild sensation of pain. It's at this point that you may very well feel that you just *can't* do another rep (nor should you). If an instructor ever tells you to work to the point where you feel "the burn," do me (and yourself!) a favor and walk out. This is the worst possible advice a leader can offer. If muscles are burning and pain is occurring, it is a sign that you are pushing too hard for your current fitness level.

Progressing gradually, holding comfortable stretches, and working until pleasantly tired is the hallmark of a good instructor (and a good participant). If it hurts early in a program, the participant is likely to give up easily and not return (that is, if she can manage to walk out after all that burning).

Fitness is developed and maintained through consistency — not (this kind of) intensity. It should be seen as a lifelong commitment to feeling good, not a painful experience to be endured.

Don't let her tell you
"No pain, no gain."
Just pick up your gym bag
And don't go there again.

I Can't Go To the Class Because I Can't Keep Up with the Instructor.

This one makes my blood boil. Not at the participant — but at the instructor.

It's not the instructor's job to force you to work at *her* level. It's her job to encourage you to work at *your own* fitness level. The class she gives is not for her to focus on improving *her* own fitness. It's for her to focus on improving *your* fitness.

Why does this make my blood boil? Because so many people are put off from exercising because a self-centered, hyperactive kangaroo of an instructor used the class as a stage to show off.

If this has happened to you, don't be put off. Try another class, with another instructor, or ask if any of your friends know of a good, well-instructed, beginner's/intermediate level class. If this is your first class, let me assure you that not all instructors are like that — nor should they be. Knowing that you struck it unlucky this time should give you the incentive to strike it lucky next time.

On the other hand, not being able to keep up in a class may be the fault of the participant, and not of the instructor. How? Well,

- ✔ The participant might have chosen a class that is too advanced for her particular fitness levels;
- ✔ The participant might have joined a ten-week class during its third week. (Guess who's left looking the klutz?);
- ✔ The class/course assumes some basic familiarity with the steps, equipment, or exercise vocabulary.

To be fair to both the instructor and the participant, if you've ended up in a class that is too difficult (either in terms of speed or choreography) and you are not happy, shop around. There are plenty of classes available.

This brings us to the end of our section on exercise, but I hope it's only just the beginning for you.

We've gone through its reasons,
We've de-bunked all its myths.
We've demystified its classes
And given you tips.

The next part's for you,
And with that very first step
You'll find a new you
Full of vigor and pep.

So lace up those sneakers,
Make a beeline for the door,
And open it wide to life's joys
Now in store.

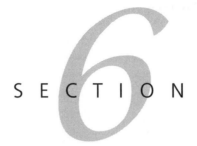

SECTION

The Finishing Line — Life After Weight Loss

Y ou've done it. All your hard work has finally paid off and you are at your goal weight. You bask in your sense of elation and success until the realization hits you that it's a whole new ballgame on this side of the fence.

While it's true that you don't want to lose any more weight, you also don't want to adopt the mentality that it's time to "go off the diet" and party-down big-time either. It's a dieter's reflex reaction, when they finally get there, to say "to blazes with it all!" Don't — 'cause if you do, you'll be back at page one of this book before you've even finished reading it.

When I was younger, I was on and off diets all the time. I would reach my goal through grit, determination, and persistence, and the minute I got there, I'd celebrate. How did I celebrate? With all those goodies that I'd just deprived myself of for months on end. Where did I end up? Back at square one.

You don't want your success experience to turn into a failure. You want it to turn into a lifetime habit, to build on and enjoy.

Since you don't want to lose any more weight, you need to come off your strict weight-reduction program. You now have a different goal — to maintain your new weight. But without a diet regimen, how are you supposed to accomplish that? Read on.

This section has been designed to provide you with the necessary tools and tips for your own DIY stay-slim program.

Chapter 20

— ◆ ◆ ◆ —

The Winner's Circle: How To Stay There For Life

Prioritizing Priorities

Just like you didn't get to the victor's stand by ignoring your needs, wants, and goals, so too, successful weight maintenance requires focusing on yourself. It's all about keeping your newly acquired healthy eating habits, your activity levels, and *yourself* a priority.

You got to this stage in the game by focusing on yourself, and you'll succeed in this finale by the same means. You are important, and what you are doing is important. Believe it and live it.

A New Perspective

Dieting might have cast a negative pall over food and what you shouldn't eat. Now you have to remind yourself of the important reasons why you *should* eat.

Instead of punching calorie totals into your calculators and exercising frugality in spending them, it's time to focus on all the good things that food gives us — like minerals, vitamins, fiber, and, wow, pleasure.

> *Of those precious few who make it to their goal weight, the overwhelming majority put it all back on again, with interest, in less than two years. Don't become a statistic — read this chapter and change your life forever.*

Since food is going to play a prominent role in the rest of your life (unless you know a better way of getting nutrition…), it makes sense to focus on putting it in a proper, and positive, perspective: i.e., eat healthy — *and* enjoy it.

Plan of Action

In practical terms, there are a number of alternatives available to help you maintain your new weight.

- ✔ Stick to the Maintenance Plan on the diet that helped you lose weight (they usually have one);
- ✔ If you weren't very happy on the diet that got you to your goal, try a different diet's Maintenance Plan;
- ✔ Continue with your weight-loss plan and have a "meal-off" every so often (depending on how often you'll be able to get away with it before the weight creeps back on);
- ✔ Once you have maintained your target for a while (and have discovered where you can and can't cheat), you can choose to stick to the fundamental principles of healthy eating (see "What Makes a Diet Healthy," page 14) and get the feel of what your body needs to break even.[1]

Writing down what you are eating can help you pinpoint any problem areas. This differs from a Food Diary because you are recording your intake not as a means of increasing self-control, but as a helpful record of cause and effect. Asking yourself, "What on earth did I eat these last two weeks to cause a three-pound gain?" can easily be answered.

Experiment

Enjoy your newfound freedom and experiment with what works for you. But be warned: When you start embarking on Experiment Number One (or with different maintenance plans or even if you're just doing your own thing), take yourself in hand as soon as those few pounds appear uninvited on the scales.

Go straight back to your tried and tested diet until they disappear again. Don't succumb to the temptation to try Experiment Number Two until those pounds have gone and you're back at target.

---

[1] Although I have discredited the "I'm Just Being Careful" diet as a weight loss program (See page 41), it can work very effectively as a weight maintenance plan. Try using Appendix 3 to find out how many calories you need per day to maintain your current weight.

A Stitch in Time Saves...Pounds

Every Skinny Minnie I know keeps two numbers engraved in her mind — the weight she considers ideal and the weight she never lets herself exceed. How far apart are those numbers? About five pounds. And it's at that magic five-pound mark that you should actively concentrate on getting them off — straight away.

Slim people notice right away when they put on a bit of weight. They feel uncomfortable and wrong. It's this feeling that will be one of the prime motivators in inspiring them to cut back before things get out of hand. Losing the weight doesn't take long, because they never get to where they need to lose much.

I have been fat and I have been thin. When I was fat, I could hardly tell when I put on another seven pounds. After all, I wore mostly elastic waistband skirts and loose-fitting tops. Then I lost weight and learned what it feels like to live inside a slimmer frame. When I put on even three pounds I feel it right away. My skirts are too tight, I feel fat, and I don't like "wearing" my body as much.

The slimmer you are, the more heightened your sense of discomfort is. Embrace this discomfort. It's your body's way of telling you that it's not happy with those extra pounds you just asked it to put on. Listen to it. Use this feeling as a wake-up call. And wake up. (No snooze buttons either…).

Weighing

If I were asked for the singularly most important tip for maintaining a new weight, it would be to **make sure you are weighing yourself regularly**. This is the ultimate honest-to-goodness check to see if what you are doing is working to keep you at an even keel.

Although during the dieting/weight reduction phase, weighing every day can be disappointing, many successful maintainers in the National Weight Control Registry say that they weigh themselves every day to help keep on track.

The reason is obvious. You want to keep a close eye on whether your chosen program is working or not — before a small one- or two-pound gain mysteriously turns into a significant six-pound one that refuses to budge.

Other Monitors

So how else do newly slender women monitor their weight? Not all swear by a daily weigh-in. Others let their clothes perform the fat-patrol function. If they can zip their skirts, they're still at the OK mark, if not…well, guess where that full-fat lasagna and chocolate fudge cake ended up?

Your clothing can be a powerful gauge of how you are doing. I've heard clients joke about how their clothes "shrunk in the closet." The reason we laugh is because we can relate.

Try leaving one item of "thin" clothing in the closet throughout the year and keep trying it on. Remember to view yourself from all sides and not just those that flatter.

Other alternative monitors are to take regular photographs and to measure yourself with a tape measure.

Pop-Up Party Time

You've been invited to a special occasion and eagerly mark it down on your calendar. You know it's coming up. And you also know that although you don't plan on abandoning every ounce of self-control, you want to be able to taste Aunty Hindy's famous cream puffs — guilt-free.

Now is the time to jump into diet-mode and out of maintenance-mode so that you can create the leeway you will need. Don't leave it till the last minute. Give yourself two pounds of credit to put in the piggy bank and you'll see that investment pay off.

This works for an anticipated vacation (or Yom Tov), too. It's not uncommon for dieters *or maintainers* to put on more than seven pounds in two weeks when those two weeks are spent in a relaxed, guard-is-down, free-for-all environment. One of the most successful antidotes is to pull the reigns in for a few weeks leading up to the vacation, to try to diminish the potential damage to your post let-it-all-go weight score.

If you have succeeded in losing four pounds before you dive into the world of food head-first, and end up putting on seven, you'll only have to face losing three when you come back. I'm not even a Math major, and that sounds good.

The 90-10 Rule

When trying to stabilize our weight, it is helpful to envision ourselves consuming healthy, nutritious, low-calorie foods ninety percent of the time, and allowing ourselves small, regular, deserved indulgences ten percent of the time.

For example, if you decide to have that heavy-duty cream cake at the Sheva Brochos for dessert, that's OK. You haven't ruined your plan or your healthy eating habits. What really matters is that over the course of time you eat sensibly, i.e., you limit your fats, increase your fiber intake, indulge in plenty of fresh fruits, vegetables, and whole-wheat, and you maintain an appropriate calorie level for your weight.

The "T" Factor

The following is another way of visualizing the correct proportions of a healthy meal:

Imagine a dinner plate with a big, black "T" written on it to cover the whole surface, like this...

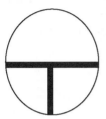

Now imagine that you are going to fill these three compartments for dinner. Choose the largest space on the plate for your vegetables, and the two smaller sections for your protein and carbohydrates. Voilà: A balanced, healthy meal — down to a "T."

Beware the Dragon of Boredom

It's not enough to just keep your tried-and-tested healthy eating habits up and running — you have to work at keeping them ignited.

By this I mean that it's important to find new ways to implement your healthy eating principles. Don't get caught in a rut eating the same things over and over. You'll soon find that boredom will set in, and that's only a short jump away from discarding all that hard work in search of something interesting to eat.

Be adventurous in your eating and in your cooking. Try a new fruit that you've never tried before. If you always eat oranges and pears but you're so bored with them that you are tempted to skip them, go and experience something different like a mango, quinoa ("*keen-wa*"), papaya, or passion fruit.

Make an effort when it comes to different grains as well. While it's true that white, long grain rice is great (although not as wholesome as brown), why not try a few different flavors like basmati, pilau, wild, or aromatic.

Your ultimate chance of success rests on your ability to teach yourself to enjoy your new style of eating. Actively enjoy it. If TCP salad turns your stomach and finds you dreading dinner, then it's time to make a new, exciting, fresh salad, like a leafy tropical mix of strawberries, mangoes, and cranberries with greens.

Calorie consciousness translated into a generally healthy way of eating must not overtake your life, but naturally fit into it. The only way to ensure long-term, happy weight maintenance is to learn not just to live with this way of eating as part of your life, but to learn to love it as well.

Invest in low-fat cookbooks and experiment. You might find a new family favorite in the bargain.

Be Flexible

Let it go at a kiddush? Succumbed to temptation when you ate out? Forgive yourself and put it behind you. Just like dieting is often a case of peaks and valleys — some weight on, some off, but the general direction remains constant — so, too, with maintenance: it means flexibility.

Move forward and be especially diligent the next few days.

Activate Yourself

In a survey done to ascertain how dieters who reach goal maintain their new weight, it was discovered that physical activity played a crucial role. The study showed that ninety-two percent of those who successfully maintained their weight loss exercised regularly. That means that *only eight percent* of those who kept off their lost weight *didn't* exercise. In comparison, sixty-six percent of those who put all their weight back on again had not exercised regularly. In other words, **dieters who exercise after reaching goal are more likely to retain their weight loss.**

Now that you've successfully lost that spare tire and extra padding, it should be easier than ever to move.

Besides the classic forms of exercise, like jogging, aerobics, swimming, etc., find other ways to move as well. Look for them and make them part of your new routine. Choose the stairs instead of the escalator or elevator; go upstairs yourself and get what you forgot, instead of asking the kids; and walk the kids to the bus stop instead of driving them. There are countless opportunities to increase your activity levels — you just have to actively look for them.

When you've integrated a new sense of activity into your day, let it become a habit that is no longer a decision, and then look for more new ways to get moving.

Never Say Never

"I'm never going to touch kugel again!" That's a shame — because you can. However, be warned. The frustration of continued deprivation might backfire in the end and send you on an uncontrolled rampage.

Now is the time to reincorporate into your lifestyle all those foods that you have had to sacrifice to get to where you are. It's better to have one small serving of those foods that are your favorites and enjoy every bit than to live a life of self-imposed deprivation.

Obviously, those foods have to be consumed with care and restraint — but they *can* be consumed nonetheless. Guilt-free. So enjoy, and bon apetit.

Focus on the Benefits Acquired

Do you remember the reasons you wanted to lose weight in the first place? (See "Focusing on Yourself," page 47.) Look back at those reasons and give yourself a well-deserved pat on the back every now and then. You can also add new benefits to your list.

Different things inspire different people. Here's a list of a few benefits that might trigger you to capture your own:

✔ **Photographs**

In terms of maintaining the new you, there are few things as powerfully motivating as seeing "before and after" photographs. Keep them. Look at them. Enjoy them. They will attest to your success forever — even after people forget how you once looked. You, yourself, may need this boost to either stop you from regressing back to that stage in your life or to propel you forward to future successes.

✔ **Old Clothes**

Keep an old dress that fit you at your largest as a tangible reminder of what you have accomplished. Need a boost? Slip it on (if it'll stay on…).

✔ **List New Abilities**

Over the last few years I have heard all sorts of people tell me about the joy they have found in seemingly simple actions. Here are some samples:

- Being able to cross their legs comfortably;
- Not having sore inner thighs from constant friction;
- Being able to cross their arms in front of their chest;
- Being able to bend over to tie their sons' shoelaces;
- Being able to dash upstairs without getting out of breath;
- Being able to go swimming (and being seen in a swimsuit) without embarrassment;
- Being able to leave the Shabbos table without feeling sluggish and overstuffed;
- Being confident enough to walk through the streets without a coat on;
- Being able to easily slip in and out of the driver's seat of a car;
- Being able to squeeze between tightly packed people or tables.

The list goes on. And it should. Write down all those little benefits so that you can read them when you need a periodic pick-me-up. Enjoy the pleasure that the simple things in life can bring.

Keep in Touch

Stay in touch with those people who supported you throughout your weight loss journey. If you've been attending a professional Weight Loss Group, stay in contact with the leader.

Sometimes Groups will offer free admission once you reach your target. Don't feel embarrassed to pop in even if you haven't been there for a while. They are there to help you. Going to Group meetings even after you have lost weight will ensure that you learn new ideas and stay motivated, and will help other people experience the joys that are now part of your life.

Surround yourself with positive, supportive friends and family who will encourage you with their "Atta girl!" enthusiasm. They'll see you through the tough patches and help you cruise forward with ease.

Step Forward

You've done it. You can speak from experience. You are proof positive that it is possible. Why not become a Weight Loss Group Leader yourself? If that seems a little too daunting, why not offer to share your story with a N'shei[2] group, or offer your services to an existing Weight Loss Group?

Not only will you succeed in strengthening others, but you'll also strengthen yourself.

Having Babies

If you managed to lose the weight after your last baby and find yourself happily expecting the next, don't despair when it comes to putting on the pounds again.

Being careful with your food intake during pregnancy is important. But trying to lose the weight after *each* baby is even more important.[3] It's all too easy to watch the weight snowball on after each baby. And it's so much easier to lose a few pounds after one baby than it is to lose fifty after several.

Don't Listen To Other People

You've probably had a lion's share of compliments on the way you now look. Don't be shocked when you hear fewer compliments and more negative comments. First of all, people stop complimenting you when they get used to seeing you slim, and second, sometimes it's hard for others to see someone succeed in an area where they themselves also desperately want to succeed.

---

[2] Ladies' gathering.
[3] Obviously, a recovery and recuperation period comes before any weight-reducing program is started, and should only be followed under a doctor's supervision.

People's jealousy over your accomplishment might induce not-so-nice comments. You might hear remarks such as, "You need to put more weight on — you've gone too far!" or, "You look so old/drawn/gaunt/haggard/anorexic/etc.!"

When I lost weight, I heard all sorts of comments (I still do). My favorite: "Your personality has changed since you lost weight. Fat people are happy people and now that you've lost weight, you're not as happy!" This, of course, was said by a fat person and, by the way, is a load of baloney 'cause I've never been happier.

It's true that there will be the few people whose opinion you can trust and might care to heed. Do you know the difference between a friend and a yenta? Whether her opinion was asked for…

So remember, as long as you are within the boundaries of your healthy range (see Appendix 2), the weight you have chosen for yourself is medically sound. This should give you the confidence to withstand all negativity. Smile, thank your "friends" for their concern, and remain steadfast in your own opinion. After all, you're the one who has to live in your body — not them. Therefore, if it feels good to you, stay in it.

Watch Out for the Downward Spiral

You're confident that you know what you are doing. You just haven't had the time or mindset to go to Group or weigh yourself very religiously. Your clothes still fit. So there doesn't seem to be any need to panic…or does there?

Tasting, testing, and nibbling at previously forbidden "fruits" can make serious inroads into your new lifestyle. It starts with just a bit here, just a bit there, and before you know it, all your good, new habits are being slowly but surely replaced by the ones you fought so hard to overcome.

If those bad habits turn into a few bad pounds, go through an emergency checklist of immediate solutions:

✔ Go back on a formal diet, or

✔ Reduce your quantities/portion sizes, or

✔ Make fruits and vegetables more prominent members of your plate, or

✔ Go back to Group (even if you now have to pay because you have exceeded the regulatory three- to five-pounds leeway), or

✔ Set yourself a deadline to get back to goal (together with reward and penalty).

Of course, you can choose to combine any of the above methods for extra assurance.

Bear in mind that you have a big advantage by taking matters in hand right away. You're not so far off track. You've reached goal before, so you can do it again. It won't take long to reclaim your thin self. Having said that, the longer you leave it, and the longer you ride the tide of the downward spiral, the longer it'll take to accomplish.

Keep Rewarding Yourself

For every month or so that you are still at goal, celebrate. It's an ongoing victory. Reinforce your sense of accomplishment so that your motivation becomes a part of your life forever.

The rewards don't have to be magnificent or expensive. A morning off to window shop; a new smooth-writing pen; a new plant…Treat them as an acknowledgement to yourself and your success.

Set Up a Club

You're not the only one out there who has successfully lost weight and kept it off. Set up a Maintainer's Club and arrange to get together, write, talk, and email each other to share tips, secrets, and experiences.

Support groups like this work because they provide a forum for people to gain from each other. No one will understand you as well as someone who has been there, done that, and lived to tell the tale.

Enjoy Being At Goal

If you don't enjoy being the size and shape you are, or you don't enjoy the things you are doing with that size and shape, you aren't going to want to continue being that size and shape for long.

This applies to the way you eat and the way you lead your life. Here are some points to help you enjoy your newly acquired status:

Reassess Your Wardrobe

If you feel like you were living at the dressmaker because of all the clothes you have had to alter while you were losing weight, maybe it's time to reassess your wardrobe.

You don't have to leave spring cleaning till Pesach. Take out all your clothes and sort them rigorously. Make piles according to:

- Clothes that don't fit and aren't worth altering (too big);
- Clothes that you haven't worn for a year;
- Clothes that you don't like (even if they fit);
- Clothes that you can't decide about;
- Clothes to give away;
- Clothes that fit and you like.

Now toss out everything you really don't want to wear anymore. You might want to enlist the help of a close friend, since choosing between keeping and discarding clothes can be a tough emotional battle. It always helps to have a friend around at times of such emotional turmoil. (Make sure you pick a close friend to help, because you are likely to ask for her honest opinion and you still want to be friends afterwards.) Once you get into the swing of it, you might even have a good giggle along the way.

Be ruthless and get rid of all unnecessary, unwanted, disliked, ill-fitting, and non-flattering clothes. It'll feel great when you're done. You'll feel clean and refreshed.

Your body has changed and your clothes need to reflect that change — for the good. Don't fall into the habit of wearing clothes that are four sizes too big and held together with safety pins. You won't feel good. The clothes won't look good. And you are not helping yourself enjoy what can so easily be enjoyed.

Now that you have made plenty of space in your closet, it's time to go shopping for the "new you." Remember, don't buy clothes too big "just in case you put the weight back on." The purpose is to enjoy the "present you" in order to ensure that the "future you" will be just as trim, slim, and thin. Take the opportunity to revel in the new you. Enjoy how your new clothes now fit and feel; how you're not ashamed to walk down the street in the summer without hiding beneath layers. Don't forget to include a new bathing suit in your new wardrobe. It's the real proof that you've made it, and a great motivator to continue to stay that way.

Enjoying the way you look and the clothes you wear will help you continue with the work you have to do to stay that way. It's an investment that is an investment in you.

Take Up New Interests

You have a new you — with new vistas, capabilities, and opportunities. Now is a great time to take up all those interesting pastimes you have dreamed of doing but felt too self-conscious of your size to actually do.

How about the following for starters:

✔ Simchah dancing;
✔ Swimming (you don't have to be embarrassed anymore);
✔ Take up a new course (computing, sewing, flower-arranging…);
✔ Biking;
✔ Hiking;
✔ Camping;
✔ Ice Skating;
✔ Bowling.

The common denominator in all of these activities should be *fun*. Enjoy moving about in your new body. It'll feel great.

Enjoy Eating

Not only must you take care to enjoy what you eat (see above, "Boredom"), but you must truly enjoy the process of eating.

Savor the colors, smells, tastes, flavors, and textures. Take your time. In this way you will activate a heightened sense of pleasure from the food you are eating. **So many people think that dieting is about depriving themselves of the enjoyment of food, but I truly believe it is about relearning how to eat so that our enjoyment is magnified.**

Part of that enjoyment is knowing when to stop. I once read a diet book that devoted a whole page to the repetition of just three words: "DO NOT OVEREAT." I can't emphasize this enough. **Eat when you are hungry. Stop when you are not.** Notice I didn't say, "Stop when you are full." This is because you should never get so full that you feel full, overstuffed, or saturated. You should feel pleasantly satisfied and posi- tively *not* hungry without any discomfort at all.

If you can learn this skill, you'll be set for life.

Conclusion

If you think, "Now that I have reached goal, I can eat whatever I want," you are right. However, you can also put all your weight right back on again as well. There's no magic wand that changes the nature of weight loss/gain once you have achieved your ideal target weight. Calories don't take on new properties just because you are now a slim size ten. Apple pie and ice cream will still cost you nearly a third of your total calorie allowance — regardless of what the scales now brag.

It was hard work getting there and it's hard work staying there. Is it worth it? You bet. But you are going to have to work at it. It isn't going to happen automatically. You have to be aware of, and on guard against, the many pitfalls and problems that can arise.

But, more importantly, **you will have to learn to like being at your goal weight and like eating and living the way you need to, in order to stay there — for good.**

Maintenance isn't about deprivation. It's about controlled consciousness. The irony is that although many people will swear that they enjoy food so much more when they are eating without the confines of a diet plan, just the opposite is true. To learn and live the skills involved in savoring each treat, as opposed to wolfing down the whole pack, will ensure that you will, in fact, live *happily* ever after.

My Secret

As we come to the end of this section and the book, I'd like to share with you a little secret. Let's call it "My Personal (Miracle) Motivator." It's what really keeps me going even when the going gets tough.

Someone once came to me and complained about how her skinny husband just didn't understand her. She had told him, "It's all right for you. You go to bed at night, every night, and wake up skinny. I go to bed every night and wake up fat."

I remember how that woman feels. We all secretly yearn for the miraculous. That we will one day just wake up and find ourselves living inside a slim, healthy body instead of waking up and finding ourselves trapped inside an overweight, cumbersome, and unhealthy one.

So here's my secret. Every day when I wake up (and I mean every day), I feel like I experience my own personal miracle of waking up inside that slim body of my dreams. Nothing gives me the same sense of joy. I just don't get tired of the magic of that feeling.

Dreams can come true. It happened to me, and it can happen to you. It might take some time, some perseverance, and some effort. But it is possible. **All you have to do is really, really want it.**

I have often said to frustrated dieters, "If I could do it for you, I would!" And I mean it. I wrote this book as the next best thing to actually doing it for you. I wrote it in the hope that what I have written will magically lift you out of your frustration with the dieting experience and transform it (and you) into a success.

I close with a heartfelt brochah to whoever holds open this page: You should follow your dieting dream out of the confines of fantasy into a new, exciting, and healthy reality.

Make your dream come true,

As only you can do.

Wishing you hatzlochah rabbah,

Chava

◆◆◆

The Last Word

Some Major Principles To Remember

✔ Dieting isn't all about willpower and waistlines. (page 11)

✔ The Bottom Line: Weight loss = fewer calories coming in than are going out. (page 17)

✔ To lose one pound you need to burn off, lose, eradicate, or zap away 3,500 calories. (pages 17, 191)

✔ The best diet is the diet that works best for you. (page 19)

✔ If you want to lose weight you either have to eat less calories or exercise more (or do a combination of both). (page 19)

✔ If it's fast, it won't last. (page 38)

✔ There is no such thing as the perfect diet. (page 43)

✔ Every diet must limit something. If it didn't, it wouldn't be called a diet. (page 43)

✔ Choosing a diet, is not a life sentence. (page 43)

✔ There is only one person responsible for how much you weigh, and that's you. (page 46)

✔ The key to success is perseverance. (pages 46-47)

✔ Confidence breeds action. (page 49)

✔ You are worth spending money on. (page 51)

✔ One of the most powerful tools in goal attainment is the energy that comes from an awareness of success. (page 52)

✔ When you reward an achievement you turn it into a success. (page 53)

✔ A false start is worse than no start at all. (page 55)

✔ The more familiar you are with a diet, the less stress or inconvenience it will feel like it is creating. (page 56)

✔ Learn to live in "day-tight" compartments. (page 78)

✔ Don't sweat the small stuff. (page 78)

✔ Learn to say no. (page 80)

✔ The aim of the game is to become in control of what you are eating, when you are eating it, and why you are eating it. (page 87)

Or in other words: Know what you are eating. Know when you are eating. Know that you are eating. (page 196)

✔ Listen to your body. (page 177)

✔ Everyone who has ever successfully lost weight and kept it off, has had failures. (page 188)

✔ Don't cry over spilt milk. (page 188)

✔ Stop when you are full. (page 197)

✔ The longer you leave it, the harder it is to begin again. (page 236)

✔ We want to remember the occasion, not the consequences. And the best occasions are about people, not about food. (page 240)

✔ The winner is not the one who never falls, but the one who can fall and pick herself up again and again, time after time. (page 260)

✔ Remember where you have come from — you never want to go back. (page 260)

✔ If you "bounce" a stretch, you risk tearing a muscle. (page 290)

✔ In exercise the rule is: If pain, no gain (page 290)

✔ There should never be any sharp or severe pain in any body part when stretching. (page 290)

✔ Before beginning any exercise regime, or even going to an exercise class, get your doctor's approval. (page 315)

✔ Don't diminish your own accomplishments by looking over the shoulder at what others are doing. (page 318)

✔ If you're doing great, take the time to feel great. (page 318)

✔ If you don't use it, you lose it. (page 328)

✔ He who has never tried and failed has never truly succeeded. (page 330)

✔ Feel the fear and do it anyway. (page 330)

✔ With exercise, one is better than none; however, three is more than three times better than one. (page 337)

✔ If an instructor tells you to work to the point where you feel "the burn," walk out. (page 340)

✔ Calorie consciousness translated into a generally healthy way of eating must not overtake your life, but naturally fit into it. (page 349)

✔ Dieters who exercise after reaching goal are more likely to retain their weight loss. (page 350)

✔ Dieting isn't about depriving yourself, it's about relearning how to eat. (page 356)

✔ Maintenance isn't about deprivation. It's about controlled consciousness. (page 356)

✔ Dreams can come true. (page 357)

✔ All you have to do is really, really want it. (page 357)

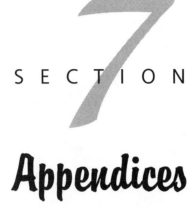

S E C T I O N

Appendices

*T*hese appendices are informative, snappy, and to the point, but you could diet successfully on a day-to-day basis without them. They're like the icing on the cake. You'll have a great party with the cake (the main body of the book), but you'll have a banquet with the appendices as the icing.

Appendix 1

◆ ◆ ◆

Reasons To Lose Weight

*D*ifferent people decide to lose weight for different reasons. For some, the trigger might be a photograph catching them at an unflattering angle ("Ugh, do I *really* look like that?"). For others, it will be their doctor's warning that all that excess weight is leading them down a dead end path (no pun intended).

Whatever the reason that is motivating you to read through this book right now, maybe you'll find an additional reason or five in the following pages to add to your burning drive, and to inspire you to realize that now really is the right time to lose those extra pounds once and for all.

I have met many dieters, newly slim people, long-term ex-slimmers, and potential would-be slimmers. In all my years of experience in the field of weight loss, I have found that there are basically nine motivating factors that will "fire up" people to try and slim down. Almost everyone is inspired by one, if not a few, of the following reasons. See if you can spot yours.

Long-Term Health Problems

Being overweight or obese is not just a cosmetic problem, it's a health hazard.

Excess weight is the Western World's number one health problem. In the United States alone, an overwhelming proportion of the population is classified as overweight. The statistics are shocking: Of the ten leading causes of death in the United States, being overweight is a risk factor for half of them. (That fact alone should scare you into action.)

Carrying those extra pounds around wherever you go puts a lot of stress on your entire body. It means it has to work harder — your heart, lungs, and bones all have to respond to the extra demands that are being placed on them. You'd soon feel the strain of carrying twenty pounds of groceries around with you all day; your body feels the same way when it has to schlep extra body weight around with it wherever it goes.

Even if you feel fine now and are not overly concerned about health-related problems, just take note that the longer you are overweight, the greater your chances are that something not-so-nice could happen to you. (No, I'm not talking about your mother-in-law coming to move in with you.) As your weight increases, so do your risk factors for any one (or more) of the following:

Heart Disease

Too much fat in the diet, too little exercise, and too much body fat all result in an increased risk of Coronary Heart Disease (CHD), the number one killer in the Western World. The American Heart Association reports that nearly seventy percent of heart disease cases are related to obesity.

And it doesn't take much extra weight to put your health at risk. If you are just twenty pounds overweight, you **double** your risk of heart disease.

The heart is a muscle. When it is overworked, it suffers. And like all "good" sufferers, it will complain.

Atherosclerosis

This condition involves the arteries becoming "clogged up" by fatty deposits, in effect narrowing the passageway for blood to travel through. (Rather like passing sherbet through a wet straw…)

To compensate, the heart pumps harder, blood pressure increases, and many parts of the body are damaged as a result. Everything from poor circulation to heart attack and stroke can be blamed on atherosclerosis.

But all is not doom and gloom. The latest medical research has shown that even if arterial narrowing has already occurred, the condition can be helped either by medical intervention or (guess what…) by reducing the amount of fat consumed and adopting a low-fat diet. (Life is full of choices…)

Hypertension (High Blood Pressure)

High blood pressure isn't just an emotional reaction to a defiant teenager, it's a condition in which the pressure exerted by the blood as it is pumped through the arteries is consistently higher than normal.

This is one test where getting a high score does not get applause.

High blood pressure increases the risk of heart attack, coronary artery disease, strokes, kidney failure, and loss of sight due to damage of the retina. (Did you really think this was going to be fun and games?)

One of the most significant risk factors for high blood pressure is being overweight. People who are twenty percent overweight (for example, you should be 130 lbs. but you're 156 lbs.) are **eight times** more likely to have high blood pressure than those who are at their correct weight.

But there is good news. You don't have to wait till you reach your ideal target weight to improve this condition. Sufferers often see marked improvements within the first two to three weeks of a weight-loss program. Even losing five to ten pounds can produce significant health gains. (Every little bit helps.)

I remember one lady in our Group who started coming to me when she was taking very heavy dosages of medication to counteract her high blood pressure. The more weight she lost, the less medication she needed, until she completely stopped any medication and brought her blood pressure back down to a normal level. It's not magic, just logic.

High Blood Cholesterol

Cholesterol is a fatty substance produced by the liver and is present in a variety of foods. (See "Clarifying Cholesterol," page 102.) In normal amounts, it is essential for many body processes, including producing hormones.

However, too much of a good thing is never a great idea, and in this case, it's downright dangerous. Among the risks associated with high blood cholesterol are high blood pressure, CHD, and strokes. According to the experts, every ten percent increase in weight increases cholesterol by twelve points. And, considering that 170 points is normal and 200 is high, you don't have to be a math professor to realize it won't take much to set off the warning bells.

Although high cholesterol levels are not *always* caused by eating foods high in cholesterol, there is no question that a diet full of fatty foods is a contributing factor. Genetics, lack of exercise, smoking, and, of course, being overweight, take most of the blame.

Diabetes

Nearly 16 million Americans have diabetes. Each year, more than 190,000 people die from it or its many complications.

Want more scary stuff?

- Diabetes is the leading cause of blindness in people between twenty and seventy-four years old;
- It's a major cause of kidney disease, which requires dialysis or a kidney transplant;
- People with diabetes are up to four times more likely than others to have heart disease or suffer a stroke;
- Diabetes causes nerve damage, which may require amputation of a toe, foot, or lower leg.

To date, there is no cure for diabetes. It requires lifelong management and medication. All diabetics require a controlled diet to regulate blood sugar levels, and need regular checkups to detect damage to the eyes, nerves, and blood vessels.

And, of course, you guessed it, this type of diabetes is more likely to occur if you are overweight, especially if your weight is being carried around your midsection (see "Waist-Hip Ratio/Body Type," page 382).

Gallstones

The gall bladder is a small, sac-like organ that, not surprisingly, stores gall. It can become clogged with gallstones, which consist mainly of cholesterol. Intense, roll-on-the-floor type of pain can result, often accompanied by inflammation and infection. Sometimes the infection can spread, causing serious complications.

This breathtakingly painful condition is prevalent in women who are overweight or are on a high-fat diet, and may require surgery.

They don't call it a gallstone attack for nothing.

Cancer

Although scientific evidence for the exact link between obesity and cancer is still unclear, statistics show a definite link.

Obese females are at greater risk of cancer of the gallbladder, breast, ovary, and uterus. Obese males have a greater risk of cancer of the colon, rectum, and prostate.

Almost **half** of breast cancer cases are diagnosed in obese women. And, although colon cancer isn't directly linked to being overweight, bad eating habits (such as high-fat, low-fiber diets) are.

Respiratory Problems

Sleep apnea is a respiratory complication that occurs when a person's sleep is constantly interrupted — not because of the baby, but because airways are partially or completely collapsed or obstructed. It is closely linked to obesity. Sometimes the condition can be so severe that the sufferer will fall asleep during the day due to exhaustion — even while driving.

Joint Diseases

Joint diseases such as osteoarthritis and gout are two painful and debilitating joint disorders that are often related to being overweight. The simple joys in life, like walking, can become a nightmare.

Osteoarthritis is a "wear-and-tear" condition that results when the cartilage that protects the ends of joints deteriorates. The joints most commonly affected are the hips and knees, which bear most of our weight. This might not sound so bad, but just count the number of times you bend your knees in a day, and it takes on a new reality.

The more weight to bear, the more (ouch, umph…) suffering involved.

Even though gout is more common in men, plenty of women suffer from it. This painful inflammation of the joints often strikes the big toe. Kidney complications are sometimes seen in people who have both gout and diabetes.

Immobility

Simply put, the heavier you are, the less likely you are to move.

This is because it requires more effort to move a greater bulk and, because we are creatures of comfort, we tend to opt for the easier, more comfortable option.

Not moving becomes increasingly synonymous with not being able to move. Muscles that are not used and kept in condition tend to atrophy, i.e., waste away. If you don't use it, you'll lose it (the ability to move, that is, not the car keys, nor the weight). So in the end, even if an obese person would wake up one morning wanting to do a low squat (and I don't suggest she does) she would not be able to.

Due to the fact that a heavy person finds it harder to move, she will also be less likely to engage in physical activities (e.g., walking, swimming, etc.) and will therefore be prone to a long-term lack of fitness.

Immobility also affects flexibility. A seriously overweight person will not be comfortable or able to bend to the floor to pick something up, or twist behind her to get her sweater. Even getting in and out of a car can be a problem.

One lady in her fifties who lost seventy pounds told me that she had thought her immobility was due to getting older, but when she had lost all that weight, she found she could move again. Small things like reaching for a pot from the bottom kitchen cupboard, or picking a paper up from the floor, became new joys.

Conclusion

The bottom line of all this is that obesity has a proven track record for messing up people's lives and sometimes even hastening their end. And being overweight is no picnic, either.

But it doesn't have to be a long-term health problem that will cause you to suffer. Short-term issues are also a pain in the neck...leg...hip...etc. If you have ever experienced one of the following, you'll know what I mean.

Short-Term Health Problems

Back Pain

Surplus weight — especially around the lower stomach area — coupled with weak abdominal muscles, can place great strain on the lower back.

Add an increased risk of poor posture (because the spine has to compensate for the excess and sometimes uneven distribution of weight) and the results are excruciating. Even a surplus of ten to fifteen pounds can result in a pain in the...back.

Varicose Veins

Excess weight causes unnecessary strain on the vascular system (blood traveling through the veins). Therefore, since legs carry all our body weight, the results can be unsightly and sometimes painful varicose veins. Support hose and potential corrective surgery might not even fix the problem.

Shortness of Breath

If you are overweight, your lungs have to work harder to supply your body with the oxygen that you need for energy.

In addition, excess fat, especially around the tummy area, exerts pressure on the diaphragm and interferes with normal breathing: It sort of gets in the way. It is not unusual for people who are overweight to suffer from shortness of breath. Not only do they have problems getting enough oxygen (you often see them panting or trying to catch their breath), they also have problems exhaling carbon dioxide. This can make them feel sleepy even when they are getting plenty of zzzzzzzzleep.

Skin Complaints

Don't think all the body's bad news is happening on the inside — outsides need to watch out, too.

Overweight people often complain of sore, rough skin and rashes. These may be the result of perspiration or lack of adequate nutrition and vitamins, or from the friction of skin surfaces rubbing together (e.g., inner thighs when walking).

I remember when I was young and fat, I always had to wear pantyhose instead of the socks my friends all wore, because my thighs would rub together when I walked and would become sore if I didn't cover them.

Infertility

It has now been medically recognized that the chances of becoming pregnant when overweight are dramatically reduced. And don't tell me you know someone who didn't have a problem; we all know that exceptions prove the rule. Most infertility specialists will advise obese clients to lose weight to increase their chances to conceive.

Pregnancy Problems

Being overweight during pregnancy exacerbates already preexisting health problems. It's like taking a magnifying glass to conditions such as varicose veins, high blood pressure, and water retention. In addition, all that extra baggage increases the possibility of complications.

In addition, the actual process of childbirth can be more awkward and difficult when one is overweight.

Conclusion

Pain, whether it's physical or emotional, is pain. And when you are suffering from it, you can't really tell whether it's long-term or short-term: It just hurts. But you know the worst thing about being overweight? You aren't really given a choice whether you want to suffer long-term or only short-term health problems. Often enough, you get both.

Appearance

No matter how many times we hear well-meaning friends tell us that we can be proud and happy to be chubby (I'm being nice…), we don't often feel that way. If we are not at, or near, a healthy body weight for our frame, we tend to feel unattractive. If we don't look good, we don't feel good. And for most of us, looking good means looking slim and feeling fit.

While we're here, let me hit one emotional gut-protest over the head before it starts: Don't feel guilty about wanting to lose weight because you want to look better.

By looking better, you will undoubtedly function better in all areas of your life — whether you are a single woman, a wife, a mother, a businesswoman, or any combination of the above. Looking better (at least for most of us) means feeling better about ourselves, having more self-esteem, taking more pride in ourselves and in our capabilities. We walk taller, we strive for more, we exert ourselves more, we grow more, and we're less afraid of the unknown.

Looking good can be a very powerful, all-encompassing cure to many debilitating "emotional handicaps." There is nothing like a low sense of self-esteem for killing good ideas ("I can't do it…"). And when it comes to motivating factors to lose all that excess weight, "looking more attractive" may be a more inspiring incentive than the prevention of death, disease, poor health, or pain. If you fall into that category, avoid the guilt trip and go for it. (In the end, you'll benefit from both — good looks *and* good health.)

As we lose weight and our appearance improves, often seemingly non-weight-related external factors also change. For example, our facial expressions (see the smile spread from ear to ear…), our tidiness (tucked in the blouse yet?), our body language (uncrossed arms), our choice of clothes (colors versus black), our posture (tall, not slumped), etc., will all mirror the increased improvement of our self-image and self-confidence.

Whether we actually *are* more attractive when we lose weight is immaterial. The truth is that we *feel* more attractive when we lose weight and therefore we *become* more attractive.

Clothes

We all know how demoralizing it is to have a closet full of clothes and nothing to wear. Let's face it. It's hard to look our best when our clothes are either too tight or utterly shapeless to hide our form. They didn't all shrink overnight. They just don't fit.

It can also be extremely depressing and frustrating when it is time to go and buy something new to wear. The pleasure of clothes shopping becomes a torture. We dread being surrounded by clothes and finding:

- That hardly anything fits;
- What does fit does not flatter;
- What does fit is not what you would have bought if you had been slimmer.

Sounds familiar?

These can be terrifically motivating factors — to fit into favorite clothes not worn for months or years because of that overly shaped shape, and to buy new clothes for a new you.

Even after losing only ten pounds, you will feel the difference in once too-snug skirts, or now-closing jackets. What a thrill it is to open the wardrobe door and stand there contemplating what to wear, knowing that everything in it not only fits, but also looks good on you.

Clients repeatedly tell me of the buzz, the terrific high, they feel when a Yom Tov outfit that didn't fit last Yom Tov fits beautifully this Yom Tov. It's great.

And having a whole new selection to choose from when shopping, in a new, slim size to boot, is an incredible feeling. Can't wait. Even if clothes shopping does not come high on your list of motivating factors *before* you lose weight, I have found that most of my successful clients, whether they lose a lot or a little, are extremely enthralled with how much easier "wardrobe management" becomes.

They often marvel that they did not realize just how much pleasure they would receive from feeling good in their clothes, and just how much this "feel good" factor was lacking in their past.

So don't dismiss the motivating factor

Of choosing slimming clothes that both fit and flatter.

Relationships

Shidduchim (Dating)

I'll be the first to testify that a person is so much more than just her body. But it is a sad fact that people can be prejudiced against a heavier person. When the time comes to look for a suitable spouse, the shidduch game can be pure torment for the overweight eligible.

Those who are prejudiced worry how the weight issues involved with childbearing will affect the girl in question. Or they may be scared to tie their son to someone who will undoubtedly be at greater risk of suffering significant health problems (that is, if she isn't suffering from them already).

It is a sad but true statement of our generation that a heavier person is not viewed to be as attractive as a slimmer person. For this reason, sometimes girls with beautiful personalities and positive outlooks don't get past the first meeting (if they even get that far). This can cause immeasurable pain and embarrassment. It can also have the negative consequence of diminishing a person's self-confidence and feelings of self-worth. If this motivates you, then use it. But remember that this is for the girls — not permission for the mothers to be overbearing with their daughters. (Moms, see "Parents," page 125.)

Husbands

Find me one man who would rather have an overweight wife than a slim one…

He might not complain (he has good character traits), he might not nag (his mother told him not to), but boy, does he appreciate his wife's efforts in looking after herself, making herself healthier, and yes, more attractive.

It is a particularly important commandment to look attractive to our husbands, and our sages tell us repeatedly just how important it is in helping to ensure that a marriage is secure and happy.

They tell us, "An attractive wife opens a husband's mind." A husband becomes more satisfied and content with his portion in life. His love for his wife, although not dependent on only the physical, is enhanced by finding her attractive — in body and in nature.

At Work

In the context of the workplace, it is worth noting that however inexcusable it is to discriminate against someone because of her size, it *can* be an issue when employers are seeking prospective employees.

Research in the field of employment has shown that when presented with the choice of two prospective employees with similar qualifications, but one is fat and one is of normal body weight, employers confessed that they would be more likely to employ the candidate of normal body weight.

Their rationale: They considered a person's state of fatness indicative of a lack of self-discipline, lack of control, and lack of self-respect. Whereas this may very well be an unfair assumption, it is worthy of consideration. We don't want to be refused a job because of our size. And, although we would rather change the attitude of the workplace, it's probably going to be easier to change ourselves instead.

In a more positive vein, when a person successfully loses weight, one of the wonderful side benefits is the increased feeling of self-confidence and that extra "spark" in their personalities. They have risen to the challenge of losing weight and are now ready to face new challenges from a positive position built upon past success experiences.

Confidence goes a long way in the workplace. Promotions do not go to the quiet, self-conscious, withdrawn employees. They go to those who show initiative, to those who inspire confidence in others because they have confidence in themselves.

Success breeds success — in weight loss as well as in the workplace. Shedding excess weight (especially if you are very overweight) is also likely to affect your work in other ways. Many people who have successfully lost weight report increased confidence in completing tasks and taking initiatives, and having more flair for leadership. They think, "I've lost weight, so surely I can tackle this as well!"

Socially

Overweight or obese people tend to be embarrassed about their bodies, their image, their size, and themselves. They may tend to be shy or seem withdrawn. This can affect them socially. Perhaps they are your stay-at-home Dear Abby type of listener, as opposed to your outgoing socialite.

If you can relate and are happy with staying at home, all's well and good. But if you feel frustrated because of your reservations, losing weight can help you increase your quality of life — both generally and socially. You could stand to shed not just excess pounds, but also feelings of inferiority, inadequacy, and self-consciousness as well.

Everyday Life

Anyone who loses a considerable amount of weight will tell you that day-to-day living becomes so much more enjoyable.

It is the seemingly small things in our daily living that so significantly increase the quality of our lives. Living life to the fullest is so much easier when we are not carrying excess weight around with us.

I know people who now find joy in:

- Being able to see their toes (welcome back…);
- Being able to sit on the floor cross-legged (Yoga, here we come…);
- Picking up a toy from the floor (instead of kicking it under the sofa);
- Sitting comfortably in an airplane's restricted seat (and being able to get out again…).

Parenthood brings with it untold pleasures. Being overweight can seriously hinder taking an active part in your children's childhood. Overweight people miss out on bike riding, chasing their toddler, giving piggyback rides, playing ball, and even just sitting on the floor playing Duplo blocks or building a train track.

These are some of life's joys and moments of pure nachas. Don't miss out.

Financial

Obesity costs the American economy more than $100 billion every year, including the cost of health care and productivity that is lost to death and disability from weight-related causes.

If your heart doesn't bleed for the American economy, let's look at what this means to us on an individual basis.

People who are overweight spend more money on medical care than people of a normal weight.

Why? Because:

- They suffer from higher rates of disease and more complications (see earlier all about that nasty diabetes and other health problems);
- They are involved in more accidents that result in injury (falling off a ladder will hurt an obese person's bones as well as her pride);
- They are hospitalized more often and tend to suffer more complications from surgery and other medical procedures (layers of fat can burst stitches, prevent healing of wounds, and increase the risk of infection);
- They may experience more difficulty in getting life insurance because of their high-risk status;
- And those who are able to get insurance will often pay higher premiums

All of this costs money. So if saving your life is not enough to make you lose weight, maybe saving your money is.

Short-Term Motivators

Ever had a wedding or Bar Mitzvah as a deadline for your diet? Then you can relate to a short-term motivator.

The problem with short-term motivators is that they are just that. Short term. You may lose the weight, but what happens after the party's over? Dieting because of short-term motivators runs the risk of putting it all back on again — probably with interest. Such shortsightedness encourages "yo-yo" dieting, which can become a lifestyle habit. (See "Yo-Yo Dieting," page 40.)

Instead, turn your short-term motivator into a "mini-goal." Lose seven pounds by niece Naomi's wedding *and either go further* (if you need to), *or maintain your loss.*

In this way, you can use short-term motivators to your best advantage.

Negative Motivators

I'm Doing it for You

As much as we might love another person, or want to please them, we will never be truly successful in losing weight when we are doing it for anyone other than ourselves.

What happens when our willpower waivers? What happens when that person is no longer around? We might want to please our parents, placate our doctor, or calm caring relatives or friends, but this is something that we have to do for ourselves. You slim for you. And only you can do it.

Not only are the short-term and negative motivators not going to work for you in the long term, but they may also create a lot of negativity in their wake. Negativity like unfulfilled expectations, frustration, guilt, lower self-esteem ("You see, I always fail"), and sadness ("My mother will be disappointed in me now").

Therefore, let's focus on the real motivators — the ones that really speak to us — the ones that inspire, intrigue, and excite us, and which will ultimately help us to reach our goal.

It's a worthwhile exercise to jot down your personal motivating factors (now) so that you can remain focused on why you started all this dieting in the first place. Having this list in front of you, in the kitchen, by your bed, or in your purse, can help you stay focused on the end results. The more specific and detailed you can be, the better.

Conclusion

If you picked up this book with a clear-cut determination to diet and you already had your motivating reason or two propelling you forward, then I hope this appendix has added even more fuel to your engine. But if you weren't really sure that you wanted or needed to diet, I hope you've been convinced by now. Because seven good reasons — avoiding long-term and short-term health problems; appearance; clothes; relationships; everyday life; and financial benefits — should be pretty persuasive stuff. After all, who doesn't want to be a healthier, happier, prettier woman? If you do, then turn the page and let's go.

Appendix 2

— ◆ ◆ ◆ —

What's A Healthy Weight For Me?

*W*hen we talk about a "healthy weight" or "healthy weight range," we mean a number or range where all those health risks (heart disease, diabetes, varicose veins, etc.) we discussed in "Appendix 1: Reasons to Lose Weight" are not even on your radar screen.

It's important to realize that *your* healthy weight is not necessarily the lowest weight that you think you can (or even would like to) reach. Rather, it's the weight where you are most likely to promote good general health and well-being.

Health care professionals use a number of key measurements to determine whether or not a person is at a healthy weight. Here are four of the most common ones.

The Height-Weight Chart

As its user-friendly name implies, this chart gives us a generous weight range (of approximately twenty pounds) to determine whether you are:

- At a healthy weight,
- Moderately overweight, or
- Severely overweight.

Although the chart is based upon different ranges, don't view the range as a license to gain weight if you are at the lower end of its spectrum. The range is generous, not to be kind to you (science generally isn't inclined that way…), but rather to take into account those people who have greater amounts of muscle and bone (as is the case for men and large-framed women).

In addition, according to today's guidelines, this healthy weight range is applicable to everyone — regardless of age. Experts now believe that the ten to fifteen pounds that many people put on in middle age, although common, are unhealthy (sorry about that).

Got two fingers? Good. Then you'll be a whiz at finding the right weight range for your height. With one finger, find your height in the left column. Glue your finger to that spot and whisk your other finger down the appropriate age column. When you get to the line your finger is on, stop, look, and read. See how easy that was? (You can move your finger now).

HEIGHT-WEIGHT TABLE[1]		
Height	**Weight in Pounds**	
	Age 19–34	Age 35 and over
5 ft. 0 in.	97–128	108–138
5 ft. 1 in.	101–132	111–143
5 ft. 2 in.	104–137	115–148
5 ft. 3 in.	107–141	119–152
5 ft. 4 in.	111–146	122–157
5 ft. 5 in.	114–150	126–162
5 ft. 6 in.	118–155	130–167
5 ft. 7 in.	121–160	134–172
5 ft. 8 in.	125–164	138–178
5 ft. 9 in.	129–169	142–183
5 ft. 10 in.	132–174	146–188
5 ft. 11 in.	136–179	151–194
6 ft. 0 in.	140–184	155–199
6 ft. 1 in.	144–189	159–205
6 ft. 2 in.	148–195	164–210
6 ft. 3 in.	152–200	168–216
6 ft. 4 in.	156–205	173–222
6 ft. 5 in.	160–211	177–228
6 ft. 6 in.	164–216	182–234

[1]Based on the U.S. Department of Agriculture tables.

The Height-Weight Chart is a useful tool to determine a suitably healthy weight for yourself dependent on your height. It is, however, rather generous in its range and is therefore not as accurate an indicator of your body's fat stores. This is where our next measuring tool, BMI, comes in....

BMI: Body Mass Index

In 1998, the National Institute of Health released new guidelines for what is considered normal weight, overweight, and obese. The guidelines are based on Body Mass Index (BMI), which is a formula that takes into account not just your weight and height, but also how much fat your body has.

I could give you the formula for you to work out your very own BMI, but, shucks, let's do it the easy way and look at a table where it's all worked out for you instead (I'm all for an easier life...).

Now all you have to do is locate your height in inches in the left hand column (your fingers are experienced by now) and follow the row across to your weight in pounds. Your BMI is at the top of the column at the intersection of your height and weight.

Once you've worked out your BMI, you can determine whether you are at a healthy weight:

- **Healthy Weight:** BMI of 19 to 24.9
- **Overweight:** BMI of 25 to 29.9
- **Obese:** BMI of 30 and up.

(There, wasn't that easier than taking out your calculator?)

Body Mass Index Table 1

To use the table, find the appropriate height in the left-hand column labeled Height. Move across to a given weight (in pounds). The number at the top of the column is the BMI at that height and weight. Pounds have been rounded off.

BMI	19	20	21	22	23	24	25	26	27	28	29	30	31	32	33	34	35
Height (inches)	**Body Weight (pounds)**																
58	91	96	100	105	110	115	119	124	129	134	138	143	148	153	158	162	167
59	94	99	104	109	114	119	124	128	133	138	143	148	153	158	163	168	173
60	97	102	107	112	118	123	128	133	138	143	148	153	158	163	168	174	179
61	100	106	111	116	122	127	132	137	143	148	153	158	164	169	174	180	185
62	104	109	115	120	126	131	136	142	147	153	158	163	169	175	180	186	191
63	107	113	118	124	130	135	141	146	152	158	163	169	175	180	186	191	197
64	110	116	122	128	134	140	145	151	157	163	169	174	180	186	192	197	204
65	114	120	126	132	138	144	150	156	162	168	174	180	186	192	198	204	210
66	118	124	130	136	142	148	155	161	167	173	179	186	192	198	204	210	216
67	121	127	134	140	146	153	159	166	172	178	185	191	198	204	211	217	223
68	125	131	138	144	151	158	164	171	177	184	190	197	203	210	216	223	230
69	128	135	142	149	155	162	169	176	182	189	196	203	209	216	223	230	236
70	132	139	146	153	160	167	174	181	188	195	202	209	216	222	229	236	243
71	136	143	150	157	165	172	179	186	193	200	208	215	222	229	236	243	250
72	140	147	154	162	169	177	184	191	199	206	213	221	228	235	242	250	258
73	144	151	159	166	174	182	189	197	204	212	219	227	235	242	250	257	265
74	148	155	163	171	179	186	194	202	210	218	225	233	241	249	256	264	272
75	152	160	168	176	184	192	200	208	216	224	232	240	248	256	264	272	279
76	156	164	172	180	189	197	205	213	221	230	238	246	254	263	271	279	287

for BMI greater than 35, go to Table 2

Body weight in pounds according to height and body mass index.

Adapted with permission from Bray, G.A., Gray, D.S., Obesity, Part I, Pathogenesis, West J. Med. 1988: 149: 429–41.

Body Mass Index Table 2

BMI → Height (inches)	36	37	38	39	40	41	42	43	44	45	46	47	48	49	50	51	52	53	54
	Body Weight (pounds)																		
58	172	177	181	186	191	196	201	205	210	215	220	224	229	234	239	244	248	253	258
59	178	183	188	193	198	203	208	212	217	222	227	232	237	242	247	252	257	262	267
60	184	189	194	199	204	209	215	220	225	230	235	240	245	250	255	261	266	271	276
61	190	195	201	206	211	217	222	227	232	238	243	248	254	259	264	269	275	280	285
62	196	202	207	213	218	224	229	235	240	246	251	256	262	267	273	278	284	289	295
63	203	208	214	220	225	231	237	242	248	254	259	265	270	278	282	287	293	299	304
64	209	215	221	228	232	238	244	250	256	262	267	273	279	285	291	296	302	308	314
65	216	222	228	234	240	246	252	258	264	270	276	282	288	294	300	306	312	318	324
66	223	229	235	241	247	253	260	266	272	278	284	291	297	303	309	315	322	328	334
67	230	236	242	249	255	261	268	274	280	287	293	299	306	312	319	325	331	338	344
68	236	243	249	256	262	269	276	282	289	295	302	308	315	322	328	335	341	348	354
69	243	250	257	263	270	277	284	291	297	304	311	318	324	331	338	345	351	358	365
70	250	257	264	271	278	285	292	299	306	313	320	327	334	341	348	355	362	369	376
71	257	265	272	279	286	293	301	308	315	322	329	338	343	351	358	365	372	379	386
72	265	272	279	287	294	302	309	316	324	331	338	346	353	361	368	375	383	390	397
73	272	280	288	295	302	310	318	325	333	340	348	355	363	371	378	386	393	401	408
74	280	287	295	303	311	319	326	334	342	350	358	365	373	381	389	396	404	412	420
75	287	295	303	311	319	327	335	343	351	359	367	375	383	391	399	407	415	423	431
76	295	304	312	320	328	336	344	353	361	369	377	385	394	402	410	418	426	435	443

Return to Table 1

Waist-Hip Ratio/Body Type

When it comes to health, it turns out that *where* you carry extra weight matters almost as much as how much you are carrying.

This is where the Waist-to-Hip Ratio (WHR = Waist ÷ Hip measurement) comes in.

A simple way of looking at WHR is to think of body types as apples or pears. Apple types are wide around the waist and tummy; pears are heavy in the hips, thighs, and buttocks. Both are very tasty, but here's the crunch…

There's good news and bad news for each type.

For apples, the good news is that they tend to have an easier time losing their "spare tire" once they begin eating sensibly and exercising regularly. The bad new is they are at greater risk for cardiovascular disease, high blood pressure, diabetes, and some cancers.

For pears, the good news is that they are less likely to suffer from heart problems. The bad news is that it is harder to shed that extra padding.

How To Find Out If You Are an Apple Or a Pear (Without Looking in the Mirror)

First, you need to measure your waist right above your navel and below your ribcage. You can find it by bending either forward or to the side. The place that creases is where your natural waist is.

Now you need to measure your hips. This will mean passing the tape measure around the widest part of your buttocks.

Here comes the math (sorry, couldn't find a chart for this one…):

Divide your waist measurement by your hip measurement. Yep, you may be dividing a smaller number by a larger number.

Is your WHR less than 1? If so, you are a pear (and you thought you were an intelligent human being…). If your WHR is 1 or more, you are a high-fiber, juicy, shiny apple.

If getting out the tape measure as well as the calculator is just too much for you, don't worry. Just know that a woman's waist measurement of over 35 inches[2] spells trouble.

Knowing whether you are an apple or a pear is valuable information, but it doesn't tell you whether you are overweight or not. You may be a small apple, or a very large pear.

---

[2] Your health risk is increased when this number is coupled with a BMI of over 25.

Risk Factors

You might decide, after working out the above measurements, that you really don't have to lose weight (i.e., you're within your "safe zone" — I can hear your sigh of relief...). But medical professionals look at the broader spectrum of your health when advising whether to lose weight or not.

They look at risk factors such as:

- High blood cholesterol;
- High blood sugar;
- High blood pressure;
- Arthritis in the knees or hips;
- Family history of weight-related health problems;
- Respiratory problems;
- Bad lifestyle habits: smoking, poor eating habits, and not exercising.

So if you fall into one or more of these categories and you are on the higher side of your healthy weight range, then maybe it's still a good idea to lose a few more pounds. If you are resisting this, then check with your doctor (he's not biased) and see who's right.

On the other hand, if you worked out your measurements and they are high (be honest), I don't need to persuade you, I'll just see you at the next appendix. However, if you are the lucky one who thinks she's all right, you have two choices. Go back and work out your measurements again (no cheating this time, please...), and then come join us, or just continue on the journey without the worry (and let's have some fun).

Appendix 3

———◆◆◆———

Calculating Calories

How Many Calories Does Your Body Need?

There are two ways to calculate how many calories we need.

There's the shortcut that's as easy-as-low-calorie-pie. And there's the more exact, detailed method for those who like accurate numbers versus well-rounded ones (we *are* trying to lose our roundness, after all…).

The Shortcut Method To Calculate How Many Calories Your Body Needs

If you consider yourself to be lightly active, multiply your current weight in pounds by 13. If you consider yourself to be active (exercising at least five times a week) multiply it by 15.

For example, Sara weighs 150 pounds and is a housewife who exercises twice a week. Her quick-as-a-jiffy total of the number of calories that she needs to maintain her weight is:

$150 \times 13 = \textbf{1,950}$

The More Scenic Long Route To Calculate How Many Calories Your Body Needs

Repeat after me: "I love math and I'm not scared — its resulting euphoria can't be compared...." It's time to stop biting those fingernails and pick up the calculator instead.

This is a three-step process. Just pretend you're following a recipe and go step by step.

Step 1: Working Out the Basic Number of Calories You Need
(We'll call it the BNC for short)

If you only know your weight in pounds, divide it by 2.2 to give you the equivalent reading in kilograms. Then you can glide your fingers across the number pad to execute the following equation:

Age	Equation
18–30	[14.7 × weight (in kilograms)] + 496
30–60	[8.7 × weight (in kilograms)] + 829
60+	[10.5 × weight (in kilograms)] + 596

Let's take Sara as an example.

Sara is forty-five years old and weighs 150 pounds. Her BNC calculation would look like this:

150 pounds ÷ 2.2 = 68.18 kilograms

68.18 kilograms × 8.7 = 593.18

593.18 + 829 = **1,422.18**[1] calories

So Sara needs 1,422 calories to keep her body ticking along at its most basic level.

If that equation blew your mind, there is a shortcut method that doesn't factor in your age but is pretty close. Multiply your current weight in pounds by 10.

In Sara's case,

150 × 10 = **1,500** calories

Step 2: Factoring in Your Activity Level

You need to know approximately how many calories you burn up each day through movement, exercise, and work, i.e., your Activity Calories. Use the following grid to guide you.

---

[1] We'll drop the pesky decimal places and just round things off as we go along.

How Active Are You?	Activity Factor	Description of Your Activities
Not at all	0.2	Very sedentary. Lots of sitting down, standing around, cooking, ironing, or typing.
Only mildly	0.3	House cleaning, walking, shopping, exercising once or twice a week.
Moderately	0.4	Very little sitting down, lots of energetic activities throughout the day. Exercises 5+ times a week.
Very	0.5	Heavily involved with sports or other vigorous activities.

Now multiply your Activity Factor (AF) by your BNC (your total from step 1) and then add that total back onto your BNC:

BNC × AF + BNC

In our home-brew case study, Sara is a housewife who doesn't get to move around very vigorously. So her activity factor would be 0.2.

Her total from step 1 was 1,422. So her calculation would be:

1,422 (BNC) × 0.2 (AF) = 284.4 Activity Calories (AC) +1,422 (BNC) = **1,706 Calories**

Step 3: Factoring in the Number of Calories We Need For Digestion
(Let's call this one NCD for short)

We need calories just to digest our food and burn it up.

So take your total from Step 2 and multiply it by 10% and then add that total back to the total from Step 2.

Sara's calculation would look like this:

1,706 (her total from Step 2) × 10% =170.6 (her NCD) +1,706 (her total from Step 2) = **1,877**

This is Sara's grand total number of calories she needs each day to maintain her current weight.

Putting It All Together

The formula for all this boils down to:

Basic Number of Calories (BNC) + Activity Calories (AC) + Digestion Calories (NCD) = Total Calories needed each day

In Sara's case, her BNC + AC + NCD was:

1,422 + 284 + 171 = **1,877**

Hey, that wasn't so bad. Almost as easy as A, B, C.

As you saw, when we used the shortcut method, we estimated that Sara would need 1,950 calories. While this number is not quite as exact as the above method, it's still a good near-guess gauge.

Happy calculating.

Appendix 4

———— ◆ ◆ ◆ ————

Debunking
Dieting Myths

*T*here must be as many dieting myths as there are diets. You know the sort of thing I mean — some well-meaning friend or relative will sidle over towards your plate and inform you that you're doing it all wrong (— and that's when you *are* keeping to the diet). These half-truths, three-quarter truths, and just plain ole non-truths can be the foundation of making or breaking your diet (not to mention your sanity).

Let's take a closer look at some of these well-espoused, sworn-by tricks and "wisdoms" and see if any of them stand up to some serious scrutiny (although we *are* allowed to smile).

I've Been on Every Diet Going and None of Them Work

There's one point in terms of following a diet that never gets high press coverage. That's probably because we don't want to hear it (still sitting on the edge of your chair?). It's also incredibly obvious — and doubly incredibly not followed: You must keep the diet for it to work.

This means conforming to its rules. This does not mean having extras because it was your best friend's simchah (and "how could I resist?"), nor does it mean finishing off the kids' leftovers of fish sticks and french fries, nor does it mean rounding up the permitted bread allowance from 2oz to three slices ('cause otherwise you'd have to weigh it).

Every diet plan[1] has been designed to work — if you work with it. Something that seems like a minor infraction not worthy of disappointing results might be all it takes to tip the scale — *not* in your favor.

Sometimes, generously proportioned people have just as generous natures. Saying no to anyone, including themselves, is hard for them. Denying themselves just a little bit of this or a dollop of that infringes on their sense of what a normal diet entails. These liberties become invisible to them as they justify that no diet *really* means no butter, no french fries, no chocolate.

Some people may not succeed on a diet because their easy-going natures prevent them from following all the rules. They will automatically view some rules as optional or impossible. Or they might not take the time to familiarize themselves with them in the first place. If you didn't learn to follow rules at school or home, you'd better start now — if you want to see positive results.

Forewarned is forearmed. A diet is not called a diet for nothing. Following it means following it — all the way along the yellow brick road to success.

I Don't Have To Diet — I'll Go To the Gym Instead

We blast this myth to smithereens in "I Need to Lose Weight, Therefore I Need to Exercise (Read: Without Dieting)," page 334.

I Won't Lose Weight If I Eat Late At Night

Since most people's bodies don't process calories differently after dark, this is a non-starter. The only ounce of truth to it may lie in the fact that most people have a tendency to relax and unwind in the evening, which might mean an automatic grab (reflex-reaction style) for the chocolates, potato chips, and nibbly-bits.

This myth is like a computer virus — a widespread infestation without any substance. Although it's often referred to in print as one of the ten commandments of dieting, we all know that there are some dodgy bible versions out these days. The truth? It's *what* you eat that packs on the pounds, not *when* you eat it (besides, doesn't that make more sense?).

---

[1] We're talking about sensible, well-balanced eating programs, not fad diets.

If Eating Less Doesn't Work, I Have To Eat Less...and Less...and Less

Been there. Done that.

See "Eat Enough," page 264.

If I Ignore My Cravings They'll Go Away

My mom always told me to ignore my kid brother and he would go away, but it never worked. So, too, with cravings — ignoring them doesn't make them go away. Got an itch for chocolate? Instead of nibbling every conceivable chocolate-alternative in the house (or scrounging from the neighbors...) and packing in extra calories, enjoy a small portion of the potion you want and stop the craving in its tracks. Sometimes all it takes is a little of the real stuff to get over the craving and get on with life. (That's why I ended up giving my brother a right hook before he would go away. Just kidding).

To Lose Weight I Must Not Eat in Between Meals

Tried it both ways. It's a more enjoyable and more successful route to snack in between meals.

See "Snack Attack," page 95.

Skipping Breakfast Saves Calories

If the human body were a calculator, this might have been true. However, missing this meal may be your first dieting mistake of the day. Your body has fasted all night (unless you are a pantry-invading insomniac) and needs fuel to get an energy fix for the day ahead. Without this kick-start, the metabolism slows down, which, in turn, will reduce the number of calories you will burn off.

In addition, such a philosophy cosmically increases the chances of overeating the next time food does make an appearance.

The Quickest and Surest Way To Lose Weight is To Fast

It may be the quickest, but it sure isn't the surest.

Our bodies need food. They're designed to absorb nutrients, vitamins, and minerals from what we ingest in order to provide revitalizing energy. If we deprive them by starvation, they suffer. This can result in lethargy, weakness, lightheadedness, headaches, and feeling generally icky (just remember how you felt last Tisha B'Av) — not real weight loss.

Do you think those magical lost pounds on the scale justify it? Just know that whatever weight you lose by fasting will just as magically reappear the minute you start eating again. Plus, those disappearing-trick numbers indicate a loss of water and muscle (the good guys), not fat.

More bad press for starvation is the oft-quoted benefit of cleansing the system. If you truly want to cleanse the system, you're better off sticking to whole grains, fruits, and veggies rather than such drastic extremist measures. Not only does fasting *not* cleanse the system, it's actually responsible for building up toxins. These are called "ketones," and they build up when carbohydrates are not available to produce energy. They can cause stress to the kidneys, increase your loss of sodium and potassium (which raises your risk of an irregular heartbeat), and give you bad breath. (Still think it's worth it?)

You Can Eat As Much As You Want of a Fat-Free Food and Still Lose Weight

There are little men who sit in advertising offices who are paid big bucks to make you think so. Unfortunately, it's just not true.

Although the product might emblazon "Fat-Free" in big bold letters all over a food product, the ingredients used to substitute the taste and feel of fat (e.g., sugar) can result in just as many (if not more) calories. (For example, two tablespoons of Skippy peanut butter will provide you with 190 calories, and two tablespoons of Skippy reduced-fat peanut butter will provide you with…you guessed it, 190 calories. See what I mean?)

Fat-free foods are not calorie-free. If they were, not only would those little men be making even more money, but you might end up being thinner too. The best rule of thumb is to check the Lie Detector, oops, I mean Nutrition Facts on the label on the back of each product. (See "Food Labels," page 112.)

Drinking Flushes Away Excess Calories

Don't count on it. For sure, the ideal is to try to keep the body well hydrated at all times, but there's no way that the wonders of water extend beyond the laws of nature — water will not bail out calories.

Let's turn things around slightly for a more positive approach.

If you make sure to drink *before* you eat, not only will you be more likely to ensure that you get your required eight cups of water each day, but you stand to take the aggressive edge off your appetite. With all that liquid swishing away inside the stomach, there is literally less room for calorie-laden food.

My Whole Family is Fat — Therefore it's My Destiny To Be Fat, Too

Genetics do provide a reason for a tendency towards obesity. However, they don't provide an excuse for it.

Genetics, metabolism, and environmental factors go a long way in determining how large your appetite is and how efficiently your body uses the food you eat. But the story doesn't end there. Although such a person born into such a family might look longingly at Little Miss Skin 'n' Bones (daughter of Mr. and Mrs. Skin 'n' Bones), she doesn't have to resign herself to a life in the fat lane.

Eating fewer calories and exercising will still work very effectively to reduce her excess weight. In the scenario of Miss Genetically Gigantic, they are even more important to ensure a long and healthy life. (See "Long-Term Health Problems," page 364.)

Conclusion

Knowing the truth behind these myths is sure to give you some clout the next time anyone starts eyeing your plate and beginning their "I know what's best for you" lecture. It also stands to provide you with some mind-blowing dinner-party conversation (discussing dieting over oily roast potatoes and fried shnitzel, of course).

But the best reason for having a realistic picture of exactly what will or will not affect your weight loss is that it can go a long way towards preventing pillow-bashing sobbing after your next weigh-in (besides the accompanying long-term health benefits). Reduced frustration brings with it positive results, which in turn make for a happy dieter.

Appendix 5

◆ ◆ ◆

Fiber: What's It Really All About?

*F*orget about which diet you are on, whether you are allowed x points, or x choices, or x grams of whichever foods. Let's put all that aside and consider one of the most basic tenets of all successful slimming; let's address a topic that gets headlines whenever we talk to professionals about weight loss: fiber.

Because whichever diet it is, if it's a sensible, long-term, healthy diet, it is bound to incorporate, promote, and encourage fiber as one of its essential ingredients.

Why is it that every health magazine, every doctor, every dietician will tell you that you should increase your intake of fiber when you are looking to lose weight? Why is it a subject that is brought up repeatedly when addressing healthy-lifestyle promotion? What is fiber, really, and why do we need it? And while we are on the subject, exactly how are we supposed to increase our intake — do we go to a store and ask for a packet of "fiber" to sprinkle over our lunches? Which foods contain fiber and exactly how much fiber is good for us?

Understanding fiber more fully — what it is, why we should have it, and how to increase it — will not only *enable* us to incorporate it into our daily lives, but will also *encourage* us to make the changes that we need to lead long, healthy, and happy lives.

This appendix on fiber is included to give you a better understanding of what fiber is and does, to ensure that you will choose the high-fiber option in your daily foods (now you know my ulterior motives…).

Due to the close connection between fiber and the digestive system, it helps to have a basic understanding of the digestive system — what it is and how it functions — before taking a closer look at fiber itself. So, notebooks at the ready, it's back to school for a Biology class…

Digestion — The "Ins" and "Outs"

A clinical definition of digestion is:

"…the process that the body goes through in order to break down the food it ingests into nutrients that the body can utilize."

In the vernacular, digestion is the way we get the good stuff out of food and into our bodies. Whatever is useless to the body is eliminated as the bad stuff.

This highly complex, incredible, automatic process starts with the food itself. How it smells and how it looks ignites the mouth's salivary glands (which produce saliva) into action. Saliva is the food's first contact with a digestive enzyme and kicks off the digestive process. The more enticing the food is, the more lip-smacking saliva we get. The body is automatically preparing itself to start the process of digestion before the food has even entered our mouths.

When we do take a bite, the chewing process further helps to break down the food before it travels through the food canal, into the stomach.

Although we are not aware of it, enzymes continue to work on the food in the stomach and break it down even further into a more digestible form. After sitting and relaxing for several hours in the stomach, the food particles are shunted down into the small intestine, which is the main site of digestion.

The small intestines make the ideal environment for digestion because of their sheer length. We're talking extreme length here — if someone would pull out her small intestines into a long line, it would measure approximately seven yards (I don't suggest you try it, at least not often, as they're devils to get back in again…). Therefore, the nutrients have plenty of time to be properly absorbed into the body while on their long trip. When all the good stuff has been squeezed out of the food, the remaining particles travel (sounds like a vacation, but it's more like an evacuation) to the large intestines. Here, the last vestiges of water are extracted, turning the remains into waste matter that is no longer useful to the body. These remnants of the digestive process are passed on to the rectum, and from there they are eliminated as feces.

What is Fiber?

Anyone who has ever set foot in Diet Land has heard of fiber. It has this vague connection to all those typically dietetic products, while leaving us groping for an exact definition. So here is its definition:

"Fiber is the name given to a number of substances that are found in the cell walls of plants."

Because fiber comes from the stuff that makes up plant cells, we'll only find fiber in plants (or, more relevant to us, from wheat and grain type foods, from stuff that grows from the ground, or grows on a tree or bush). Animal products like meat or milk contain no fiber at all. (Now fiber is starting to make nutritional sense....)

There are two forms of fiber: Insoluble fiber and soluble fiber.

What is Insoluble Fiber?

Insoluble means "cannot be dissolved in water." Like a hungry magnet, insoluble fiber will attract and hold onto any water it does find on its travels.

What is Soluble Fiber?

Soluble fiber dissolves in water to form a thick, gummy liquid. (We'll get to the positively gripping part about why this is such a truly magnificent dieting tool in a moment.)

What Does Fiber Do? (Apart From Lounging Around Our Digestive Systems on His Deckchair)

What Does Insoluble Fiber Do?

Because insoluble fiber has the tendency to retain water, it acts just like a bath sponge (the sort that hides between Moby Dick and Ducky Duck on the bathtub's ledge). Case in point: Have you ever seen how quickly a bowl of oatmeal absorbs milk, as opposed to the slow rate at which cornflakes absorb it?

Insoluble fiber soaks up and holds onto water in the bowel (part of the large intestine). The end result is a larger and softer bulk passing through the large intestines. Bowel movements are easier and more regular.

Because the partly digested food is larger and softer as a result of ingesting insoluble fiber, this stimulates the action of the digestive tract muscles in the large intestine. This is called "peristalsis," which is a wave-like motion, squashing and pushing the food along the intestine (rather like getting a sausage out of its skin). In real what-this-means-to-my-tummy terms, it means that the process of elimination is carried out more efficiently and effectively.

In short, insoluble fiber speeds up the food's journey through the body so that the process of digestion is carried out efficiently (i.e., no sightseeing tours along the way). This is a very desirable end product (no pun intended).

What Does Soluble Fiber Do (for a Living)?

Soluble fiber effects absorption in the small intestine. This is beneficial to the body because it is primarily in the small intestine that nutrients are absorbed. This process is carried out more efficiently in the presence of soluble fiber, because the nutrients are absorbed more systematically and regularly, instead of sporadically — i.e., the nutrients are absorbed at the right time and in the right quantities.

Health Benefits

Besides the benefits of fiber to your average "I'd love to be two dress sizes smaller" dieter, there are general health benefits applicable to every Sora, Rivka, or Rochel.

Health Benefits of Insoluble Fiber

- By moving food quickly through the intestines, insoluble fiber may help prevent or relieve digestive disorders such as constipation.
- It also helps to prevent diverticulosis (infection caused by food getting stuck in small pouches in the wall of the colon).
- Another dividend of this wonder substance is that it bulks up stools and makes them softer, thereby reducing the risk of developing hemorrhoids and lessening the discomfort of existing piles (anyone who's ever lived to tell the tale after one of these complaints knows how unpleasant they can be).
- Increasing the amount of insoluble fiber in the diet also decreases the amount of time that harmful food waste spends inside the body[1] and reduces the risk of infection or cell changes due to carcinogens[2] that are produced when some foods, particularly meat, degrade.

Due to the fact that low-fiber foods (for example, meat) stay in the body longer, there is considerable time for putrefaction (unhealthy fermentation — bubble, bubble, toil and trouble…) to occur. Therefore, if you like meat, make sure you also eat high-fiber foods. (It is interesting to note that a high-meat, low-fiber diet can increase the time it takes for digestion to occur from twenty-four to seventy-two hours.)

- By improving intestinal regularity, insoluble fiber becomes an important safeguard against cancer of the colon (large intestine).
- Insoluble fiber can reduce the risk of bowel cancer. In the UK and Ireland, bowel cancer is the second biggest cancer killer. Although it doesn't get as much press as smoking, it's still a big-time killer. Research shows that eating foods rich in fiber can reduce the risk of bowel cancer.

---

[1] The digestive process involves extracting the "good" i.e., nutrition, minerals, and vitamins, etc., from food, and eliminating or "getting rid" of the "bad" waste products that are not required by the body. Waste products that are left inside the body for extended periods (i.e., in the case of constipation or intestinal disorders) can cause considerable long-term health disorders.
[2] Cancer-producing substances.

Health Benefits of Soluble Fiber

- Soluble fiber is good news for people with diabetes. It helps to control their blood sugar levels (and therefore minimize their need for medication). Rapid absorption of glucose in the small intestine can lead to a sudden surge of sugar in the blood. Soluble fiber slows down and regulates the rate at which the glucose is absorbed into the blood. (Sweet news.)

- The aforementioned regulation process also has a benefit for people without diabetes. Since glucose (the body's energy provider) is regulated, a person will avoid high/low swings in her energy levels. This is good because regulating the level of sugar in our blood means that we can remain alert and energized (bouncy, bright-eyed, and bushy-tailed) for longer periods.

- Soluble fiber seems to lower the amount of cholesterol circulating in our blood and may be why a diet rich in fiber appears to give us some protection against heart disease.

- Soluble fiber helps prevent gallstones. This is because the digestive system is working more efficiently and the bile salts are being properly used and removed from the body instead of accumulating in excessive quantities.

- Soluble fiber helps to prevent diverticular diseases and other intestinal disorders such as Irritable Bowel Syndrome and Colitis. This is due to the decreased transit time in the intestines, which in turn prevents the unhealthy build-up of bacteria and harmful carcinogens (they even sound nasty).

Conclusion

The right combination of insoluble and soluble fiber is a powerful tool for healthier living. The improvement of the overall digestion process also brings with it other benefits. To quote Patrick Holford in *The Optimum Nutrition Bible*,

> *Improving digestion is the cornerstone to good health. Energy levels improve, the skin becomes softer and clearer, body odour reduces and the immune system is strengthened.*

Now, doesn't that sound like it's worth it?

Since we have been formally introduced to fiber, it's time to make friends and encourage him to come and live with us. He can do more than help you with the washing up; he brings a whole bunch of benefits to our weight loss, so you might just want him to stick around long-term.

Benefits To a Weight Loss Program

Fiber can help us lose weight for the following reasons:

✔ High-fiber foods take longer to eat than low-fiber foods with the same corresponding number of calories. (It takes longer to munch an apple than it does to gobble a small piece of chocolate.) This therefore creates the (real) impression that we're eating tons of food and still managing to lose weight. (Husbands usually gawk at fiber-conscious dieters' plates).

Psychologically, if something takes a long time to eat, then we feel that there must have been a lot of it, and we are therefore more likely to feel satisfied.

✔ High-fiber foods lower levels of insulin. An increase in the hormone insulin stimulates appetite. If this hormone is lowered, so are our feelings of hunger. Furthermore, because the appetite has not been stimulated, it is easier to feel satiated sooner. This makes fiber a great all around hunger-reducer.

✔ Fiber helps us to feel fuller for longer after mealtimes. This is because soluble fiber helps to slow down and regulate the process of breaking down food in the stomach. The food stays in the stomach longer, which means that we feel satiated for longer and we will be less likely to snack in between meals (that's the theory, anyway…).

✔ More energy (read: calories) is used up during the digestion and absorption of high-fiber foods. This is because the body requires energy to break down food in the digestive process. It utilizes the food we ingest to provide this energy. Different foods require different amounts of energy/calories to break them down into substances that are easily absorbed by the body. If we eat high-fiber foods, we will be using more calories in the process of digestion and will therefore be left with fewer calories to store. (Excess stored calories convert into fat.)

✔ If we fill up on foods rich in insoluble fiber and low in fat, like whole-wheat bread, etc., we will have less room for less beneficial foods, i.e., those foods high in fat/sugar (you know the list…).

✔ The wonderful thing about eating more fiber is that it automatically helps us eat a healthy diet. Most food that is high in fiber is naturally low in fat and full of vitamins, minerals, and other substances that protect our health and make us feel on top of the world. When we reduce fat in the diet and replace it with whole grains, fruits, and vegetables, the amount of vitamins and minerals in the diet per 1,000 calories is significantly increased.

How Much Fiber Does a Person Need?

Most individuals consume between 7g and 15g of fiber daily. Although 12g is the minimum recommended intake, many people find that they can eat even more than this without any ill effects. It is safe to go up to 35g daily. The Department of Health has recommended that we try and increase our fiber intake. We need about 20–35g of fiber each day (from a mix of soluble and insoluble fiber). Very few people are currently consuming this level of fiber, so we can all afford to eat more high-fiber foods.

Fiber Contents of Foods

Insoluble fiber is found mainly in wheat products like bran-based cereals (All-Bran, Fruit 'n' Fiber, Weetabix, Shredded Wheat, and wheat germ[3]), and also in whole-wheat flour, whole-wheat bread,[4] whole-wheat pasta and many fruits. Vegetables (like green beans and potatoes) are also excellent sources, as are the skins of fruits and vegetables.

It is worth noting that most fruits and vegetables contain more fiber when they are not peeled (as there are more of these cellulose-based plant cells inherent within the peel). For example, a potato baked with its skin on has double the amount of fiber as the same good old potato without his jacket on. For this reason, it is worth opting to eat whole grains versus refined grains.[5]

Soluble fiber is found in peas, beans, lentils, oats, oatmeal, barley, rye, fruits (such as apples and oranges), and vegetables (such as carrots).

Most high-fiber foods contain both soluble and insoluble fiber. For example, most grains and veggies are two-thirds insoluble and one-third soluble; fruit tends to be fifty-fifty, and the fiber in oatmeal, barley, and legumes is about sixty-five percent soluble.

---

[3] Look for cereals with 3–6g of fiber per serving.
[4] Whole-wheat bread with at least 2g of fiber per serving is a good choice.
[5] Refined grains typically have parts of the grain, such as the husk, removed.

Below are listings for the amount of fiber present in different foods.

Charts Showing the Amount of Fiber (in grams) In Certain Foods

Food	Fiber (grams) in 100g of food	Usual Portion Size	Fiber Content in Usual Portion Size
Bread & Flour			
Bagel	2.6	1 bagel (50g)	1.3
Pita bread (white)	2.2	1 pita (60g)	1.3
Pita bread (whole-wheat)	7.8	1 pita (60g)	4.7
White bread	2.6	1 slice (35g)	0.9
Whole-grain bread	7.5	1 slice (35g)	2.6
Cereals			
All Bran	26.7	30g	8.0
Cornflakes	3.0	30g	0.9
Oatmeal	7.2	60g	4.3
Porridge oats	8.6	50g	4.3
Weetabix	10.1	1 biscuit (18.8g)	1.9
Grains			
Barley, pearl (raw)	7.3	28g	2.0
Bran	39.6	28g	11.1
Brown rice (cooked)	1.8	1 cup (195g)	3.5
Cornmeal (whole grain)	7.3	1 cup (122g)	8.9
Oat bran (cooked)	2.6	1 cup (219g)	5.7
Wheat germ, toasted (plain)	15.0	1 cup (100g)	15.0
White rice (cooked)	0.4	1 cup (158g)	0.6

Fruits			
Apple	3.0	1 apple (100g)	3.0
Apricots	2.5	1 cup (148g)	3.7
Banana	2.4	1 cup, sliced (150g)	3.6
Blackberries	5.3	1 cup (144g)	7.6
Figs (dried)	9.2	2 figs (38g)	3.5
Kiwi	3.1	1 kiwi (100g)	3.1
Orange	2.4	1 orange (141g)	3.4
Pear	2.6	1 pear (154g)	4.0
Plum	1.5	1 plum (66g)	1.0
Prunes	5.7	100g	5.7
Raisins	4.0	1 cup, packed (165g)	6.6
Raspberries	6.8	1 cup (123g)	8.4
Strawberries	2.3	1 cup (152g)	3.5
Tangerine	2.3	1 tangerine (100g)	2.3
Beans			
Baked beans	7.2	75g	5.4
Chickpeas (canned)	4.1	100g	4.1
Lima beans/Butter beans (cooked)	7.0	50g	3.5
Vegetables			
Beets (cooked and drained)	2.0	½ cup (85g)	1.7
Broccoli	3.0	1 cup (71g)	2.1
Cabbage	2.3	1 cup, shredded (70g)	1.6
Carrots	3.2	1 cup, grated (100g)	3.2
Cauliflower	2.5	1 cup (100g)	2.5
Corn on the cob	1.3	100g	1.3

Eggplant (cooked and drained)	2.5	1 cup, cubed (100g)	2.5
Peas, frozen (boiled)	5.1	100g	5.1
Potato (Jacket)	2.8	1 potato (200g)	5.5
Tomatoes	1.1	1 cup, chopped/sliced (180g)	2.0
Nuts			
Almonds (dry-roasted)	13.7	1 cup (138g)	18.9
Almonds (oil-roasted)	11.2	1 cup (150g)	17.6
Coconut	9.0	1 cup (80g)	7.2
Peanuts (dry-roasted)	6.4	50g	3.2
Pistachios	10.8	1 cup (128)	13.8
Other			
Lentils (cooked)	7.8	½ cup (100g)	7.8
Matzah (plain)	2.9	1 matzah (28g)	0.8
Peanut Butter (crunchy)	6.6	2 Tbsp. (32g)	2.1
Pickles (sweet)	1.1	1 cup, sliced (170g)	1.9
Pickle (sour)	1.2	1 large, 4" long (135g)	1.6
Rye Crispbread (Ryvita)	16.7	1 cracker (9g)	1.5
White pasta (cooked)	1.3	1 cup (140g)	1.8
Whole-wheat flour	12.2	1 cup (120g)	14.7
Whole-wheat pasta (cooked)	4.5	1 cup (140g)	6.3

Diagram 3 : *Food Combinations of Increased Fiber*

A Typical Low-Fiber Diet

5g Fiber:	Food	Grams of Fiber
	2 Slices white bread	1.8
	30g Cornflakes	0.9
	½ Cup white pasta	0.9
	1 Rye crispbread (Ryvita)	1.5
	Total	5.1

The Minimum Recommended Amount of Fiber

12g Fiber:	Food	Grams of Fiber
	2 Slices whole-grain bread	5.2
	1 Weetabix biscuit	1.9
	1 Baked potato	5.5
	Total	12.6

A High-Fiber Diet

21g Fiber:	Food	Grams of Fiber
	75g Baked beans	5.4
	2 Weetabix	3.8
	Pear	4.0
	Broccoli, 1 cup	2.1
	Strawberries, 1 cup	3.5
	2 Plums	2.0
	Total	20.8

How Do We Increase Fiber in Our Diet?

When we increase fiber in our diet, it is important not to be too enthusiastic (although that may be hard once you've read all these great things about fiber). An excessive and dramatically sudden increase in fiber intake brings its own problems. If you have been ignoring that blue box of Bran Flakes or yellow Weetabix sitting on your breakfast table, and have therefore been eating a typical Western low-fiber diet of about ten grams a day, **you must increase the levels of fiber gradually.** If you triple your intake overnight, you may suffer the triple discomfort of intestinal distress, flatulence, and possibly diarrhea (don't say I didn't warn you).

It is also important to make a concerted effort to drink more than you usually do when you increase your fiber content. Although we've just espoused fiber's great quality of reducing constipation, the opposite results may occur when you increase your fiber intake without the corresponding necessary increase in water. (This is due to the water-retentive qualities of insoluble fiber we mentioned in the beginning of this appendix.)

It is worth noting that certain forms of fiber in *very* large quantities can also interfere with the absorption of certain vitamins and essential minerals (such as iron and calcium). In addition, small children have small stomachs and feel full quickly. They can therefore feel full before they have eaten enough food to provide the energy and nutrients they need for growth and development. **Therefore, a high-fiber diet is not suitable for children under the age of five years.**

Conclusion

- Fiber goes a long way in relieving digestive disorders, preventing unnecessary and potentially dangerous health problems (like cancer, diverticulosis, gallstones, etc.), and reducing the risks of hemorrhoids and piles.
- It's good news for diabetics as fiber helps to regulate energy swings and lowers cholesterol levels.
- And, most pertinent to this book, it plays an extremely important role in the area of weight loss.

In a nutshell (nuts being high in fiber, of course), increasing fiber is a relatively easy, inexpensive, wholesome way to stay healthy, become healthier, and live life to the fullest. Make a lifestyle change. Choose fiber for life.

Appendix 6

— ◆ ◆ ◆ —

Drinking

*W*e humans don't store our liquids very well. This means that, unlike camels, we need a new supply every day. We need enough to replace what we use to breathe, perspire, urinate, and defecate. On average, this totals somewhere between one and one half to three quarts a day. On hot summer days, or when you are engaged in exercise, you will need more.

The body itself will take a degree of responsibility for making some of this total requirement (about fifteen percent) through digestion and other metabolic processes. The remaining balance comes from what we eat and drink.

Although we tend to think of food as food and drink as drink (that's because food *is* food and drink *is* drink…), there is still a water content present in food. For example, fruits and vegetables are full of water. Lettuce is ninety percent water; even a hamburger contains more than fifty percent water, a bagel twenty-nine percent, and butter and margarine ten percent. (Only oils have no water.) So some of that necessary total will come from our food.

But it doesn't take many brain cells to figure out that the best way to get enough liquids is to drink them.

So How Much Do I Need To Drink Each Day?

The Formula

Divide your weight in half to get the appropriate number of fluid ounces you should drink every day.

Weight ÷ 2 = Daily fluid ounces needed

For example, Rachel weighs 140 pounds.

140 ÷ 2 = 70 fluid ounces

Using typical 8oz cups, that's approximately nine cups per day.

A Word About What Not To Drink

Although all liquids might well fill your glass or cup and look, smell, and feel like a refreshing drink, some are more liquid than others.

At zero calories, water is hands-down the best liquid on the market. But juices, diet sodas, etc., are all good alternatives.

However, watch out for caffeine in drinks such as tea, coffee, Coke, and some other soft drinks (for example, Mountain Dew). Be careful, as well, with the alcohol content in beer, wine, and spirits. These all come under the banner of *diuretics* — namely, chemicals that make you urinate more abundantly. They force the body to rid itself of valuable water (and minerals). It's like trying to fill a bucket with a hole in it: The liquid goes in, but a lot of it goes back out again as well. And we definitely don't want that to happen, 'cause liquid (especially water) is, quite literally, vital to our survival.

- It aids the digestive process;
- Our metabolism depends upon it;
- Our body temperature is regulated by it;
- Potentially toxic waste products are eliminated through it;
- Our joints are lubricated by it;
- The electrical messages sent between cells that allow us to see, think, and feel, are carried by it; and
- Our breathing is affected by it, etc.

Not to mention (one last time…), it's a dieter's dream. It fills you up without any calories. So don't wait till you're thirsty to drink (by then you've already lost the amount of water equal to about one percent of your body weight), rather…

Grab a cup
'n' freshen up,
Glass in handy
You'll feel dandy.

I'll have mine on the rocks, with a slice of lemon, please…. Cheers.

Appendix 7

———— ◆◆◆ ————

Dieting And Kids

*W*ith so many obese and overweight adults hanging around, it's hardly any wonder that the number of overweight children is at an all-time high.

According to the American Heart Association, by age twelve, as many as seven out of every ten American children have fatty deposits in their arteries. Nowadays, we even have cholesterol guidelines for children.

Overweight children are at a higher risk of lifelong obesity. Statistics are scary. An overweight six-month-old baby has a fourteen percent risk of becoming an overweight adult. An overweight seven-year-old has a forty-one percent risk; for an adolescent, the risk is a staggering eighty percent.

With all those doom and gloom numbers, shouldn't we, as parents, purge the house of ice cream, french fries, soda, and cookies? After all, we care. We were partners in giving them life and we want them to live long enough to enjoy it. But this is where the picture gets a little cloudy…

Life isn't simple for us, and it isn't simple for kids either. There are a number of points to ponder when considering what action to take in the case of an overweight youngster.

Physical Factors

Changing Height

Since most kids do a fair amount of growing in their early years, it's safe to presume that their height is constantly in a state of flux. It therefore becomes a more complex issue to define the right weight for each child.

Inaccurate BMI[1] Readings

Children may weigh more and have artificially inflated high BMI readings because their bodies have a greater proportion of muscle to fat.

Growth Spurts

I know, kids will spurt all sorts of things at us before they're finished, but let's overlook all that and concentrate on their sporadic growth spurts. They may find themselves suddenly needing more calories to fuel an oncoming growth spurt. It's not unusual for a child to gain thirty or forty pounds and then shoot up ten or twelve inches. A calorie-restricted diet would suppress their natural caloric intake and leave their bodies depleted in the number of calories needed for natural growth.

Changing Shape

Kids' bodies can change so often and so drastically that it's hard to qualify them as being overweight. Because of this, their bodies need extra calories to grow. They may well be temporarily overweight at a given stage, but, given six months, this acne-prone, gangly, ugly duckling may turn into a beautiful swan. (Start praying.)

Activity Levels

Kids are generally more active than adults. (When was the last time you had Phys Ed scheduled from 1–3pm on Mondays and Wednesdays, or ran all the way home from school?) Kids actually use their higher calorie intake. However, their exact caloric needs are difficult to quantify, given their varied yet constantly active lifestyle.

---

[1] See "BMI," page 380.

Emotional Factors

Choose Your Battlefield

Part of an adolescent's struggle to assert their own identity may involve conflicts in the home. This is a pleasant way of saying adolescence is like hormones — take a deep breath and know that they'll pass one day.

As dieting can be an emotionally charged area, you might want to consider whether all those fireworks are really worth it.

If you are already involved in power-struggle issues, choose your battles wisely. Remember, he who wins the battle, doesn't necessarily win the war.

Hormones

Hormones may be responsible for some of those tears, door-slams, and vocalizations. But they are also responsible for more body changes. Not only do those changes need calories, but they also involve laying down extra fat deposits, especially in girls. Again, the adolescent's body is trying to decide what shape it wants to be — we are not always sure if she is fat or just developing.

Self-Esteem

Self-esteem is all the rage these days. Maybe that's because it's in short supply. Let's not fall into the trap of creating a failure-experience for our children. This can so easily happen if we don't know what we are doing when we are encouraging them to diet.

For example, do you really know:

> ✔ That your child is actually overweight?
> ✔ What she should ideally weigh?
> ✔ How exactly she can achieve this ideal weight?
> ✔ How long it's going to take to achieve it? (Children need closure.)

They need success-experiences more than ever when they are young. We want to build them, not break them.[2]

---

[2] And certainly don't criticize her appearance. Be especially careful if your child is a preteen daughter. If your daughter thinks you are criticizing her appearance, she may believe that you find **her** unacceptable too. She may deal with her crushed feelings by becoming anorexic (see next appendix) in a heroic effort to please you, or she may rebel and become even fatter as an expression of anger and defiance. Included in this is the all-important "Don't make one child feel different from every other child" rule, i.e., don't give one child a diet plate while everyone else dives into fried chicken and chocolate cake. The psychological harm by far outweighs any physical good.

Stress for Mom

If you are a skinny mom and you've never been on a diet, do you really feel confident in your capacity to advise your child? If you are an overweight mom, then you'll probably agree that it's hard enough to diet for yourself — do you really think you can manage to diet for her too?

Adolescent Immaturity

Sometimes children can be so…childish. They may lack the maturity, balance, dedication, and ability to take on dieting. They are volatile. Their emotions often lead. They can be moody (don't we know it…). They can become easily disenchanted. Not a good line-up for solid success.

Mental Health

There is a risk element that young people may take dieting too seriously. They might even make a religion out of it. There are enough commandments in the Torah without your kids feeling stifled by an extra thousand or so. Take care, because they might not be able to differentiate the importance between the two.

Responsibility

If you still go ahead and decide that it's a good idea for young Shnocky or his sister to start a diet, make sure he or she thinks so too. If the kids don't take ultimate responsibility for what they are or aren't eating, it isn't going to work.

This means that if they are only doing it in order to please you (or Bubbie, or Auntie Gertrude), your child could be headed for a short-term success but a long-term failure.

Peer Pressure

Let's make sure we take into account how the cool dude's going to feel if he can't have pizza with his friends on a motzei Shabbos, or how the little girl's going to feel with her carrot and celery sticks for a snack when all her friends have Bamba and cookies.

Conclusion

Does all this mean I am not in favor of putting kids on diets? Yes. Does all this mean you're trapped, sitting on your hands, unable to actually *do* anything to help your kid? No, there's still a lot you can do.

Talk

Rather than bulldozing your way and dictating to your children how they have to change their eating habits, try to build bridges of trust and cooperation by talking instead. Keep the lines of communication open. Ask them how they feel about their body/shape/size/weight. Do they want to do anything to change it? How much does it bother them?

Find out if emotional stress or unhappiness is contributing to your child's weight gain. Children may substitute food for friends when they are lonely. Overeating when bored, angry, depressed, anxious, or otherwise stressed can also be contributing factors. Finding out and overcoming a child's problems via communication not only makes the child happier, but also avoids sowing the seeds of potential eating disorders.

Educate

It's important for you to give them a healthy relationship with food. You can start by giving them a healthy relationship with themselves. Let them grow up to be confident, secure, happy people who are able to make informed decisions.

At the same time, educate them in food matters. Serve healthy, high-nutrient foods and periodically explain which foods are good for them, which are not, which can be eaten freely, and which they should try to limit — and why. Encourage them to see food in a positive context: It fuels the body and provides nourishment, it keeps us healthy, etc.

Focus on health being the priority, not appearance. Make sure they understand that personal worth depends on character, not on looks.

Don't dictate, just educate.

Teach by Example
(This one's gonna hurt…)

There's no stronger message we can give our kids than "do as I do" versus "do as I say." If they see us eating healthy foods and developing healthy eating habits, they'll automatically follow and strive to emulate our ways. If they see us getting fatter and fatter as the years go on, or constantly jumping from diet to diet, or giving up on ourselves, don't be surprised when the apple doesn't fall far from the tree.

Make family meals healthy for everyone. Instead of collapsing on the sofa after dinner, go for a walk or bike ride with the kids.

Striving to ensure that the whole household has access to nutritious, wholesome, healthy food and snacks, and that food is seen as a means to an end (and not an end in itself), will be invaluable tools for all your children — those who are overweight and those who are not.

We need to have the right attitudes toward food in order to ensure that our children will also have the right attitudes. We can't make our own dieting a religion. On the other hand, we can't say and live, "Being fat is fine, healthy, and a happy way to be." We mustn't worship our bodies, but we also don't want to worship our food… In this way, we are at least setting the groundwork for our children to develop their own positive, healthy attitudes on food and weight loss.

When Will My Child Be Old Enough To Diet?[3]

Answer? When your child is grown up enough to prepare food in the kitchen for herself. When she asks you to help her lose weight.[4] When you think your kids are old enough, mature enough, and emotionally stable enough to succeed and to take responsibility for their own diets. (You can help, but you shouldn't feel that the main burden falls on your shoulders.) Then and only then should you offer your help and encouragement to set them up with an appropriate formal diet plan.

Even after your teen has chosen a diet plan, you need to reassess the situation often — because the life of a teenager is anything but routine. After she is on a diet, let her take responsibility for what she eats. Offer your support instead of your services. Keep an eye on things from a distance and encourage, but don't intrude.[5]

Children (of all ages) need love, warmth, encouragement, space to grow, guidance, friendship, and an example to follow. The trick is knowing that they need all of these things at all stages of life, but that at different stages, these things have to be delivered in different ways. (And you thought *dieting* was complicated....)

Our aim as parents is to nurture our children's souls as well as their bodies. We have to always focus on the children's ultimate good in the long run. We need to feed our children's sense of self-esteem as well as their bodies. In this way, when they *are* old enough to want to change the way they eat, they will have the best tools at their disposal to ensure optimum success.

---

[3] In a child's younger years, if there has to be a focus on weight, then the goal of weight control should be just that: control, *not weight loss*. Instead of trying to help a child reduce his/her weight, let height catch up to weight by maintaining a slow rate of weight gain. The only exception is if the child is so overweight that it presents a health hazard. In such a case, the matter should be discussed with a physician.
[4] They have to want it. It's not enough for you to want it for them. I have had plenty of mothers ask me to put their daughters on a diet plan. When I asked if this request was coming from the daughters or from the mothers themselves, almost every one answered that it was coming from the mothers. What chance does a diet like that have of succeeding? Fat chance (pun intended).
[5] Don't nag about food or weight. Your child will resent you and withdraw, probably to a hidden stash of food. If you try to police what your child eats, you may inadvertently create depression, shame, and feelings of abandonment, anxiety, or even a life-threatening eating disorder.

Appendix 8

———◆◆◆———

Eating Disorders – When Dieting Goes Too Far

*E*ating disorders are not a natural outcome of dieting. You don't get an eating disorder because you went on a diet. Eating disorders are not just a fad, a phase, or a trivial eccentricity. They are abnormal, psychological disorders that have serious consequences for mental and physical health.

The purpose of this appendix is to increase your awareness of the three main eating disorders and their potential signs; to understand the reasons why eating disorders occur; and what to do about them if they do show up. In this way, when dieting issues become distorted and harmful, you will be able to recognize the early warning signs and take appropriate action.

Anorexia

Anorexia (officially called "Anorexia Nervosa") is the relentless, obsessive pursuit of thinness — to the point of self-starvation. An anorexic typically weighs eighty-five percent or less of her ideal body weight (equivalent to a BMI[1] of 17.5 or less). She is terrified of becoming fat,[2] is endlessly preoccupied with food, demonstrates strange eating habits or rituals, and stops menstruating.

[1] See "BMI," page 380.
[2] An anorexic will often irrationally view herself as fat even when she is painfully thin.

The condition often includes depression, irritability, low self-esteem, and compulsive, peculiar rituals associated with food.

Bulimia

Bulimia (officially called "Bulimia Nervosa") is a disorder that includes a vicious cycle of first dieting, then bingeing, followed by purging. A bulimic person will typically:

- ✔ Diet to the point where she becomes extremely hungry;
- ✔ Binge eat, i.e., she will eat excessive amounts of food while feeling out of control (This gorging is usually done in secret.);
- ✔ Purge her body of the extra calories by self-induced vomiting, misuse of laxatives, or diuretics[3] in order to avoid weight gain.

Clinically speaking, a person with this condition binges at least twice a week and eats large amounts of food in a relatively short period of time.

Even though bulimics put up a brave front, they are often depressed, lonely, ashamed, and dissatisfied. Their behavior may also involve impulsive shoplifting, sexual promiscuity, and alcohol or drug abuse. Unlike the excessively thin anorexic, the bulimic is usually within a normal weight range.

Additional telltale signs of bulimia:

- ✔ She makes excuses to visit the bathroom after meals;
- ✔ She develops a "chipmunk" type of face that involves swelling around the jaw and cheeks, in addition to scraped knuckles — resulting from induced vomiting;
- ✔ She suffers from dental enamel erosion due to the repeated contact with the acidity of vomit;
- ✔ Huge amounts of food mysteriously disappear.

---

[3] Drugs that cause increased urination.

Binge Eating Disorder

The sufferer will binge on large amounts of food frequently and repeatedly but will not purge herself of the intake afterwards. Most binge eaters are overweight or obese and may therefore suffer from weight-related disorders (such as type 2 diabetes, high blood pressure, etc.)[4]

Who Gets Eating Disorders?

These disorders usually appear in bright, attractive, conscientious young women between the ages of twelve and twenty-five. (Approximately ninety percent of the sufferers are female, and the occurrence of these conditions is proportionally greater in the Western World.)

What Causes Eating Disorders?

There are many triggers that may cause an eating disorder and no one simple answer will cover everyone. Some or all of the following factors may contribute to developing these conditions:

Personality Factors

Some personality types are more vulnerable to eating disorders than others. For example, people with eating disorders tend to be perfectionists. They see the world as black and white with no shades of gray. Everything is either good or bad, a success or a failure, fat or thin. If fat is bad and thin is good, then thinner is better and thinnest is best — even if thinnest is sixty-eight pounds, in a hospital bed, on a life support machine.

Another personality trait that is commonly found in those who have an eating disorder is obsessive-compulsive behavior.

Emotional Factors

Those with eating disorders often have very low self-esteem, are approval-seeking, and display traits of anxiety and nervousness.

Some see their eating habits as a means of finding their identity. They think, "I am successful at dieting. I diet, therefore I am."

---

[4] See Appendix 1.

Family Factors

Sometimes people with eating disorders have families who are overprotective, strict, and emotionally aloof. These families may have high expectations of achievement and success and an intolerance of imperfections. The family may emphasize the importance of appearance, or tease about the sufferer's size or shape.

Society Factors

Whether we like it or not, whether we believe it or not, our society champions the statement that thinness is the ideal. It is viewed as attractive, and associated with power and success. Our society is affluent. Food is plentiful. In the Orthodox Jewish world, there is limited access (or at least a social stigma attached) to drugs, cigarettes, and alcohol. But food? It's there morning, noon, and night. And it's kosher. In this way, food becomes an accessible tool to wrestle with the different control and self-identity issues.

Triggers

A condition may remain dormant until a life-change in circumstances triggers it into action. Triggers often happen at times of transition, shock, or loss, where increased demands are made on people who are already unsure of their ability to meet expectations. Stages such as puberty, starting a new school, beginning a new job, death, divorce, marriage, family problems, criticism, graduation into a chaotic, competitive world, etc. are all potential triggers.

Physical Consequences of Eating Disorders

All the above eating disorders are serious. Deadly serious. These conditions, especially anorexia, can kill if left untreated.

The following symptoms may arise from eating disorders:

- Irregular heartbeat (may lead to cardiac arrest and death);
- Liver damage (may result in death);
- Dehydration and malfunctioning kidneys (may result in death);
- Menstruation stops (may lead to infertility and osteoporosis);
- Muscles wither (causing weakness and inability to move);
- Inefficient digestion (resulting in constipation and bowel problems);
- Permanent depletion of bone calcium (may result in broken or fractured bones);
- The sufferer feels constantly cold and has an unwell appearance;
- The immune system is weak;
- Anemia and malnutrition may develop.

Where To Find Help

If you are in crisis, go to a hospital emergency room or call a crisis hotline. The number can be found in the phone book's Yellow Pages under "Crisis Intervention."

If you are not in crisis, the best plan of action is to find a counselor, physician, and treatment team you can trust (including psychologists and other mental health therapists who have been trained to work with these desperately needy people). Asking your family doctor for an evaluation and referral is an effective first step. Don't let embarrassment stop you from telling the physician all the details. Unfortunately, physicians (even pediatricians) have heard it all before.

If your income is limited, or if your insurance will not cover treatment for eating disorders, look for community service agencies in the "Counselors" section of the yellow pages, or talk to your local social worker. She'll know whom to contact for funds and counseling.

Help and Treatment

What is the Best Treatment for an Eating Disorder?

There are many factors that contribute to the development of an eating disorder. Since every person's situation is different, the best treatment must be custom tailored for each individual.

✔ The most radical treatment may be hospitalization, in order to prevent death, suicide, and medical crisis.

Weight restoration is vital to improving health, mood, and cognitive functioning. (Note: An anorexic's fear of weight gain, especially forced weight gain in the hospital, is a huge obstacle to treatment and recovery.)

✔ Medication is another form of treatment that may be necessary to relieve depression and anxiety.

✔ Dental work to repair enamel damage and minimize future problems may need to be considered.

✔ Individual counselling is a must, to develop healthy ways of taking control of one's life. In addition, group counselling may help the sufferer learn how to manage relationships effectively, and family counselling may be needed to change old patterns of behavior and create healthier new ways of interaction.

✔ Nutrition counselling might be helpful to debunk food myths and design healthy meals.

✔ Support groups (both for the sufferer and the family, respectively) may prove useful in breaking down the perceived walls of isolation and alienation.

Are You At Risk? Take a Self-Test

The following questionnaire (reproduced with permission from ANRED, Anorexia Nervosa and Related Eating Disorders[5]) can help you decide if you have an eating disorder or if you are at risk of developing one. Checkmark any statements that apply to you.

✔ Even though people tell me that I'm thin, I feel fat.

✔ I get anxious if I can't exercise.

✔ My menstrual periods are irregular or absent.

✔ I worry about what I will eat.

✔ If I gain weight, I get anxious and depressed.

✔ I would rather eat by myself than with family or friends.

✔ Other people talk about the way I eat.

✔ I get anxious when people urge me to eat.

✔ I don't talk much about my fear of being fat because no one understands how I feel.

✔ I enjoy cooking for others, but I usually don't eat what I've cooked.

✔ I have a secret stash of food.

✔ When I eat, I'm afraid I won't be able to stop.

✔ I lie about what I eat.

✔ I don't like to be bothered or interrupted when I'm eating.

✔ If I were thinner, I would like myself better.

✔ I like to read recipes, cookbooks, calorie charts, and books about dieting and exercise.

✔ I have missed work or school because of my weight or eating habits.

✔ I tend to be depressed and irritable.

✔ I feel guilty when I eat.

✔ I avoid some people because they bug me about the way I eat.

✔ When I eat, I feel bloated and fat.

✔ My eating habits and fear of food interfere with friendships or family relationships.

✔ I binge eat.

✔ I do strange things with my food (cut it into tiny pieces, eat it in special ways, eat it on special dishes with special utensils, make patterns on my plate with it, secretly throw it away, hide it, spit it out before I swallow, etc.)

✔ I get anxious when people watch me eat.

✔ I am hardly ever satisfied with myself.

---

[5] http://www.anred.com

✔ I vomit or take laxatives to control my weight.

✔ I want to be thinner than my friends.

✔ I have said or thought, "I would rather die than be fat."

✔ I have stolen food, laxatives, or diet pills from stores or from other people.

✔ I have fasted to lose weight.

✔ I have noticed one or more of the following: cold hands and feet, dry skin, thinning hair, fragile nails, swollen glands in my neck, dental cavities, dizziness, weakness, fainting, rapid, or irregular heartbeat.

As strange as it seems in our thin-obsessed society, none of the above behaviors is normal or healthy. The more items you have checked, the more serious your problem may be.

The sufferers of these conditions *suffer*. Big time. They didn't bring their illnesses upon themselves by being overzealous in their dieting campaign. The seeds of psychological imbalances were there from the start.

Because eating disorders invariably revolve around food, dieting (and with it, healthy weight control) has been tarnished by its brush. This has warped our vision.

It's important to distinguish between the two. One is a mental disease — it's dangerous, accompanied by serious health consequences, and is out of control. The other is a means of *taking control* of one's life through a healthy dose of self-esteem, self-respect, and a positive, balanced, educated perspective on food, weight, and life.

Index

－◆ ◆ ◆ －

A

acrobatics, 304
Aerobics, 284
    classes, 305, 339
alcohol, 97
analyzing yourself/your lifestyle, 19
Anorexia, 417
Atkins' diet (New Diet Revolution), 25
attitudes, Chapter 2

B

back pain, 273, 368
bands, 293
Bar mitzvahs. See weddings
barbells, 293
being careful, 41
binges, 120
    Binge eating disorder, 419
BMI (Body Mass Index). *See* tables
body conditioning, 309. *See also* strength
  training
body sculpting. *See* body conditioning
boredom
    in general, 64, 80
    on a diet, 43
    with your job, 66
Boxercise, 307
bread, 243. *See also* sandwiches
breakfast
    erev Shabbos, 147
    Purim day, 210
    skipping it, 391
Bulimia, 418
butter, 101

C

calories
    and activity levels, 18, 386
    and age, 17 footnote 4
    and metabolism, 17 footnote 5
    and weight, 17 footnote 6, Appendix 3
    defined, 17 footnote 3, 113
    from fats, 100, 113
    pounds, 17, 191
    too few results in, 264
    weight loss equation, 17
cancer, 366
carbohydrates, 14,194
cardio, cardiovascular, CV, 284

celebrations, 65, 81
cereal, 96, 156
challah, 162, 182
Chanukah, 198
Charley horse, 289, 311
cheese, 101
chicken soup, 163
children. *See* kids
chocolate, 99, 179
    before a fast, 195
cholent, 169
cholesterol, 102, 114, 240
Circuit class, 308
coleslaw, 249
Cooldown, 309
croutons. *See* soup nuts

D

delegating, 143
dessert, 165, 170. *See also* ice cream
Diabetes, 271, 366. *See also* exercise and
  diabetes
diet cookies (meal replacement), 36
diet group leaders, 133, 134, 136, 340, 341
diet group, 133
diet pills, 37
dieting partner, 132
drink(s), 174, 186, 314
    before a fast, 195,
    enough 265. *See also* 393, Appendix 6
dumbbells, 293

E

eating
    after a fast, 197
    at night, 390
    disorders, Appendix 8
    how to eat, 120
    out. *See* weddings. *See also* restaurants
    why do we?, Chapter 3
endorphins, 275, 285
erev Shabbos, Chapter 6
erev Yom Kippur, 192
exercise
    and appearance, 275
    and Arthritis, 272
    and body fat, 274
    and bones, 272, 285
    and breast cancer, 271

and cholesterol, 270
and Colon cancer, 271
and constipation, 271
and depression, 275
and Diabetes, 271
and Dyslexia, Dyspraxia, 277
and heart disease, stroke, heart attack, 270
and high blood pressure, 270
and incontinence, 333
and menopause, 276
and muscles, cartilage, ligaments, and tendons, 272
and Osteoporosis, 272, 285
and PMS, 276
and pregnancy, 331
and the back, 273
and the heart, 270
and varicose veins, 271
and weight loss, 18, 274, 334
as a mitzvah, 279
as a stress reducer, 72, 275
burns off calories, 18, 334
clothing, 320
eating and drinking beforehand, 313, 314
equipment, 320-323
insomnia, 315
nausea, 314
reasons to, Chapter 14
which exercises do what, Chapter 15
exercise to music, 306

F

fad diets, 38
false starts, 54
fasting, 192-196, 392
fats
and calories, 100
before a fast, 195
finding them, 248
monosaturated, 100
polyunsaturated, 100
saturated, 99
fiber, 114, 218, Appendix 5
fish, 157
Fit for Life diet, 35
flexibility. *See* stretching
food diary, 108, 256
formulas (meal replacement), 36
french fries, 94
friends, 128
fruit, 14, 160, 165, 166, 170, 174, 263

G

gallstones, 366
glucose, 194. *See also* sugar
gluteals, 307
grapes, 194

H

Hay diet (food combining), 34
healthy diet, 13, 14
heart disease, 270, 364
high blood cholesterol, 270, 365
honey, 98,182
hunger
and shopping, 110
and tasting, 149
erev Shabbos, 146
as a reason to eat, 61, 70
husbands, 130

I

ice cream, 101,185
impact, 286
high and low, 305, 340

J

Jazzercise, 306

K

kiddush, 167
Kiddushes. *See* weddings
kids
and dieting, Appendix 7
for emotional support, 127
for physical support, 143
kugel, 164

L

labels (food), 111
liquid diets (meal replacement), 36
loneliness, 64, 76
lunchtime, 151

M

margarine, 101
matzah balls, 184
measuring yourself, 107-108
meat, 102
cooking it, 119
medicine, copyright page, 67, 86
Melaveh Malkah, 171
menu plan, 175, 181
milk, 95
mind-body exercise, 296
mitzvah to guard your health, 279
motzei Yom Kippur 197

O

obesity, 38, 364
Ornish diet (Eat More, Weigh Less), 30
Osteoporosis, 272, 285

P

parents, 125
pasta, 157
pelvic floor, 286, 333
percent daily value (%DV), 115, 116

Pesach, 213
photographs, 107, 257
Pilates, 300
posture. *See* stretching
preparation
    attitudes. *See* attitude
    practical, 54
protein, 14, 247
    before a fast, 194
Purim, 203

R

Rec-check (Rectus Abdominus check), 332
RDA. *See* percent daily value
recipes
    cheesecake, very low-fat, 220
    eggplant dip, 209
    healthy potato kugel, 164
    rice stew, 215
    rugelach, 202
    salad dressing, 92
    spaghetti bolognaise, 215
    swiss roll, 201
re-motivation, Chapter 12
restaurants, Chapter 11. *See also* weddings
rewards, 51
rice cakes, 154

S

salad dressing, 92, 248-250
salads 92,155, 248-250
Salsa Aerobics, 306
salt (sodium), 96
sandwiches
    open face options 153
    options, 154, 226
scales, 50, 106
Scarsdale diet, 23
Seudah Shilishis, 170, 180
Shabbos day, 167
Shabbos night, 161
Shabbos, Chapter 7
Shavuos, 219
Sheva brochos. *See* weddings
shopping, 110
sleep
    erev Shabbos, 142
    erev Yom Tov, 176
Slimming World diet, 31
snacks, 95-96,179
sneakers, 321
social pressures, 65, 80
socializing, 65, 81
soup nuts/croutons, 183
soup, 93, 155, 206, 216
spices, 97
Spinning, 287, 309
Step Aerobics, 287, 306

strength training, 292
stress, 64, 72, 275
    and Purim, 206
stretching, 287, 311
substitutes, 104
success, 188
sugar, 98
    before a fast, 194-195
summer vacations, Chapter 10
    camping out, away from civilization, 235
    family camps, bungalow colony, 228
    hotel, fully catered, 232
support, Chapter 5

T

tables
    BMI (Body Mass Index), 379
    fiber contents of food, 401
    height-weight, 377
Tai Chi, 300
Tanis Esther, 207. *See also* fasting
tasting, 105, 149
tayvah/desires, 62, 71
tennis, 304
Three-Quarters rule, 163
tired, 66, 84
travelling, 235
tubes, 293
Twerski, Dr. Rabbi A.J., foreword, 38
tzimmes, 184

U

varicose veins, 368. *See also* exercise and
    varicose veins
vegetable oil, 100-101
vegetables, 14, 91, 155,163, 245, 263

W

Warm-up, 301
Water Aerobics, 308
weather, 68, 87
weddings. *See* socializing, celebrations, and
    restaurants
weighing food, 117
weighing yourself, 106, 347
weight lifting. *See* strength training
Weight Watchers diet, 21
weights, 292-293
whole grains, 14, 91
willpower, 46
worry, 64, 77

Y

Yoga, 299
yoghurt, 101
Yom Tov, Chapter 8, Chapter 9
yo-yo dieting, 40

Z

Zone diet, 27

About the Author

Chava Goldman holds a BA in Business Administration and is a qualified Weight Management Consultant. She has run her own Diet and Exercise Consultancy for nearly a decade and has designed and currently supervises a Weight Management Group. Over the years, Chava has helped many women reach and maintain their dieting goals. She also advises fellow diet consultants from around the world.

Chava is also one of the premier Orthodox Jewish aerobics instructors in the world. She is a fully qualified RSA Aerobics and Body Conditioning Instructor, specially trained in Advanced Choreography and Antenatal and Postnatal Exercise. Chava regularly teaches classes (sometimes with nearly one hundred participants) to high schools, seminaries, and married ladies. She runs an Ante/Postnatal Exercise course for qualified instructors and will soon be training future aerobics instructors.

In addition, Chava has written a weekly column for a national newspaper on diet and exercise issues for the Jewish woman and is currently a freelance journalist and guest lecturer. The British Government recently commissioned her to write a short guide to dieting and exercise for Anglo Jewry.

Chava also loves photography, writing poetry, painting and creating modern art.

She somehow fits all this around her very busy schedule as a mother of a whole lot of lively children and as a wife of a husband in full-time Torah learning.

Chava says the secret to her busy schedule is to be well organized and not to breathe — there's no time for that!

If you want Chava to:

- Speak at your next conference, fund-raising event, educational evening, or social;
- Lead a fun, upbeat, and inspiring aerobics session to raise funds for your charity;
- Train a group of your fellow aerobics instructors in Ante/Postnatal exercise or advanced choreography;
- Answer your dieting/exercise questions;
- Write an article on dieting, exercise, or on a variety of other subjects, for your publication,

then leave a message or fax for Chava toll free at 1-866-372-2823 (in the USA).

Or send her an email to *Lightenup@Lightenup1.co.uk*

She will try to respond to your message as soon as possible.

Future Project

If you have an inspirational story (short or long), an encouraging personal experience, or a motivating one-liner, connected with dieting or exercise, that you would like to share, perhaps we can include it in an upcoming book. (Of course, your privacy will be protected.) So please send it by email to *Lightenup@Lightenup1.co.uk*